Tumors
of the
Pituitary Gland

Atlas
of
Tumor Pathology

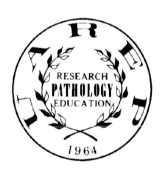

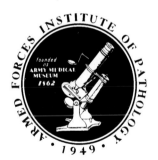

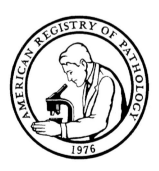

ATLAS OF TUMOR PATHOLOGY

Third Series
Fascicle 22

TUMORS OF THE PITUITARY GLAND

by

SYLVIA L. ASA, M.D., Ph.D.
Associate Professor of Pathology
University of Toronto
Pathologist, Mount Sinai Hospital
Toronto, Ontario, Canada

Published by the
ARMED FORCES INSTITUTE OF PATHOLOGY
Washington, D.C.

Under the Auspices of
UNIVERSITIES ASSOCIATED FOR RESEARCH AND EDUCATION IN PATHOLOGY, INC.
Bethesda, Maryland
1998

Accepted for Publication
1997

Available from the American Registry of Pathology
Armed Forces Institute of Pathology
Washington, D.C. 20306-6000
ISSN 0160-6344
ISBN 1-881041-44-1

ATLAS OF TUMOR PATHOLOGY

EDITOR
JUAN ROSAI, M.D.
Department of Pathology
Memorial Sloan-Kettering Cancer Center
New York, New York 10021-6007

ASSOCIATE EDITOR
LESLIE H. SOBIN, M.D.
Armed Forces Institute of Pathology
Washington, D.C. 20306-6000

EDITORS' NOTE

The Atlas of Tumor Pathology has a long and distinguished history. It was first conceived at a Cancer Research Meeting held in St. Louis in September 1947 as an attempt to standardize the nomenclature of neoplastic diseases. The first series was sponsored by the National Academy of Sciences-National Research Council. The organization of this Sisyphean effort was entrusted to the Subcommittee on Oncology of the Committee on Pathology, and Dr. Arthur Purdy Stout was the first editor-in-chief. Many of the illustrations were provided by the Medical Illustration Service of the Armed Forces Institute of Pathology, the type was set by the Government Printing Office, and the final printing was done at the Armed Forces Institute of Pathology (hence the colloquial appellation "AFIP Fascicles"). The American Registry of Pathology purchased the Fascicles from the Government Printing Office and sold them virtually at cost. Over a period of 20 years, approximately 15,000 copies each of nearly 40 Fascicles were produced. The worldwide impact that these publications have had over the years has largely surpassed the original goal. They quickly became among the most influential publications on tumor pathology ever written, primarily because of their overall high quality but also because their low cost made them easily accessible to pathologists and other students of oncology the world over.

Upon completion of the first series, the National Academy of Sciences-National Research Council handed further pursuit of the project over to the newly created Universities Associated for Research and Education in Pathology (UAREP). A second series was started, generously supported by grants from the AFIP, the National Cancer Institute, and the American Cancer Society. Dr. Harlan I. Firminger became the editor-in-chief and was succeeded by Dr. William H. Hartmann. The second series Fascicles were produced as bound volumes instead of loose leaflets. They featured a more comprehensive coverage of the subjects, to the extent that the Fascicles could no longer be regarded as "atlases" but rather as monographs describing and illustrating in detail the tumors and tumor-like conditions of the various organs and systems.

Once the second series was completed, with a success that matched that of the first, UAREP and AFIP decided to embark on a third series. A new editor-in-chief and an associate editor were selected, and a distinguished editorial board was appointed. The mandate for the third series remains the same as for the previous ones, i.e., to oversee the production of an eminently practical publication with surgical pathologists as its primary audience, but also aimed at other workers in oncology. The main purposes of this series are to promote a consistent, unified, and biologically sound nomenclature; to guide the surgical pathologist in the diagnosis of the various tumors and tumor-like lesions; and to provide relevant histogenetic, pathogenetic, and clinicopathologic information on these entities. Just as the second series included data obtained from ultrastructural (and, in the more recent Fascicles, immunohistochemical) examination, the third series will, in addition, incorporate pertinent information obtained with the newer molecular biology techniques. As in the past, a continuous attempt will be made to correlate, whenever possible, the nomenclature used in the Fascicles with that proposed by the World Health Organization's International Histological Classification of Tumors. The format of the third series has been changed in order to incorporate additional items and to ensure a consistency of style throughout. Close cooperation between the various authors and their respective liaisons from the editorial board will be emphasized to minimize unnecessary repetition and discrepancies in the text and illustrations.

To its everlasting credit, the participation and commitment of the AFIP to this venture is even more substantial and encompassing than in previous series. It now extends to virtually all scientific, technical, and financial aspects of the production.

The task confronting the organizations and individuals involved in the third series is even more daunting than in the preceding efforts because of the ever-increasing complexity of the matter at hand. It is hoped that this combined effort—of which, needless to say, that represented by the authors is first and foremost—will result in a series worthy of its two illustrious predecessors and will be a suitable introduction to the tumor pathology of the twenty-first century.

Juan Rosai, M.D.
Leslie H. Sobin, M.D.

ACKNOWLEDGMENTS

The preparation of this Fascicle has been possible only because of the help and contributions of many individuals. Firstly, I offer humble thanks to Dr. Kalman Kovacs, who shared his wealth of knowledge with me over many years of training and collaboration, who taught me lessons of critical thought, and who personifies the love of pituitary. Dr. Kovacs and his wife and collaborator, Dr. Eva Horvath, co-authors of the Second Series Fascicle, provided me with a superb model upon which to build.

I owe a debt of gratitude to Dr. William Singer who taught me many secrets about the pituitary, and to Dr. Arthur I. Cohen whose longstanding interest in this fascinating gland has been both academic and personal. The help and support of these two men has allowed me to pursue studies in this field.

Many pathologists, endocrinologists, and neurosurgeons have contributed the material that was used for this work, whether by sending cases for a consultative opinion, or by contributing interesting slides and photographs for this specific purpose. Special thanks are due to Dr. Juan M. Bilbao and Dr. H. P. Higgins (St. Michael's Hospital, Toronto), Dr. Shereen Ezzat, and Dr. Harley S. Smyth (Wellesley Hospital, Toronto), whose contributions of photographs are acknowledged throughout the book, and to Dr. Robyn L. Apel (Brisbane, Australia) and Dr. Elvio Silva (M.D. Anderson Cancer Center, Houston, Texas) who contributed unusual cases for the purpose of illustration. I thank Dr. C. Bergeron, Dr. S. Carpenter, Dr. C. Coire, Dr. J. Deck, Dr. R. Flemming, Dr. G. From, Dr. S. Handy, Dr. R. Josse, Dr. I. MacKenzie, Dr. P. Muller, Dr. S. Nag, Dr. J. Provias and Dr. R. Silver (Toronto, Ontario), Dr. M. Brennan, Dr. M. Dietrich, Dr. T. Draisey, Dr. M. Oxley, Dr. S. Raphael, Dr. A.R. Sellars (Windsor, Ontario), Dr. G. Davidson and Dr. D. Killinger (London, Ontario), Dr. S. Govatsos and Dr. E. Ur (St. John's, Newfoundland), Dr. W. Halliday (Winnipeg, Manitoba), Dr. J.M. Hughes (Cooperstown, New York), Dr. N. Inderadjaja (Kortrijk, Belgium), Dr. J.O.L. Jorgensen (Aarhus, Denmark), Dr. B. Lach (Ottawa, Ontario), Dr. A. Lee (Burlington, Massachusetts), Dr. D.G. Lowe (London, England), Dr. J. Marks (Westmead, NSW, Australia), and Dr. P. Snyder (Philadelphia, Pennsylvania), for contributing cases over the years. As well, students and residents have brought interesting material for teaching rounds; they have taught me many lessons over the years.

Two anonymous reviewers offered detailed comments and suggestions for valuable improvements to the original draft; I thank them for their time, effort, and knowledge.

The technical support of many is also appreciated. Again, it is not possible to name all who have helped, but I must acknowledge the patience of Lily Ramyar who provided the technical expertise behind many of the photographs and electron micrographs in the following pages. The secretarial work of Colette Devlin is also gratefully acknowledged.

This work would not have been possible without the generous support of Dr. Kenneth P. H. Pritzker and the members of the Department of Pathology and Laboratory Medicine of the Mount Sinai Hospital, and Dr. David Murray and the Department of Pathology of St. Michael's Hospital.

Most importantly, I would like to express my deepest appreciation to my partner and best friend, Dr. Shereen Ezzat, for his unwavering support, both intellectual and emotional, that allowed me to complete this formidable task.

Sylvia L. Asa

Permission to use copyrighted illustrations has been granted by:

Appleton & Lange:
     Pathol Ann 1984;19:275–315. For figure 1-12.

Blackwell Scientific:
     Functional Endocrine Pathology, 1991. For figure 1-11.

Excerpta Medica:
     Diagnosis and Treatment of Pituitary Tumours. International Congress Series
          No. 303. For figure 3-5.

Novartis Medical Education:
     The Ciba Collection of Medical Illustrations, 1970. For figures 1-1, 1-2, and 1-3.

Contents

TUMORS OF THE PITUITARY GLAND

1
THE NORMAL PITUITARY GLAND

GROSS ANATOMY

The human pituitary gland, or hypophysis, is a small bean-shaped organ that lies in the sella turcica, or hypophysial fossa, a concave structure in the superior aspect of the sphenoid bone at the base of the brain (figs. 1-1–1-3). The gland is well protected by the bony sella. Lateral to the sella are the cavernous sinuses which contain the internal carotid arteries and the oculomotor, trochlear, abducens, and first division of the trigeminal nerves; inferior and anterior is the sphenoid sinus; superior is the hypothalamus; and superoanteriorly is the optic chiasm. The bilaterally symmetric gland has two distinct parts, the adenohypophysis and the neurohypophysis. As their names suggest, these two parts are structurally and functionally different. The adenohypophysis is a red-brown epithelial gland; the neurohypophysis is a firm, grey neural structure that is composed of axons of hypothalamic neurons and their supporting stroma.

The adult human pituitary gland measures approximately 13 mm transversely, 9 mm antero-posteriorly, and 6 mm vertically (figs. 1-4, 1-5). It weighs approximately 0.6 g. The female pituitary is somewhat larger than the male gland; this can be documented on magnetic resonance imaging where a difference of up to 2 mm in height is seen (8). The pituitary of pregnant and postpartum women is larger (8,9) and heavier (6); the increased size is due to marked prolactin cell hyperplasia during pregnancy and lactation, which may increase the weight to 1 g or more. Postlactational

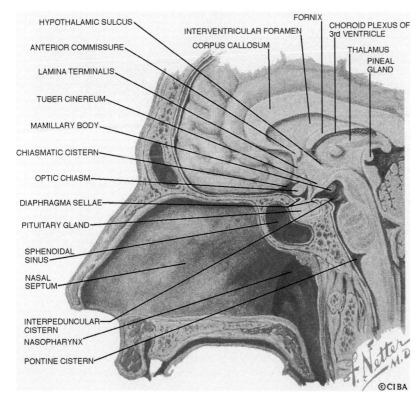

Figure 1-1
ANATOMY AND RELATIONS OF THE PITUITARY GLAND
Sagittal section through the midline shows the pituitary gland within the sella turcica, attached to the hypothalamus by the pituitary stalk. The gland is situated immediately posterior to the sphenoid sinus. (Plate 4 from Section I. In: Netter FH, Forsham PH, eds. The CIBA collection of medical illustrations. Vol. 4, Endocrine system and selected metabolic diseases. CIBA, New York: Colorpress, 1965.)

1

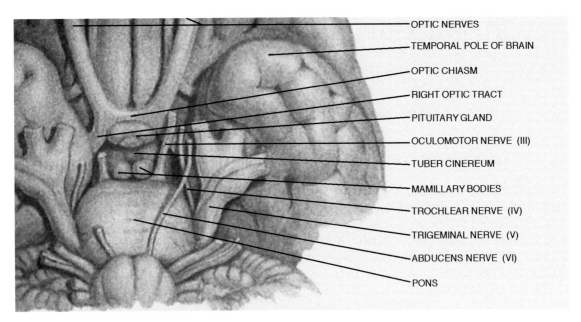

Figure 1-2
ANATOMY AND RELATIONS OF THE PITUITARY GLAND

A view of the base of the brain shows the pituitary gland immediately posterior to the optic chiasm and anterior to the tuber cinereum. (Plate 4 from Section I. In: Netter FH, Forsham PH, eds. The CIBA collection of medical illustrations. Vol. 4, Endocrine system and selected metabolic diseases. CIBA, New York: Colorpress, 1965.)

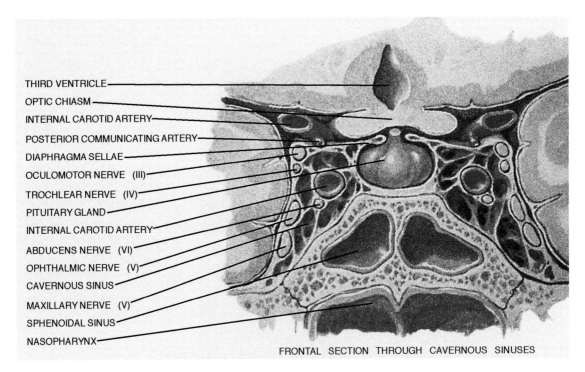

Figure 1-3
ANATOMY AND RELATIONS OF THE PITUITARY GLAND

Frontal section shows the relationship of the pituitary gland to the cavernous sinuses and their contents. (Plate 5 from Section I. In: Netter FH, Forsham PH, eds. The CIBA collection of medical illustrations. Vol. 4, Endocrine system and selected metabolic diseases. CIBA. New York: Colorpress, 1965.)

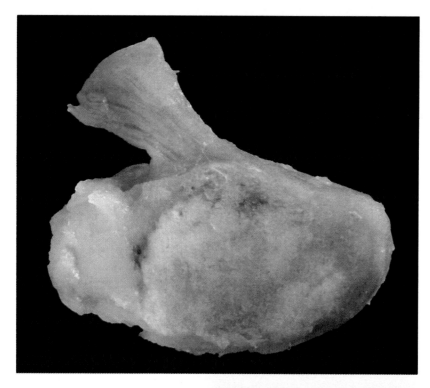

Figure 1-4
GROSS APPEARANCE OF THE
NORMAL PITUITARY GLAND
Sagittal section showing the anterior lobe (lower right), posterior lobe (lower left), and pituitary stalk (top).

Figure 1-5
GROSS APPEARANCE OF THE
NORMAL PITUITARY GLAND
Horizontal cross section showing the anterior (lower) and posterior lobes (upper).

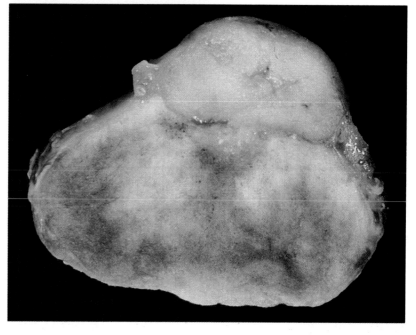

involution occurs but the gland does not return to its pregestational size and the pituitaries of multiparous women are heavier than those of nulliparous women (2). There is a slight to moderate size and weight reduction with advancing age in both sexes (8,13).

The neurohypophysis is composed of nerve fibers from hypothalamic nuclei that project downward to give rise to the median eminence or infundibulum, the neural stalk or infundibular stem, and the posterior lobe of the gland or infundibular process.

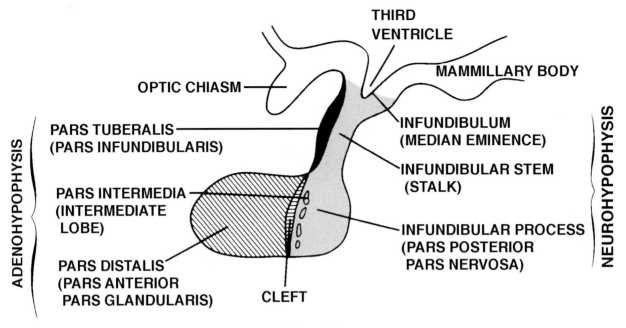

Figure 1-6
ANATOMIC COMPONENTS OF THE PITUITARY GLAND
(Figure 3 from Fascicle 21, 2nd Series.)

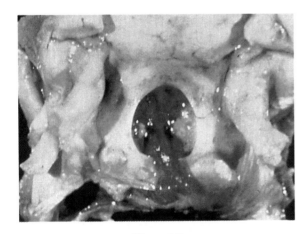

Figure 1-7
NORMAL DIAPHRAGMA SELLAE

Gross view of a normal sella as viewed from above shows an intact diaphragm and pituitary gland. (Plate IA from Fascicle 21, 2nd Series.)

The adenohypophysis comprises about 80 percent of the pituitary. It is composed of three parts: the pars distalis, the pars intermedia, and the pars tuberalis (fig. 1-6). The pars distalis constitutes the largest portion of the gland; it is generally known as the anterior lobe or the pars glandularis. The pars intermedia or intermediate lobe is rudimentary in the human pituitary;

it is the vestigial posterior limb of Rathke's pouch (see Embryology) and is found in an underdeveloped form adjacent to the residual cleft of the gland. The pars tuberalis is an upward extension of adenohypophysial cells that surround the lower hypophysial stalk; it is also known as the pars infundibularis.

The hypophysis is enveloped by dura mater, a layer of dense connective tissue that lines the sella turcica. The diaphragma sellae, a reflection of the dura which constitutes the roof of the sella turcica, has a small central opening for the hypophysial stalk, the connection to the hypothalamus (fig. 1-7). The sellar diaphragm protects the pituitary from the pressure of cerebrospinal fluid (CSF). Defective development or absence of this structure causes the empty sella syndrome in which increased CSF pressure results in enlargement of the sella turcica and compression of the pituitary (figs. 1-8–1-10); in severe cases, the entire gland may be found as only a thin layer of tissue at the bottom of the sella turcica. This lesion is usually unassociated with functional hypophysial abnormalities (3,12), however, 5 percent of patients have hyperprolactinemia, which may be caused by a coexistent prolactin-producing pituitary adenoma but is often idiopathic and

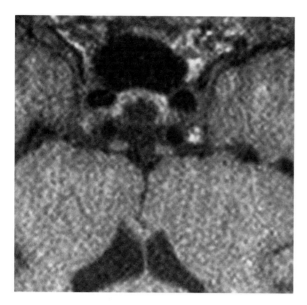

Figure 1-8
EMPTY SELLA SYNDROME:
RADIOLOGIC FINDINGS

Magnetic resonance imaging (MRI) identifies an enlarged sella turcica in which the pituitary parenchyma is
compressed at the bottom; the space is filled with cerebrospinal fluid. (Courtesy of Dr. S. Ezzat, Toronto, Canada.)

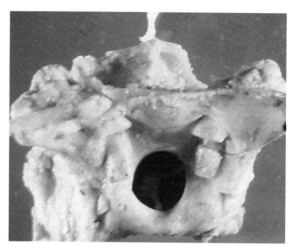

Figure 1-9
EMPTY SELLA SYNDROME

A widely opened sellar diaphragm allows increased pressure from cerebrospinal fluid to compress the pituitary.
(Plate 1B from Fascicle 21, 2nd Series.)

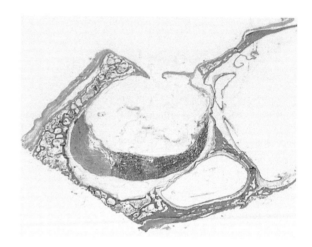

Figure 1-10
EMPTY SELLA SYNDROME

In the "empty sella syndrome," the pituitary gland is
attenuated along the bottom of the enlarged sella. (Plate 1C
from Fascicle 21, 2nd Series.)

has been attributed to distortion of the infundibular stalk and reduction in hypothalamic tonic
inhibition (10).

Other minor anatomic variations in the size
and shape of the hypophysis and its relation to
surrounding structures appear to have no endocrine significance (6).

Vascular Supply

Blood is supplied to the human hypophysis by
a complex portal system that originates in the
hypothalamus (fig. 1-11). This hypophysial portal circulation carries hypothalamic stimulatory
and inhibitory hormones from the infundibulum
to adenohypophysial cells, thereby playing a
major role in the regulation of adenohypophysial
hormone secretion (4,5,7,15–17).

The arterial supply of the median eminence
and posterior pituitary is derived from two or, in
some individuals, three paired arteries which
arise from the intracranial portions of the internal carotid arteries: the superior, middle, and
inferior hypophysial arteries. The superior hypophysial arteries branch into an external and an
internal plexus. The external plexus is composed
of small arteries that surround the upper half of
the stalk and give rise to a mesh of capillaries.
The internal plexus forms the gomitoli, unique
vascular structures which measure 1 to 2 mm in
length and 0.1 mm in width. They are composed
of a central muscular artery surrounded by a
spiral of capillaries; the arteriole feeds the capillaries through small orifices surrounded by muscular sphincters. Flow through these complex

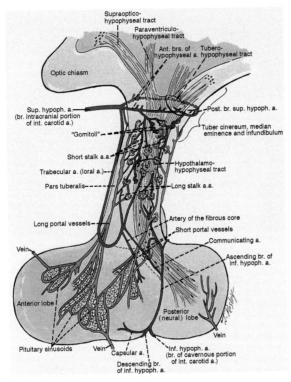

Figure 1-11
SCHEMATIC REPRESENTATION OF THE
BLOOD SUPPLY OF THE
HYPOTHALAMUS AND PITUITARY

(Plate XVII from Scheithauer BW. The hypothalamus and neurohypophysis. In: Kovacs K, Asa SL, eds. Functional endocrine pathology. Boston: Blackwell Scientific Publications, 1991:170–244.)

structures in the infundibulum and proximal hypophysial stalk proceeds through the portal vessels to adenohypophysial capillaries. Although the function of the gomitoli is not certain, their structure suggests that they regulate the rate of blood flow to the anterior pituitary, thereby influencing the transport of hypothalamic regulatory hormones to the adenohypophysis. In some individuals, the middle hypophysial arteries form the trabecular or loral arteries, which descend along the external surface of the pituitary stalk in the subarachnoid space and give rise to the subcapsular artery and the artery of the fibrous core; these arteries may provide a minor contribution to the blood supply of the adenohypophysis, then return upwards along the pituitary stalk as the long stalk arteries to anastomose with the neurohypophysial capillary bed. The inferior hypophysial arteries enter the sella just beneath its

diaphragm and supply the pituitary capsule, the neural lobe, and the lower pituitary stalk. In the intralobar groove, they divide into ascending and descending branches which form an arterial circle about the neural lobe. A branch to the lower pituitary stalk, the communicating artery, anastomoses with the trabecular arteries. Notably, the capillaries of the neurohypophysis are fenestrated and lie outside the blood-brain barrier.

Early studies suggested that the long portal vessels which arise in the infundibulum carry 70 to 90 percent of the blood flow while only 10 to 30 percent originates in the short portal vessels which link the infundibular stem or process to the adenohypophysis (7). However, it is now recognized that blood flow occurs within the neurohypophysial capillary bed, resulting in mixing of blood derived from different portal vessels (4,5). The adenohypophysis receives the majority of its blood from portal vessels via the neural lobe, but, in addition, some arterial blood is directed to it via two branches of the inferior hypophysial artery, the capsular artery, which serves the connective tissue of the pituitary capsule and penetrates to the superficial cell rows of the adenohypophysis and the artery of the fibrous core. In some individuals, the middle hypophysial artery may vascularize the adenohypophysis directly (11).

The venous drainage of the pituitary is to the cavernous sinus and from there to the inferior petrosal sinuses bilaterally. It has been reported that the volume of veins leading away from the adenohypophysis and neurohypophysis to the cavernous sinus is considerably smaller than that of the portal vessels entering the gland. This observation led to the recognition of the neurohypophysial capillary bed as a dynamic pool in which the short portal vessels also serve as efferent channels. The reversal of blood flow in this system implies that secretory products of the adenohypophysis enter the neurohypophysis and the median eminence and thereby help regulate hypothalamic factors (4,5).

Pituitary capillaries are lined by fenestrated endothelium with a thin subendothelial space. Hormones released by adenohypophysial cells pass through the basement membrane of their cell of origin, the capillary basement membrane, the subendothelial space, and the endothelial cell layer to reach the bloodstream.

Nerve Supply

The nerve supply of the pituitary is unique and crucial in the regulation of pituitary function (1). Despite this fact, the human adenohypophysis has no direct nerve supply, apart from small sympathetic nerve fibers that are associated with and presumably innervate capillaries. Thus, neural connections may affect blood flow to the adenohypophysis but apparently have no direct role in the regulation of adenohypophysial hormone secretion.

The posterior lobe, in contrast, is composed almost exclusively of axons and nerve fibers that arise from the hypothalamus. It is these neural connections that are required for the normal secretion of the two hormonal productions of the posterior pituitary, oxytocin and vasopressin, as well as for the transport of the other hypothalamic peptides that regulate adenohypophysial function (1,14).

The hypothalamo-hypophysial tract consists primarily of nerve fibers from the supraoptic and paraventricular nuclei and carries vasopressin and oxytocin to the posterior lobe of the pituitary, where the hormones are released into capillaries. The tubero-infundibular tract, originating from neurosecretory neurons which produce hypophysiotropic hormones, projects from several nuclei to the median eminence where the hormones are released into the hypophysial portal vascular system.

EMBRYOLOGY

The adenohypophysis derives from Rathke's pouch, an endodermal invagination of the primitive oral cavity. At the third week of gestation, endoderm from the roof of the stomodeum thickens and begins to invaginate; by 5 weeks, Rathke's pouch is a long tube with a narrow lumen and a thick wall composed of stratified cuboidal epithelium (fig. 1-12). By 6 weeks, the connection with the oropharynx is totally obliterated and Rathke's pouch establishes direct contact with the downward extension of the hypothalamus that gives rise to the infundibulum. The two tissues are enclosed by the cartilage anlage of the sphenoid bone, which separates them from the stomodeum, and the sella turcica is formed by 7 weeks (18).

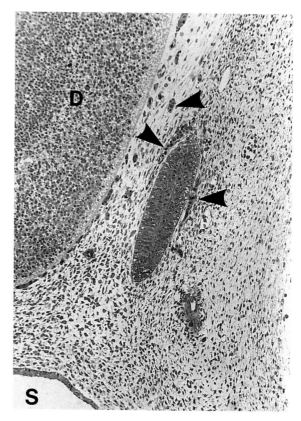

Figure 1-12
RATHKE'S CLEFT IN A FETUS
AT 5 WEEKS OF GESTATION
Columnar cells line Rathke's cleft and the connection with the stomodeum (S) has been obliterated. Blood vessels (arrows) adjacent to the primitive diencephalon (D) and the pituitary anlage are the precursors of the hypophysial portal system. (Fig. 1a from Asa SL, Kovacs K. Functional morphology of the human fetal pituitary, Pathology Annual 9 (part 1) 1984:275–315.)

It was suggested that Rathke's pouch arises from the ventral neural ridge in the pharyngeal region, thus sharing with the hypothalamus and posterior pituitary a common neuroectodermal origin (26, 38). The use of avian allografts, biologic markers, and serial sections of early chick embryos has provided indirect evidence for this theory; however, further proof is required for its validation.

As the cells of Rathke's pouch proliferate, the anterior portion forms the pars distalis and pars tuberalis whereas the posterior wall lies in direct contact with the posterior lobe anlage and becomes the pars intermedia (18). The growth of the anterior limb extends laterally and follows a triradiate pattern: the lateral borders become the lateral wings of the adult gland and the midline portion becomes the anteromedial mucoid wedge. By midgestation, the medial cleft becomes a residual lumen and growth of the pars nervosa reverses the convexity of the posterior wall of the cleft to a concave structure. The border between Rathke's pouch and the pars nervosa becomes indistinct; it consists of remnants of the obliterating lumen, a few cystic cavities lined by cuboidal or columnar epithelium. This represents the rudimentary pars intermedia of the human hypophysis.

The pituitary grows rapidly in early fetal life: the mean weight at 10 to 14 weeks of gestation is 3 mg, at 25 to 29 weeks 50 mg, and at term approximately 100 mg (23,24).

The pituitary portal vascular system begins to form before 7 weeks of gestation and by 12 weeks the anterior pituitary and median eminence are well vascularized. Portal vessels are recognized at 11.5 to 14 weeks, are well developed by 15 to 16 weeks, and are fully established by 18 to 20 weeks (34,35).

Remnants of the developing adenohypophysis may be deposited along the route followed by Rathke's pouch. The most common site is the roof of the nasopharynx. This so-called "pharyngeal pituitary" is found in most individuals (20,31) and contains all the hormone-producing cell types found in the normal gland; it is thought to have transsphenoidal vascular connections to the sellar hypophysis to maintain homeostatic feedback mechanisms (21). Ectopic adenohypophysial tissue has also been described in a suprasellar location in up to 20 percent of people (27). These ectopic foci are usually of incidental interest only, but they may be the site of adenoma formation that can confound the clinical diagnosis (30) or they may be detected with sophisticated imaging techniques and mimic a tumor (22). Salivary gland rests are relatively common if carefully sought, and are thought to be continuous with Rathke's cleft (28,37).

Aplasia of the pituitary is usually associated with severe congenital malformations, and forms part of the Cornelia de Lange syndrome (19). Aplasia or hypoplasia may be associated only with evidence of hypopituitarism, including adrenal and thyroid aplasia or hypoplasia (25, 29,32). Dystopia of the gland is the result of failure of union of the adenohypophysis and neu-

rohypophysis (33). Duplication of the pituitary gland has also been reported, usually in association with other craniofacial malformations (36).

MICROSCOPIC AND FUNCTIONAL ANATOMY

Hypothalamus and Neurohypophysis

The hypothalamic nuclei that give rise to the neurohypophysis are divided into four anatomic areas: the preoptic, supraoptic-lateral, tuberal, and mamillary regions (fig. 1-13). Whereas the nuclei are topographically discrete in many species and may be demarcated in the human fetus, they are poorly defined in the mature human hypothalamus (46). Structure-function correlations are difficult because of the cellular heterogeneity of many hypothalamic nuclei. Any given hypothalamic hormone is often produced in more than one nucleus, and in many cases a single nucleus may express more than one hormone. The physiologic roles of many nuclei remain unknown. Nevertheless, this area is responsible for the production of the neurohypophysial hormones, oxytocin and vasopressin, and for the hypophysiotropic hormones that are released into the hypophysial portal vasculature and regulate adenohypophysial function, including growth hormone-releasing hormone (GRH), somatostatin (or somatotropin release-inhibiting hormone [SRIH]), dopamine and other putative prolactin-inhibiting substances, corticotropin-releasing hormone (CRH), thyrotropin-releasing hormone (TRH), gonadotropin-releasing hormone (GnRH), and numerous other peptides that can affect adenohypophysial function (46).

The most anterior nuclei are the paired medial and lateral nuclei that are associated with autonomic function, particularly temperature control and olfaction. The suprachiasmatic nucleus, in the preoptic area dorsal to the optic chiasm and anterior to the supraoptic nucleus, is an area that is essential for gonadotropin release and sexual behavior in lower animals. This sexually dimorphic nucleus, which decreases in volume and cell number with age, is thought to play a role in the sexual differentiation of the brain which, in the absence of male gonadal hormones, remains female, but if exposed to male gonadal hormones at a critical stage in development, becomes male (64,110). It

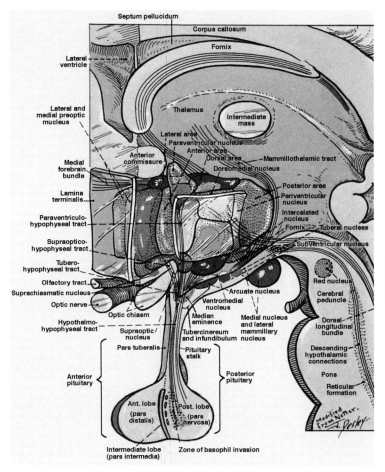

Figure 1-13
SCHEMATIC REPRESENTATION OF THE HYPOTHALAMIC REGION AND PITUITARY, THE DISPOSITION OF ITS NUCLEI, AND PRINCIPLE FIBER TRACTS
(Plate XVIII from Scheithauer BW. The hypothalamus and neurohypophysis. In: Kovacs K, Asa SL, eds. Functional endocrine pathology. Boston: Blackwell Scientific Publications, 1991:170–244.)

may also play a role in maintaining circadian rhythms; it is associated with fibers of the supraoptic commissure, and receives afferent fibers from the retina and the lateral geniculate bodies. The anterior hypothalamic nucleus is composed of small neurons which mediate parasympathetic effects.

The lateral hypothalamic nuclei are composed of large neurons which receive fibers from and contribute efferent fibers to the median forebrain bundle. The paraventricular nuclei, which are adjacent to the third ventricle ventromedial to the fornix, are composed mainly of large "magnocellular" neurons and contain a number of "parvicellular" neurons as well. The supraoptic nuclei, which overlie the optic tract, are the other paired magnocellular nuclei of the hypothalamus; they have no significant parvicellular component. These nuclei are major sites of oxytocin and vasopressin synthesis; efferent fibers from these nuclei terminate in the posterior lobe of the pituitary. Patients with traumatic or surgical stalk section

and those with longstanding hypopituitarism have atrophy of these nuclei with a marked reduction in the number of magnocellular neurons and stalk nerve fibers (105,118); the parvicellular component of the paraventricular nuclei remains.

The dorsomedial and ventromedial nuclei, situated between the tuber cinereum and paraventricular nuclei, are involved in autonomic function, hunger and satiety, and emotional behavior. Stimulation of the dorsomedial and destruction of the ventromedial nuclei produces rage in experimental animals. Destruction of the ventromedial nucleus results in obesity (53,83); conversely, destruction of the ventrolateral nucleus, known as the "feeding center," causes anorexia and cachexia (53). These nuclei have afferent connections from olfactory and retinal fibers, the reticular formation, and the nucleus of the solitary tract which receives input from the vagus. Afferent fibers from the cortex enter by way of the thalamus.

Ventral to the third ventricle and paraventricular nuclei lies the arcuate (infundibular) nucleus which is another important component of the hypophysiotropic region and plays a major role in the modulation of anterior pituitary function. The subventricular nucleus on the floor of the third ventricle posterior to the arcuate and anteromedial to the tuberal nuclei is a parvicellular nucleus, which undergoes marked hypertrophy to become a magnocellular nucleus in postmenopausal women (95,103), in young women with postpartum hypopituitarism and gonadal atrophy (114), in hypogonadal men and women, during starvation (65), after hypophysectomy (66), and in late pregnancy. The neurons develop a distinctive nucleolar change considered a manifestation of the feedback effect, likely a lack of estrogens (95,102,104), which is also observed in neurons of the arcuate nucleus (114).

The tuberal nuclei, irregularly grouped masses of large neurons inferior to the lateral nuclei, give rise to efferent fibers of the hypothalamus; after stalk section, they exhibit a slight increase in coarsely granular basophilic cytoplasmic material (105). The posterior hypothalamic nucleus, situated between the third ventricle and the mamillothalamic tract superior to the mamillary bodies, produces sympathetic effects when stimulated; it has been implicated in temperature regulation and its large neurons are thought to be the source of hypothalamic efferent fibers which descend to the reticular formation of the brainstem.

The paired mamillary nuclei and other minor nuclei in the supramamillary area, including the nucleus intracalatus, form the posterior hypothalamus. These nuclei integrate incoming information from the limbic system and the midbrain tegmentum and send out efferent fibers to the anterior thalamic nucleus and the brainstem.

The neurohypophysis is composed of nerve fibres, axon terminals, and stromal cells or pituicytes, modified glia thought to originate from the ependyma. The neural elements contain neurosecretory material, which can be demonstrated histologically with the Gomori chrom alum hematoxylin, aldehyde fuchsin, or aldehyde thionin stains (fig. 1-14). Immunohistochemistry with neuron-specific enolase or neurofilament antibodies reliably detects the neuronal elements; antibodies to glial fibrillary acidic protein or S-100 protein the

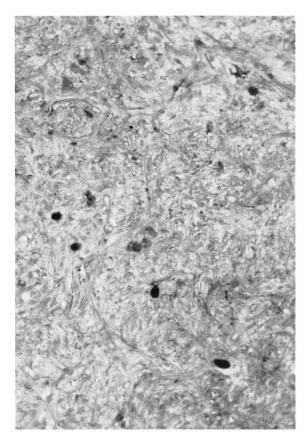

Figure 1-14
POSTERIOR LOBE OF THE PITUITARY
Neurosecretory material is identified with the aldehyde thionin stain in axonal terminals of the posterior lobe.

pituicytes; and antisera to oxytocin, vasopressin, and their carrier proteins, the neurophysins, the neurosecretory material. The ultrastructural features of the neurohypophysis (fig. 1-15) have been described in detail (51,100,101,111).

Adenohypophysis

In contrast with the hypothalamus, the cell types of the adenohypophysis are highly characterized with respect to structure and function. Although acidophils, basophils, and chromophobes are recognized with conventional hematoxylin and eosin staining (fig. 1-16) and a number of specialized histochemical stains have been devised to identify individual cell types (fig. 1-17), accurate classification is based on both immunohistochemical localization of hormone products and ultrastructural morphology (75);

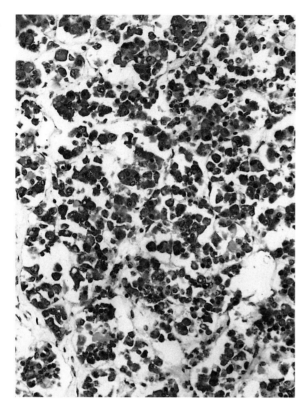

Figure 1-19
NORMAL GROWTH HORMONE CELLS
Growth hormone-immunoreactive cells comprise the majority of cells in the lateral wings. These middle-sized ovoid or polyhedral cells show strong diffuse cytoplasmic positivity for immunoreactive growth hormone.

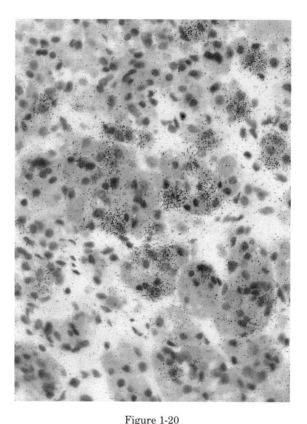

Figure 1-20
NORMAL GROWTH HORMONE CELLS
In situ hybridization shows strong positivity in the cytoplasm of clusters of acidophils that produce growth hormone.

as medium-sized, spherical or oval, acidophilic cells with central, spherical nuclei. Their cytoplasm stains with eosin, phloxine, and orange G but not with periodic acid–Schiff (PAS), lead hematoxylin, erythrosin, or carmoisine. Immunohistochemistry reveals intense positivity for GH throughout the cytoplasm (fig. 1-19) (77). Occasionally, smaller cells contain GH positivity in a globular structure which represents the Golgi complex; these may be sparsely granulated, actively secreting cells. A subset of somatotrophs also contains the α–subunit of glycoprotein hormones (69,113). By in situ hybridization, GH mRNA is localized to both densely granulated acidophils and to occasional chromophobes (fig. 1-20).

By electron microscopy, somatotrophs are spherical or oval cells with centrally located spherical nuclei and cytoplasm of relatively low electron density (fig. 1-21) (69). The prominence of the rough endoplasmic reticulum and Golgi regions vary with the secretory activity of the cell; active cells generally have well-developed, lamellar rough endoplasmic reticulum and a large Golgi complex whereas less active ones tend to have less conspicuous synthetic organelles. In the majority of somatotrophs, the cytoplasm is occupied by spherical, evenly electron dense secretory granules which range in size from 150 to 800 nm in diameter (average, 350 to 500 nm). Ultrastructural immunocytology confirms the presence of GH in secretory granules and within the Golgi region of actively secreting cells.

Somatotrophs are the second cell type to develop in the fetal gland after corticotrophs (44, 45,50): at 8 weeks, GH immunoreactivity is abundant and somatotrophs are recognizable by ultrastructural criteria. The incidence, distribution, morphology, and hormone content of somatotrophs are remarkably constant in the postnatal human pituitary. They do not appear to be affected by age, sex, various disease states, or drug

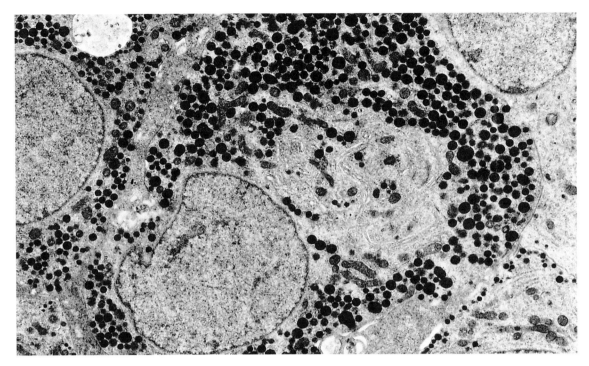

Figure 1-21
SOMATOTROPH

A somatotroph in the nontumorous pituitary is large, round to ovoid, and contains numerous electron-dense secretory granules that range from 250 to 700 µm in diameter. Short profiles of rough endoplasmic reticulum are scattered throughout the cytoplasm. The juxtanuclear Golgi complex is prominent and harbors forming secretory granules.

therapies. Even in glands containing GH-producing adenomas the nontumorous somatotrophs show no evidence of suppression and cannot be distinguished from those in normal glands (69). An exception to this morphologic uniformity is the case of longstanding hypothyroidism in which some degranulation of somatotrophs may occur; this change is much less than the almost complete degranulation of somatotrophs due to hypothyroidism which has been documented in rodents (119).

Lactotrophs. The number of cells containing prolactin shows wide variation related to age, sex, and parity. In adult men and nulliparous women they constitute approximately 9 percent of adenohypophysial cells whereas in multiparous women, they represent up to 31 percent of the cell population (47). While some of these cells are mammosomatotrophs, the majority in the mature gland are lactotrophs. Prolactin cells are randomly distributed throughout the anterior lobe, however, they are most numerous in the posterolateral portions of the gland. Using con-

ventional stains, they are usually sparsely granulated chromophobes but some are densely granulated acidophils which are indistinguishable from somatotrophs. The Herlant erythrosin and Brookes carmoisine stains allow selective visualization of densely granulated lactotrophs, however, these techniques are not sensitive enough to detect sparsely granulated forms.

Immunohistochemistry clearly reveals the two populations of prolactin-containing cells (77). Polyhedral or elongated cells with abundant cytoplasm almost completely filled with dense granular prolactin positivity are frequently found close to capillaries randomly distributed throughout the anterior lobe (fig. 1-22). The more numerous sparsely granulated cells, in contrast, are found predominantly in clusters at the posterolateral portion of the gland; they are elongated or angular, with long cytoplasmic processes and strong immunoreactivity for prolactin in the juxtanuclear globular Golgi complex (fig. 1-23). It has been postulated that the densely granulated cells store prolactin whereas

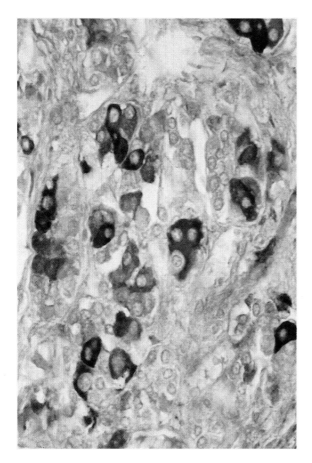

Figure 1-22
NORMAL PROLACTIN CELLS

Strong positivity for prolactin is seen within the cytoplasm of polyhedral cells which have elongated cell processes. Some of the processes surround adjacent immunonegative cells that correspond to gonadotrophs.

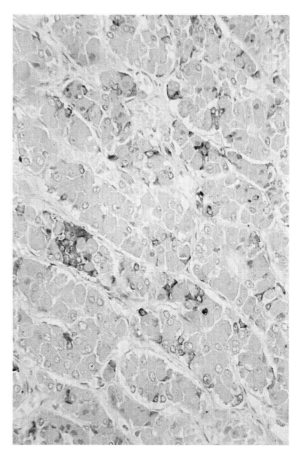

Figure 1-23
NORMAL PROLACTIN CELLS

At low magnification, prolactin cells are scattered throughout the gland and show variable patterns of immunoreactivity. The majority are densely granulated, with elongated cell processes that interdigitate with adjacent cells. Occasional cells have juxtanuclear globular immunopositivity, consistent with sparsely granulated forms that do not store prolactin but rather are immunoreactive in the Golgi region.

the sparsely granulated cells are actively secreting forms. Some of the acidophilic cells that resemble somatotrophs but contain prolactin are mammosomatotrophs.

By electron microscopy, the several cell types that produce prolactin are readily distinguishable (69). Densely granulated cells are rare in the adult pituitary but are more common in childhood and adolescence; many of these are mammosomatotrophs (see below). They have ovoid or elongated cell bodies, well-developed rough endoplasmic reticulum, and a prominent Golgi complex containing forming granules. The cell cytoplasm is almost completely filled with spherical, oval, or irregularly shaped large granules that have evenly electron dense cores and measure up to 650 nm in diameter. The majority of lactotrophs in the

adult gland are sparsely granulated, elongated or polygonal cells (fig. 1-24) which may have multiple cell processes extending from the center of acini to the basement membrane and intimately surrounding gonadotrophs. They contain richly developed rough endoplasmic reticulum found in parallel arrays and occasionally forming concentric structures known as "Nebenkern" formations. The Golgi apparatus is prominent and contains pleomorphic immature secretory granules. The few secretory granules range from 150 to 250 nm in diameter. Granule extrusions are common in prolactin-secreting cells and are found not only at the basal cell surface but also on the lateral cell borders, distant from capillaries and

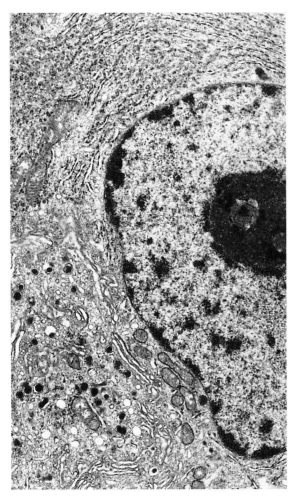

Figure 1-24
NORMAL LACTOTROPH

A lactotroph in the nontumorous pituitary has a well-developed rough endoplasmic reticulum which forms concentric whorls. A prominent Golgi complex is seen in a juxtanuclear location and harbors forming pleomorphic secretory granules. The cytoplasm is otherwise sparsely granulated.

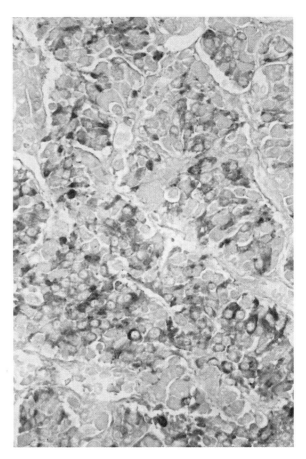

Figure 1-25
PROLACTIN CELL HYPERPLASIA

In the third trimester of pregnancy, there is prolactin cell hyperplasia; cells containing immunoreactive prolactin comprise almost 50 percent of the cell population of the gland.

basement membranes; the term "misplaced exocytosis" is used to designate this form of granule extrusion which is the ultrastructural hallmark of prolactin secretion. Immunocytology localizes prolactin in secretory granules of sparsely and densely granulated cell types; positivity can also be found in the Golgi region of sparsely granulated forms.

Lactotrophs are the last cells to differentiate in the human fetal pituitary. Prolactin immunoreactivity is scant but detectable at 12 weeks of gestation (45) and appears to be localized in mammosomatotrophs, bihormonal cells which

seem to be the sole source of prolactin until 24 weeks of gestation (44). Differentiated lactotrophs are found after that time and undergo a striking hyperplasia in the late third trimester (45), analogous to that seen in late gestation and during lactation in the pituitary of the mother (47,99); this marked hyperplasia of prolactin cells has been attributed to stimulation by estrogens. During pregnancy and lactation, the weight of the pituitary gland may increase to more than 1 g and almost 50 percent of the total pituitary cell population is composed of prolactin-containing cells (fig. 1-25). Exogenous estrogens are known to induce only mild hyperplasia of lactotrophs in the human pituitary; the increased cell population is composed predominantly of sparsely

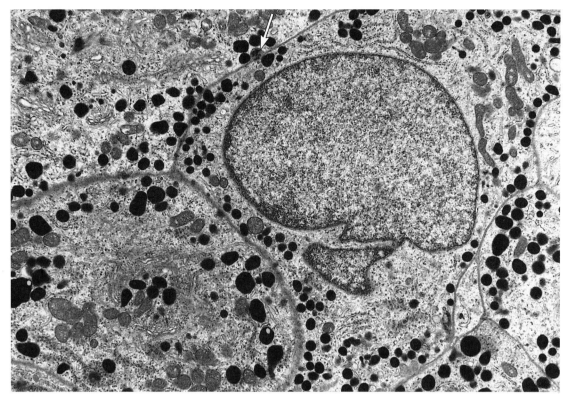

Figure 1-26
NORMAL MAMMOSOMATOTROPH
Occasional cells resembling densely granulated somatotrophs exhibit atypical features consistent with prolactin secretion: the secretory granules are highly pleomorphic and there is misplaced exocytosis, i.e., extrusion of secretory material along the lateral cell border (arrow).

granulated cells (98). Suppressed lactotrophs are found in some pituitary glands containing prolactin-producing adenoma or in patients treated with dopamine agonists. These inactive cells have a reduced nuclear volume, an irregular indented nucleus with coarse clumped heterochromatin, a small amount of cytoplasm with poorly developed organelles, and secretory granules which measure 50 to 300 nm; the granules contain immunoreactive prolactin and have an increased relative cytoplasmic volume due to the markedly reduced total cytoplasmic volume. These suppressed lactotrophs are identifiable only with immunocytology at the electron microscopic level; they cannot be characterized on the basis of their ultrastructural features alone.

Mammosomatotrophs. Bihormonal cells containing both GH and prolactin have been recognized in the nontumorous adenohypophysis only recently (59,69,84,85). Mammosomato-

trophs cannot be recognized using conventional histologic techniques; they are acidophils that are indistinguishable from somatotrophs. Immunohistochemistry reveals intense GH staining within these densely granulated, polyhedral cells. Prolactin is also identified but staining is usually less intense.

By electron microscopy, these cells resemble densely granulated somatotrophs (fig. 1-26). They are large and polyhedral with ovoid nuclei. They have abundant electron lucent cytoplasm which contains a well-developed rough endoplasmic reticulum and a prominent Golgi apparatus. The mitochondria vary from ovoid to rod shaped; they have a light matrix and lamellar cristae. The distinctive feature of these cells is their unique population of secretory granules. Some are small, spherical or slightly ovoid, electron dense granules which measure 150 to 400 nm; they have tightly fitting limiting membranes. The larger

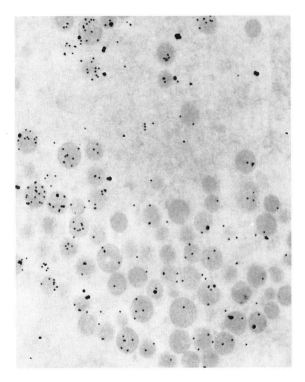

Figure 1-27
NORMAL MAMMOSOMATOTROPH
The double immunogold technique documents the presence of both growth hormone (small gold particles) and prolactin (large gold particles) in the same cell and within the same secretory granules.

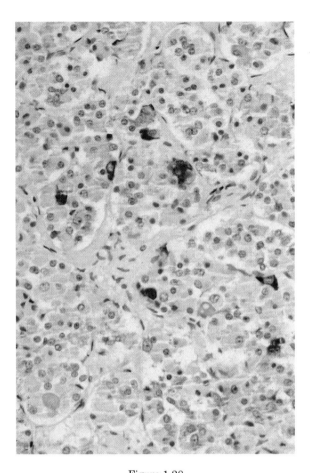

Figure 1-28
NORMAL THYROTROPHS
Cells containing immunoreactive ß-TSH are scattered singly throughout the normal pituitary.

granules are irregular, often extremely elongated structures which can measure from 350 to 2000 nm; they contain secretory material of variable electron density and are bound by a loosely fitting membrane. These secretory granules frequently show the misplaced exocytosis that characterizes prolactin-secreting cells. Ultrastructural immunocytology using the double immunogold technique documents the presence of both GH and prolactin in a single cell, frequently within the same secretory granule (fig. 1-27).

Mammosomatotrophs are the precursors of lactotrophs in the developing adenohypophysis (44). They are numerous during gestation, after which they appear to be a fluid cell population that fluctuates from somatotrophic differentiation to bihormonal cells to lactotrophs depending on the endocrine environment (59); for example, they have been shown to be a source of the increase in lactotrophs during pregnancy (108).

Thyrotrophs. The least common cell type in the adenohypophysis is the thyrotropin (TSH)-containing cell which comprises approximately 5 percent of the total adenohypophysial cell population. Thyrotrophs are usually found singly or in small clusters in the anteromedial portion of the gland. These medium-sized cells are chromophobic or basophilic when stained with conventional dyes and are PAS positive; they stain with aldehyde fuchsin and aldehyde thionin. The immunoperoxidase technique reveals granular positivity for α-subunit and β-TSH in their cytoplasm. The former is not specific enough to identify this cell type since it is also detected in gonadotrophs and somatotrophs; in contrast, the latter identifies these characteristically angular cells with long cytoplasmic processes that establish contact with the basement membrane (figs. 1-28, 1-29).

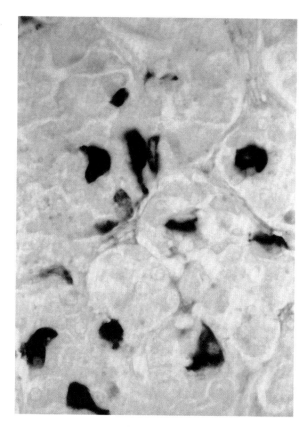

Figure 1-29
NORMAL THYROTROPHS
These cells have angular cell bodies with elongated processes.

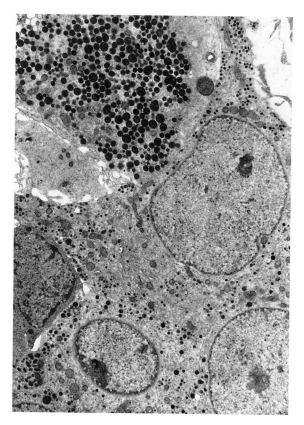

Figure 1-30
NORMAL THYROTROPH
A normal thyrotroph has an ovoid nucleus, well-developed cytoplasm, and elongated cell processes. The secretory granules are small, ranging from 100 to 200 nm in diameter. The profiles of the rough endoplasmic reticulum are short and a juxtanuclear Golgi complex is well developed.

Marked angularity and well-developed cytoplasmic processes also characterize the ultrastructural morphology of thyrotrophs (figs. 1-30, 1-31) (69). The nucleus is spherical and often eccentric. The cytoplasm contains short, slightly dilated cisternae of rough endoplasmic reticulum and a globular Golgi complex. The small, spherical secretory granules measure 100 to 200 nm in diameter and characteristically are found preferentially lined up at the cell membrane; more densely granulated cells may have granules scattered throughout the cytoplasm.

Immunoreactive TSH is detected in the fetal pituitary at approximately 12 weeks of gestation but the ultrastructural characteristics of thyrotrophs are not recognized until several weeks later (44,45). The numbers of thyrotrophs do not appear to vary with age; however, this cell type exhibits morphologic changes that reflect alterations in the hormonal milieu. In patients with primary hyperthyroidism, thyrotrophs are few and small; their ultrastructural features are not well documented (69). In patients with untreated primary hypothyroidism, thyrotrophs are released from the negative feedback effects of thyroid hormones and TSH secretion is increased. The number and size of thyrotrophs are increased; the enlarged cytoplasm is less strongly positive using the PAS, aldehyde fuchsin, and aldehyde thionin stains, and TSH immunoreactivity is faint but diffuse. Large PAS-positive lysosomes are prominent. By electron microscopy, these "thyroidectomy cells" or "thyroid deficiency cells" have abundant, dilated rough endoplasmic reticulum and large Golgi complexes but only a few secretory granules (fig. 1-32) (69). In patients with longstanding hypothyroidism, nodular hyperplasia and ultimately thyrotroph adenomas may develop (70). There is

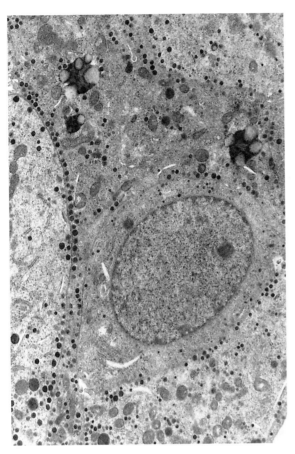

Figure 1-31
NORMAL THYROTROPH
This thyrotroph has elongated cell processes and small secretory granules that line up along the cell membrane. Lysosomes are common in this cell type.

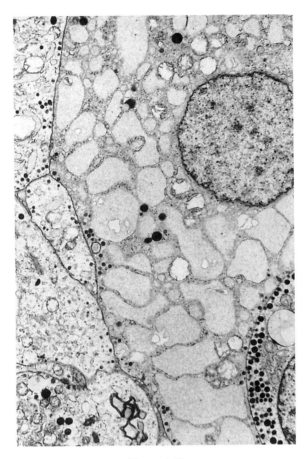

Figure 1-32
THYROIDECTOMY CELL
In patients with chronic hypothyroidism the thyrotrophs undergo striking changes characterized by a marked dilation of rough endoplasmic reticulum. Secretory granules are small and few and tend to line up along the cell membrane.

evidence from rat models that at least some of the thyroidectomy cells derive from a subset of altered somatotrophs (72); the morphologic changes are reversible in the experimental animal.

Corticotrophs. A single cell type in the human pituitary is responsible for the production of the proopiomelanocortin (POMC) molecule and its various derivatives, including adrenocorticotropic hormone (ACTH), melanocyte-stimulating hormone (MSH), lipotropic hormone (LPH), and endorphins. Corticotrophs comprise approximately 15 to 20 percent of the adenohypophysial cell population. Most of these cells are found in clusters in the central mucoid wedge; occasional scattered cells are also found in the lateral wings of the anterior lobe. Corticotrophs are also the predominant cell type in the poorly developed intermediate lobe of the human pituitary where they are found lining scattered vestigial follicular structures. By light microscopy, these medium-sized cells have varying degrees of cytoplasmic basophilia and stain strongly with PAS (fig. 1-33); the affinity is attributed to the carbohydrate moiety present in ACTH precursors. They also stain with lead hematoxylin. The presence of a large unstained perinuclear lysosomal vacuole known as the "enigmatic body" may be helpful in identifying these cells by light microscopy. The most reliable method of identifying corticotrophs is the immunoperoxidase technique which reveals strong granular cytoplasmic positivity for ACTH (fig. 1-34). Most corticotrophs are also immunoreactive for MSH, LPH,

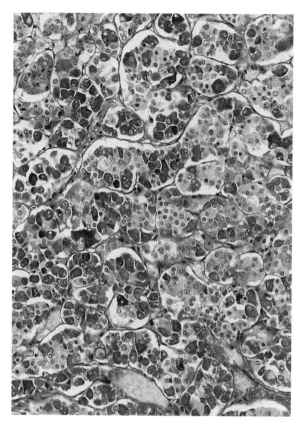

Figure 1-33
CORTICOTROPH CELLS
The PAS stain documents the presence of corticotrophs in the normal pituitary. Some of these cells have clear cytoplasmic vacuoles corresponding to the "enigmatic body."

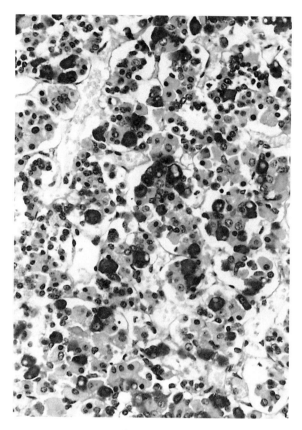

Figure 1-34
NORMAL CORTICOTROPHS
The cytoplasm of spherical or polyhedral cells contains immunoreactive 1-39 ACTH. The unstained cytoplasmic vacuoles adjacent to the nucleus represent "enigmatic bodies" which are complex lysosomes.

endorphins, and other fragments of the POMC molecule, which are derived by differing post-translational processing (107).

By electron microscopy (fig. 1-35), corticotroph cells are oval or slightly angular medium-sized cells with spherical or oval eccentric nuclei and a spherical nucleolus, which is usually attached to the nuclear membrane. The cytoplasm has highly variable electron density. The rough endoplasmic reticulum is moderately developed and is widely dispersed throughout the cytoplasm. Numerous free ribosomes are found. The Golgi apparatus is spherical or flattened and is often displaced by the "enigmatic body." This large structure is membrane bound and has an electron dense periphery which exhibits acid phosphatase activity, confirming its lysosomal nature (68). Mitochondria are spherical or ovoid, with lamellar or tubular cristae

and a moderately electron dense matrix. Variable numbers of intermediate filaments of the cytokeratin type (90), previously described as type I microfilaments, are found in small bundles, usually adjacent to the nucleus; they measure about 7 nm in width and show no periodicity. They vary considerably in amount and are not numerous under physiologic conditions. The secretory granules are usually numerous and extremely variable in size, shape, and electron density: they may be spherical, flattened, dented, heart shaped, or teardrop shaped. They measure from 150 to 700 nm in diameter, most between 150 and 400 nm. While secretory granules may be found lined up along the cell membrane, exocytosis is not recognized in this cell type. Immunoelectron microscopy identifies the various POMC-derived peptides in the secretory granules of corticotrophs, and there is no evidence

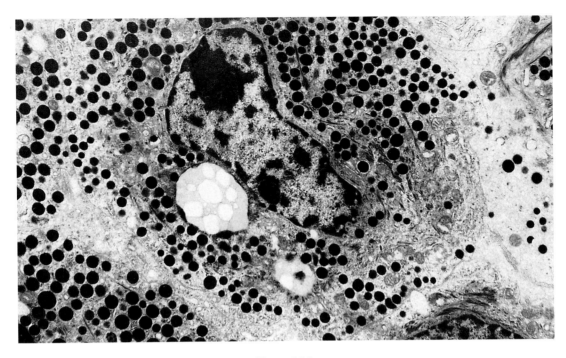

Figure 1-35
NORMAL CORTICOTROPH
The normal pituitary corticotroph contains dispersed profiles of rough endoplasmic reticulum; numerous secretory granules of variable size, shape, and electron density; and conspicuous juxtanuclear complex lysosomes. In a perinuclear location are small bundles of intermediate filaments representing keratin.

that the morphologic differences in granule populations reflect their hormone content (77).

Corticotrophs are the first cell type to differentiate in the fetal pituitary (44,45): at 6 weeks of gestation, cells with ultrastructural features of corticotrophs are present and by 7 weeks, ACTH immunoreactivity is detectable. Since these cells are found in significantly decreased numbers in anencephaly (41) it has been suggested that after autonomous differentiation they are dependant on hypothalamic factors for normal growth and development. Their numbers do not vary with age or changes in the hormonal environment, with the exception of chronic CRH excess which can increase the number of ACTH-containing cells (43,52). However, corticotrophs do develop specific morphologic features that reflect changes in endocrine homeostasis.

Exposure to glucocorticoid excess, either by exogenous corticosteroid administration or due to any cause of endogenous glucocorticoid hypersecretion including ectopic secretion of ACTH, causes corticotrophs to undergo a distinctive but reversible morphologic alteration known as

Crooke's hyaline change (fig. 1-36). The cells accumulate a glassy, homogeneous, pale acidophilic substance in the cytoplasm; PAS-positive (fig. 1-37) and ACTH-immunoreactive secretory granules are displaced to the perinuclear rim and the cell periphery (77). The hyaline material is composed of keratin filaments and stains with antibodies directed against low molecular weight keratin proteins (fig. 1-38) (90). By electron microscopy, Crooke's hyaline material is composed of intermediate filaments that resemble the smaller bundles seen in nontumorous corticotrophs. The web of microfilaments can be so extensive that it occupies almost the entire cytoplasm, leaving only a small juxtanuclear Golgi region and a small rim of secretory granules adjacent to the cell membrane (fig. 1-39).

Today one rarely sees patients with inadequately treated adrenal insufficiency. Nevertheless, this abnormality does give rise to a characteristic morphologic appearance of corticotrophs which become hypertrophied, with large nuclei, prominent nucleoli, and a poorly granulated vacuolated cytoplasm. The ultrastructural appearance

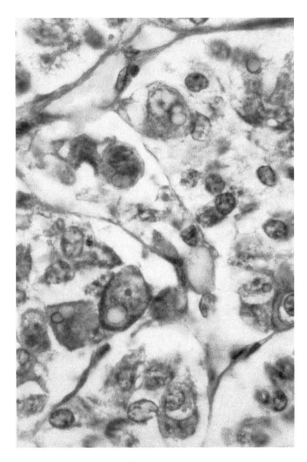

Figure 1-36
CROOKE'S HYALINIZATION
Pituitary corticotrophs subjected to glucocorticoid excess develop a characteristic cytoplasmic hyalinization that pushes the PAS-positive secretory material to the cell periphery. The complex lysosomes known as "enigmatic bodies" are present as clear vacuoles in the cytoplasm.

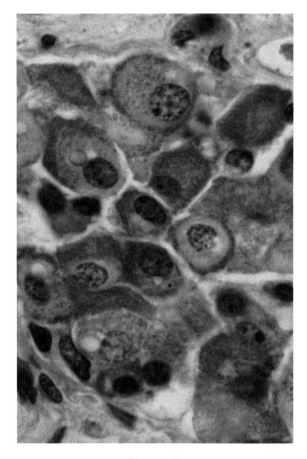

Figure 1-37
CROOKE'S HYALINIZATION
Pituitary corticotrophs subjected to glucocorticoid excess develop cytoplasmic hyalinization that pushes the ACTH-positive secretory material to the periphery of the cell. The clear vacuoles correspond to complex lysosomes known as "enigmatic bodies."

of these "adrenalectomy" cells in the human pituitary has not been well documented, however, in adrenalectomized rats, the markedly enlarged cells contain abundant dilated rough endoplasmic reticulum and Golgi membranes and a variable number of secretory granules (106). In cases of longstanding Addison's disease, nodular hyperplasia of corticotrophs and corticotroph adenomas may be present (97).

The pars intermedia corticotrophs also are strongly PAS positive and exhibit intense immunostaining for ACTH and other POMC derivatives. The border between the pars intermedia and the pars distalis is often indistinct; occasionally a thin layer of connective tissue is noticeable between these two portions of the adenohypo-

physis. On the posterior aspect of the pars intermedia, basophil cells are frequently identified, often in clusters within the neuropil of the pars nervosa, and they can spread deeply into the neural lobe (figs. 1-40, 1-41). This process, known as "basophil invasion," is more frequent and pronounced with advancing age; it has been reported to be more prominent in men than women. Its functional significance is not known and it is not associated with any recognized endocrine abnormalities. It may be that cleavage of the POMC molecule is different in this cell population (62), and the hormonal activity of these cells is not recognized. By electron microscopy, corticotrophs of the pars intermedia are smaller, denser, and contain fewer intermediate

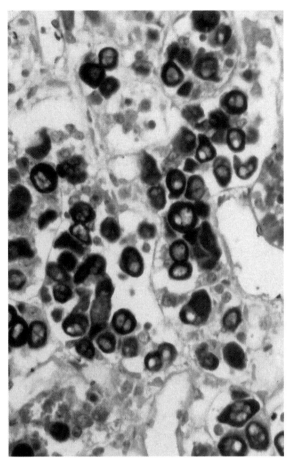

Figure 1-38
CROOKE'S HYALINIZATION
The cytoplasm of cells exhibiting Crooke's hyalinization contains strong diffuse positivity for low molecular weight cytokeratins. The nucleus and juxtanuclear "enigmatic bodies" are not immunoreactive.

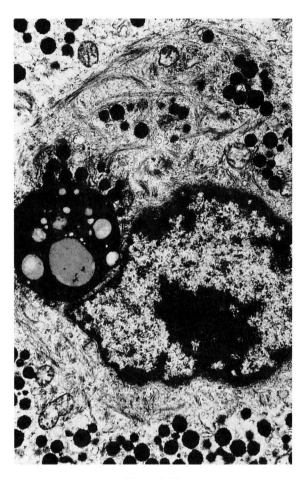

Figure 1-39
CROOKE'S CELL
The rough endoplasmic reticulum and Golgi complex are inconspicuous. The perinuclear cytoplasm is filled with intermediate filaments that represent accumulations of low molecular weight cytokeratins. This filamentous web has trapped secretory granules and a large complex lysosome. The remainder of the secretory material is pushed to the periphery of the cell.

filaments than corticotrophs of the pars distalis. They are also apparently less sensitive to the feedback effect of glucocorticoids, since they do not accumulate the keratin filaments of Crooke's hyaline in response to glucocorticoid excess.

Gonadotrophs. These cells, which produce the gonadotropins follicle stimulating hormone (FSH) and luteinizing hormone (LH) represent approximately 10 percent of the human adenohypophysial cell population. In rats, the number of gonadotrophs containing each hormone varies with age, sex, and hormonal status (69); in humans there is likely also variation in cell number, immunoreactivity, and morphology, but the details have not been reported. Gonadotrophs

are scattered throughout the pars distalis and comprise the major constituent of the pars tuberalis, where they undergo squamous metaplasia with advancing age (43). They stain with basic dyes, the PAS technique, aldehyde thionin, and aldehyde fuchsin. Immunohistochemistry localizes cytoplasmic positivity for α-subunit, β-FSH, and β-LH (fig. 1-42) in these cells; often β-FSH and β-LH are found in the same cell, indicating that one cell type is capable of producing both gonadotropins. There are, however, differences in the number of cells containing the two hormones, indicating that some gonadotrophs contain only one gonadotropin.

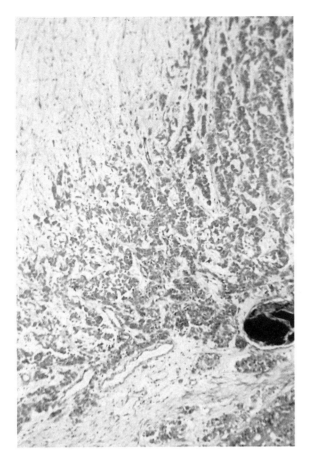

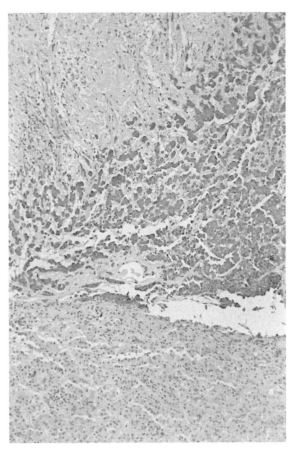

Figure 1-40
BASOPHIL INVASION
Basophils stained with PAS infiltrate the posterior lobe (left) from the cystic spaces that represent the residual Rathke's cleft or vestigial intermediate lobe. Scattered PAS-positive cells are also seen in the anterior lobe (bottom right).

Figure 1-41
BASOPHIL INVASION
The basophilic epithelial cells that infiltrate the posterior lobe are immunoreactive for ACTH, as shown, as well as other POMC-derived peptides.

The ultrastructural features of gonadotrophs reveal a single cell population (fig. 1-43). These are large oval or elongated cells with spherical nuclei that are found at one pole of the cell (69,70). They have abundant, slightly dilated rough endoplasmic reticulum profiles which often contain a flocculent electron lucent substance. The globoid Golgi complex is prominent. Mature secretory granules are scattered throughout the cytoplasm and are composed of two distinct populations that may show sexual dimorphism: in men, smaller secretory granules with an average diameter of 250 nm predominate, whereas in women, most secretory granules measure 300 to 600 nm in diameter. Ultrastructural immunocytology localizes β-FSH and β-LH within the same cells and, in some cases, within the same secretory granule.

Gonadotrophs are found in close proximity to the basement membrane. They are also intimately associated with lactotrophs which extend cell processes around gonadotrophs. There are intercellular junctions between the two cell types (69), suggesting paracrine interactions which are not well understood.

Gonadotrophs are present in sex-related dimorphic numbers in the fetal adenohypophysis (45). Between 15 and 25 weeks of gestation, pituitaries of female fetuses contain more gonadotrophs than do pituitaries of male fetuses. Throughout gestation, cells containing β-LH predominate in males whereas the number of cells containing β-FSH and β-LH are almost equal in females. This dimorphism correlates with differences in the levels of hypothalamic GnRH at the

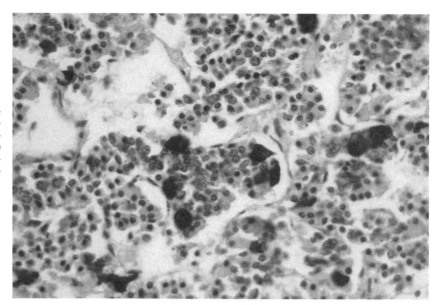

Figure 1-42
NORMAL GONADOTROPHS
Cells containing immunoreactive ß-FSH are scattered throughout acini of the nontumorous pituitary. These round cells have evenly dispersed cytoplasmic immunoreactivity for α and ß gonadotropic subunits.

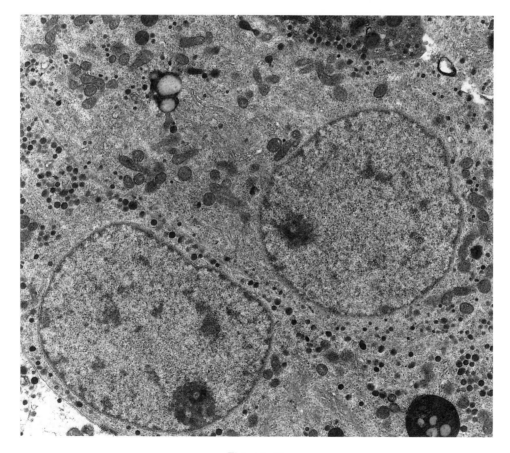

Figure 1-43
NORMAL GONADOTROPHS
These large round to elongated cells have ovoid nuclei with occasional nucleoli. Short profiles of rough endoplasmic reticulum are scattered throughout the cytoplasm. They are dilated and frequently contain electron-lucent material. The Golgi complex is usually well developed and in a juxtanuclear location. Secretory granules are highly variable in size, shape, and electron density and lysosomes are prominent.

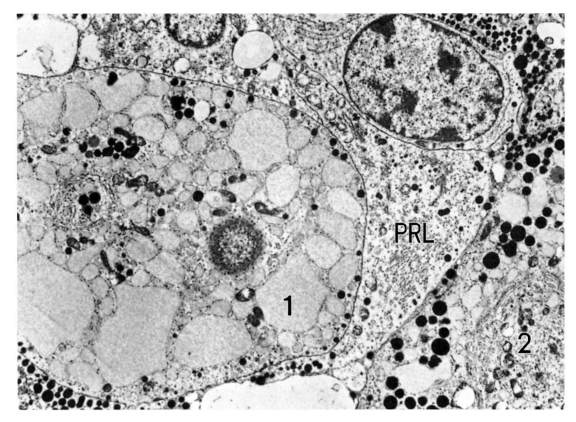

Figure 1-44
GONADECTOMY CELLS
Two stimulated gonadotrophs (1, 2) exhibit marked dilation of the rough endoplasmic reticulum that contains granular contents of low electron density. The prominent ring-like Golgi complex is seen in a juxtanuclear location. Secretory granules are few and relatively large. A prolactin cell (PRL) is sandwiched between the two gonadectomy cells. (Figure 30 from Fascicle 21, 2nd Series.)

same stages of gestation (41). In the adult pituitary, no such dimorphism of gonadotroph numbers has been identified.

Gonadotrophs of the pars distalis undergo morphologic changes which reflect changes in their hormonal environment; in contrast, the gonadotrophs of the pars tuberalis usually show signs of functional inactivity. In patients treated with pharmacologic doses of estrogen, the gonadotroph cells are small and dense (98). During pregnancy, the number of cells immunoreactive for β-FSH, β-LH, or both is significantly reduced (99). Gonadotrophs are also reduced in number, size, and immunoreactivity in Kallmann's syndrome, an uncommon variant of hypothalamic hypogonadism due to GnRH deficiency and associated with anosmia (78). Castration leading to prolonged lack of the negative feedback effects of gonadal steroids results in stimulation of gonadotrophs which then secrete FSH and LH in higher quantities; these stimulated "gonadectomy cells," "gonadal deficiency cells," or "castration cells" are larger and more numerous than normal gonadotrophs (69). Their vacuolated cytoplasm may displace the nucleus to the periphery, giving the cell a "signet ring" appearance. Electron microscopy reveals that this vacuolation is due to accumulation of markedly dilated rough endoplasmic reticulum. The Golgi complex is enlarged and secretory granules are present in reduced numbers (fig. 1-44).

Prominence of large active gonadotrophs has been associated with prolactin-producing pituitary adenomas in women (69). The factors underlying this change are not understood.

Follicular Cells. Follicles are found throughout the adenohypophysis as lumina that are lined mainly by agranular or poorly granulated cells

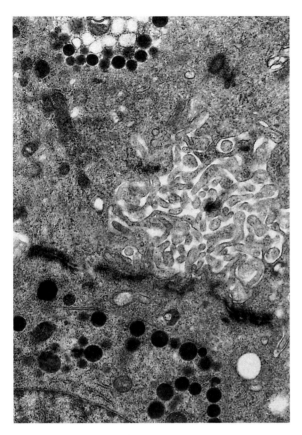

Figure 1-45
PITUITARY FOLLICLE
Pituitary cells containing secretory granules surround a
lumen lined by well-formed microvilli and tight junctions of
the macula adherens type.

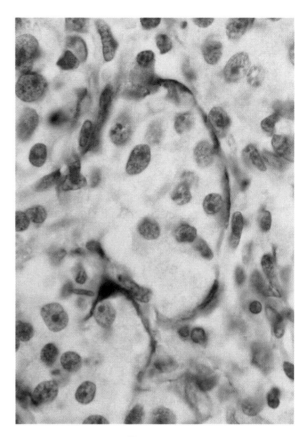

Figure 1-46
FOLLICULO-STELLATE CELL
This cell is identified by its immunoreactivity for S-100
protein. The long branching cytoplasmic processes surround
a cluster of adenohypophysial cells.

joined at their apex by junctional complexes (71).
By electron microscopy, granulated adenohypophysial cells can be seen to form follicles around
damaged cells (fig. 1-45); the surrounding cells
form specialized intercellular attachments and undergo degranulation and dedifferentiation. These
"follicular cells" can derive from somatotrophs,
lactotrophs, or corticotrophs. The follicular cells
form specialized junctions, macula adhaerens, between each other and with adjacent granulated
adenohypophysial cells; in contrast, granulated
adenohypophysial cells form only the less prominent zonulae adhaerentes. Follicles are found in
areas with increased cell destruction, particularly surrounding tumors (69). It is assumed they
play a role in isolating and processing cell debris.

Folliculostellate Cells. Immunocytochemical studies have localized S100 protein to a specific subtype of cells in the normal human pitu-

itary gland (63,73). These cells are agranular
and are not immunoreactive for the classic adenohypophysial hormones. Some are immunoreactive
for glial fibrillary acidic protein (GFAP). They have
a characteristic stellate morphology, with long,
branched cytoplasmic processes embracing granulated adenohypophysial cells (fig. 1-46). Because
of confusion with the follicular cells described
above, some authors have suggested that these
cells be called "stellate cells" (63). They are believed
to have a supportive role similar to that played by
the S100-positive sustentacular cells of the adrenal medulla and paraganglia. In addition, they are
thought to play a role in paracrine regulation (49)
and were recently shown to produce interleukin-6,
a cytokine which may participate in local regulation of hormone secretion (115). These cells
have also been implicated as the source of fibroblast growth factor in bovine pituitaries (58).

Folliculostellate cells are not found in the pituitaries of anencephalics (55). They are numerous in the compressed adenohypophysis at the periphery of adenomas. Some investigators have found no S100-reactive sustentacular cells within pituitary adenomas, providing a possible diagnostic criterion to discriminate between adenomas and normal or hyperplastic pituitary tissue (73); however, other investigators have found S100-containing cells within tumors of several types (81,87). They are also found in large numbers at the periphery of other pituitary lesions, such as abscesses, amyloid deposits, and in the residual hypophysis after surgery, but not adjacent to metastatic tumor deposits, infarcts, or Rathke's cleft cysts (91).

Null Cells. The nontumorous pituitary contains cells that cannot be conclusively identified by ultrastructural criteria. These may represent resting cells, or uncommitted or committed stem cells. In the fetal pituitary gland, cells with features of the glycoprotein hormone cell line can be identified prior to the recognition of differentiated thyrotrophs or gonadotrophs (44); α-subunit immunoreactivity is present in fetal glands at the same stage of gestation and β-subunits are not yet detected (45). It has been suggested that these primitive cells, which resemble null cells, may be precursors of the glycoprotein hormone cell line; they may be the cell of origin of some null cell adenomas.

Oncocytes. Oncocytes are large polyhedral cells which have abundant acidophilic granular cytoplasm due to the presence of numerous mitochondria (70). These cells may stain purple with trichrome stains that use aniline blue, leading to misinterpretation as basophils. The phosphotungstic acid–hematoxylin method demonstrates mitochondrial abundance. By electron microscopy, the cytoplasm of oncocytes is almost filled with dilated, spherulated mitochondria, but scattered secretory granules attest to the hormonal activity of these cells. Oncocytic cells may be found in the normal human adenohypophysis (76). The number of these cells appears to increase with advancing age, a phenomenon also found in other organs including thyroid, parathyroid, and salivary glands.

Other Cells. Unclassified plurihormonal cells have been identified in the nontumorous pituitary. Colocalization of GH, α-subunit, prolactin, and TSH has been reported in cells which have ultrastructural features of somatotrophs or mammosomatotrophs, and in cells which resemble thyrotrophs (69). Studies of the rat pituitary suggest a role for these plurihormonal cells in some pathologic states; for example, some somatotrophs transform into a population of thyroidectomy cells in hypothyroidism (72). Cells producing POMC derivatives with ultrastructural features of corticotrophs may produce gonadotropins or other hormones in the rat nontumorous pituitary (89); conversely, cells with gonadotroph morphology may contain ACTH as well as gonadotropins (88).

Cytodifferentiation in the Adenohypophysis

The process of cytodifferentiation in adenohypophysial cells has a highly specific pattern and temporal sequence; the factors underlying this process have only recently been investigated. Several putative transcription-activating proteins have been identified in the adenohypophysis and have been implicated as key elements in the definition of cell-specific phenotypes and the regulation of hormone gene expression (fig. 1-47). For example, a member of the helix-loop-helix family of transcription factors, corticotroph upstream transcription element-binding (CUTE) protein, is an important determinant of cell-specific expression of the POMC gene in the pituitary and other sites (112); its activity is exerted in synergy with another element that binds the POMC promoter, a bicoid-related pituitaryhomeobox 1 factor, Ptx1 (80). Pit-1, a 291-amino acid protein which belongs to the homeobox family of developmental regulatory proteins, binds the promoter sequences and activates the structurally related GH and prolactin genes in rats and humans (96). In addition, the gene encoding the β-subunit of TSH contains sites that bind Pit-1, though with lower affinity than sites in the GH or prolactin gene 5'-flanking regions (109). Studies of human pituitary adenomas have shown that the *pit-1* gene is selectively expressed in adenohypophysial cell types responsible for GH, prolactin, and β-TSH synthesis (48,60,92). Differentiation or maintenance of somatotroph, lactotroph, and thyrotroph phenotypes are dependent on expression of a functional *pit-1* gene; mutations in the *pit-1* gene result in hypopituitarism (82,93,94). A putative thyrotroph-specific factor

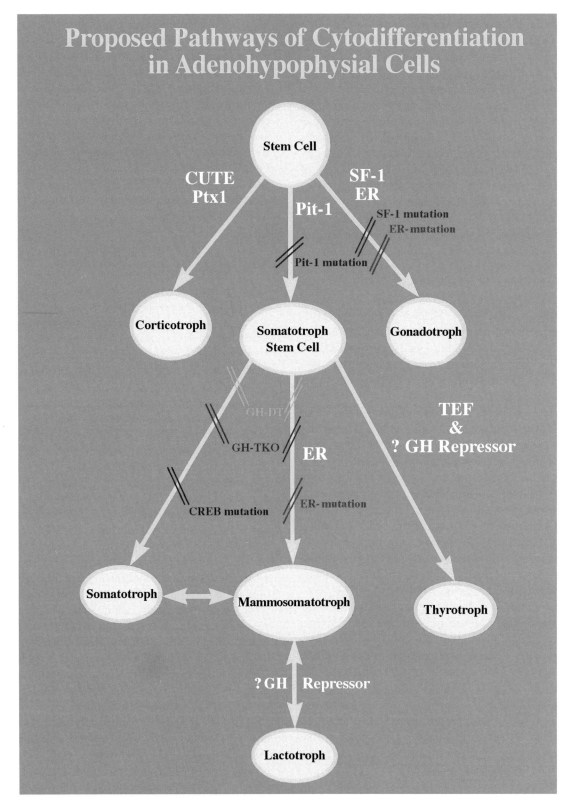

Figure 1-47
PROPOSED PATHWAYS OF CYTODIFFERENTIATION IN ADENOHYPOPHYSIAL CELLS

has been described: thyrotroph embryonic factor (TEF) is a trans-acting factor that belongs to the leucine zipper gene family of transcription factors and is thought to activate the expression of the human β-TSH gene (56). Expression of the estrogen receptor correlates with expression of prolactin or gonadotropins (54,61,120); this cell-specific expression suggests that the estrogen receptor may be the factor responsible for the development of prolactin expression in *pit-1*-expressing somatotrophs. The nuclear receptor steroidogenic factor-1 (SF-1), a member of the steroid receptor superfamily (67,79), is a transcription factor that regulates expression of the cytochrome P450 *CYP11A* and *CYP11B* genes in steroidogenic tissues and is involved in their differentiation (86). SF-1 is expressed by and is localized in gonadotropin-containing cells but not in other cell types of the pituitary (40) and is necessary for the differentiation of pituitary gonadotrophs (74).

Future studies of the molecular regulation of hormone gene expression will, no doubt, clarify the ability of adenohypophysial cells to maintain cytologic differentiation or undergo multidirectional differentiation, both functional and morphologic.

Localization of Other Peptides in the Adenohypophysis

A number of hormones not initially thought to be of pituitary origin have been found in adenohypophysial cells (Table 1-2) (46). Several hypothalamic hormones, including GRH, somatostatin, TRH, and GnRH, have been detected in adenohypophysial cells. While these may be internalized from hypothalamic sources, the data suggest production by de novo synthesis in adenohypophysial cells. Angiotensin II as well as renin and angiotensin converting enzyme have been localized in pituitary gonadotrophs. Immunoreactive bombesin/gastrin-releasing peptide (GRP) and calcitonin gene-related peptide (CGRP) have been found in the pituitary gland, however, cell localization has not been demonstrated. Cholecystokinin (CCK) is found in the adenohypophysis but in a form which differs from that present in other CCK-synthesizing tissues; no immunocytochemical localization has been reported but CCK has been found in large amounts in corticotroph adenomas and it appears, therefore, that pituitary CCK derives from corticotrophs. Galanin has been localized in

Table 1-2

PEPTIDES IN THE ADENOHYPOPHYSIS

Type	Peptide
Adenohypophysial hormones	Growth hormone (GH)
	Prolactin (PRL)
	ACTH and other POMC-derived peptides
	Thyrotropin (TSH)
	Gonadotropins (FSH and LH)
Hypothalamic hormones	GH-releasing hormone (GRH)
	Somatostatin
	TSH-releasing hormone (TRH)
	Gonadotropin-releasing hormone (GnRH)
Other hormones	Angiotensin II, renin
	Bombesin/gastrin-releasing peptide (GRP)
	Calcitonin gene-related peptide (CGRP)
	Cholecystokinin (CCK)
	Galanin
	Gastrin
	Neuropeptide Y (NPY)
	Neurotensin
	Substance P
	Vasoactive intestinal peptide (VIP)
Cytokines	Interleukin-6
Growth factors	Insulin-like growth factors (IGFs) I and II
	Epidermal growth factor (EGF)
	Fibroblast growth factor (FGF)
	Transforming growth factors (TGFs) TGF-α
	Inhibins and activins (TGF-β family)
	Chondrocyte growth factor*
	Ovarian growth factor*
	Glial growth factor*
	Adipocyte growth factor*
	Mammary growth factor*

* As yet uncharacterized.

corticotrophs of the nontumorous human pituitary, including Crooke's cells and cells of basophil invasion in the posterior lobe, and in some corticotroph adenomas; in contrast, in rats, galanin mRNA is found in estrogen-induced pituitary tumors and galanin has been localized in prolactin- and GH-producing cells as well as some TSH-containing cells. The reason for this species-specific regulation is unknown. Gastrin is present in the neurohypophysis, but there appears to be species-specific variation in the adenohypophysial expression of this hormone as well: the human adenohypophysis contains only traces of gastrin which is localized to corticotrophs and corticotroph adenomas. Neuropeptide Y (NPY) immunoreactivity and mRNA are found in the pituitary and have been localized in adenohypophysial cells consistent with a subset of thyrotrophs. Neurotensin is thought to be present in gonadotrophs. Immunoreactive substance P has been found in the rodent anterior pituitary where it is localized in gonadotrophs and lactotrophs, but in the guinea pig it is found in thyrotrophs. Vasoactive intestinal peptide (VIP) is synthesized in pituitary lactotrophs.

Cytokines are known to modulate pituitary function and some have been shown to be pro-duced in the hypothalamus; only a few have been conclusively shown to be expressed in the adenohypophysis itself. Interleukin-6 has been demonstrated in stellate cells within the pituitary (115) and in GH and ACTH cells (116). Interleukin-2 mRNA has been detected in cultured human corticotroph adenomas (39); it remains uncertain whether this cytokine is produced by nontumorous human adenohypophysial cells.

Growth factors are also known to be produced by adenohypophysial cells. A number of these have been described: insulin-like growth factors (IGFs) I and II, epidermal growth factor (EGF), fibroblast growth factor (FGF), transforming growth factors (TGFs), a chondrocyte growth factor, an ovarian growth factor, a glial growth factor, an adipocyte growth factor, a mammary growth factor, and a number of others (57,117).

REFERENCES

Gross Anatomy

1. Asa SL, Kovacs K, Melmed S. The hypothalamic-pituitary axis. In: Melmed S, ed. The pituitary. Boston: Blackwell Scientific Publications, 1995:3–44.
2. Asa SL, Penz G, Kovacs K, Ezrin C. Prolactin cells in the human pituitary. A quantitative immunocytochemical analysis. Arch Pathol Lab Med 1982;106:360–3.
3. Bergeron C, Kovacs K, Bilbao JM. Primary empty sella: a histologic and immunocytologic study. Arch Intern Med 1979;139:248–9.
4. Bergland RM, Page RB. Can the pituitary secrete directly to the brain? (Affirmative anatomical evidence). Endocrinology 1978;102:1325–38.
5. Bergland RM, Page RB. Pituitary-brain vascular relations: a new paradigm. Science 1979;204:18–24.
6. Bergland RM, Ray BS, Torack RM. Anatomical variations in the pituitary gland and adjacent structures in 225 human autopsy cases. J Neurosurg 2968;28:93–9.
7. Daniel PM, Prichard MM. Observations on the vascular anatomy of the pituitary gland and its importance in pituitary function. Am Heart J 1966;72:147–52.
8. Elster AD. Modern imaging of the pituitary. Radiology 1993;187:1–14.
9. Elster AD, Sanders TG, Vines FS. Size and shape of the pituitary gland during pregnancy and post partum: measurement with MR imaging. Radiology 1991;181:531–5.
10. Gharib H, Frey HM, Laws ER Jr, Randall RV, Scheithauer BW. Coexistent primary empty sella syndrome and hyperprolactinemia. Report of 11 cases. Arch Intern Med 1983;143:1383–6.
11. Gorczyca W, Hardy J. Arterial supply of the human anterior pituitary gland. Neurosurgery 1987;20:369–78.
12. Jordan RM, Kendall JW, Kerber CW. The primary empty sella syndrome. Analysis of the clinical characteristics, radiographic features, pituitary function and cerebrospinal fluid adenohypophysial hormone concentrations. Am J Med 1977;62:569–80.
13. Lurie SN, Doraiswamy PM, Husain MM, et al. In vivo assessment of pituitary gland volume with magnetic resonance imaging: the effect of age. J Clin Endocrinol Metab 1990;71:505–8.
14. Scheithauer BW. The hypothalamus and neurohypophysis. In: Kovacs K, Asa SL, eds. Functional endocrine pathology. Boston: Blackwell Scientific Publications, 1991:170–244.
15. Sheehan HL, Davis JC. Pituitary necrosis. Br Med Bull 1968;24:59–70.
16. Stanfield JP. The blood supply of the human pituitary gland. J Anat 1960;94:257–73.
17. Wislocki GB. The vascular supply of the hypophysis cerebri of the rhesus monkey and man. Res Publ Assoc Nerv Ment Dis 1938;17:48–68.

Embryology

18. Asa SL, Kovacs K. Functional morphology of the human fetal pituitary. Pathol Ann 1984;19[pt 1]:275–315.

19. Björklöf K, Brundelet PJ. Typus degenerativus amstelodamensis (Cornelia de Lange first syndrome). Congenital hypopituitarism due to a cyst of Rathke's cleft? Acta Pediatr Scand 1965;54:275–87.

20. Boyd JD. Observations of the human pharyngeal hypophysis. J Endocrinol 1956;14:66–77.

21. Ciocca DR, Puy LA, Stati AO. Identification of seven hormone-producing cell types in the human pharyngeal hypophysis. J Clin Endocrinol Metab 1985;60:212–6.

22. Colohan AR, Grady MS, Bonnin JM, Thorner MO, Kovacs K, Jane JA. Ectopic pituitary gland simulating a suprasellar tumor. Neurosurgery 1987;20:43–8.

23. Daikoku S. Studies on the human foetal pituitary. 1. Quantitative observations. Tokushima J Exp Med 1958;5:200–13.

24. Daikoku S. Studies on the human foetal pituitary. 2. On the form and histological development, especially that of the anterior pituitary. Tokushima J Exp Med 1958;5:214–31.

25. Ehrlich RM. Ectopic and hypoplastic pituitary with adrenal hypoplasia. J Pediatr 1957;51:377–84.

26. Ferrand R, Pearse AG, Polak JM, Le Douarin NM. Immunohistochemical studies on the development of avian embryo pituitary corticotrophs under normal and experimental conditions. Histochemistry 1974;38:133–41.

27. Hori A. Suprasellar peri-infundibular ectopic adenohypophysis in fetal and adult brains. J Neurosurg 1985;62:113–5.

28. Kato T, Aida T, Abe H, et al. Ectopic salivary gland within the pituitary gland. Case report. Neurol Med Chir 1988;28:930–3.

29. Kauschansky A, Genel M, Walker Smith GJ. Congenital hypopituitarism in female infants. Its association with hypoglycemia and hypothyroidism. Am J Dis Child 1979;133:165–9.

30. Lloyd RV, Chandler WF, Kovacs K, Ryan N. Ectopic pituitary adenomas with normal anterior pituitary glands. Am J Surg Pathol 1986;108:546–52.

31. Melchionna RH, Moore RA. The pharyngeal pituitary gland. Am J Pathol 1938;14:763–71.

32. Moncrieff MW, Hill DS, Archer J, Arthur LJ. Congenital absence of pituitary gland and adrenal hypoplasia. Arch Dis Child 1972;47:136–7.

33. Priesel A. Uber die dystopie der neurohyophyse. Virchows Arch Pathol Anat Physiol Klin Med 1927;266:407–15.

34. Räihä N, Hjelt L. The correlation between the development of the hypophysial portal system and the onset of neurosecretory activity in the human fetus and infant. Acta Pediatr Scand 1957;72:610–6.

35. Rinne UK. Neurosecretory material passing into the hypophysial portal system in the human infundibulum, and its foetal development. Acta Neuroveg 1963;25:310–24.

36. Roessmann U. Duplication of the pituitary gland and spinal cord. Arch Pathol Lab Med 1985;109:518–20.

37. Schochet SS Jr, McCormick WF, Halmi NS. Salivary gland rests in the human pituitary. Light and electron microscopical study. Arch Pathol 1974;98:193–200.

38. Takor T, Pearse AG. Neuroectodermal origin of avian hypothalamohypophysial complex: the role of the ventral neural ridge. J Embryol Exp Morphol 1975;34:311–25.

Microscopic and Functional Anatomy

39. Arzt E, Renner U, Lechner K, Stelzer G, Müller OA, Stalla GK. Expression of interleukin-2 mRNA in human corticotropic adenoma cells in vitro [Abstract]. J Endocrinol Invest 1991;14(suppl 4):188.

40. Asa SL, Bamberger AM, Cao B, Wong M, Parker KL, Ezzat S. The transcription activator steroidogenic factor-1 is preferentially expressed in the human pituitary gonadotroph. J Clin Endocrinol Metab 1996;81:2165–70.

41. Asa SL, Kovacs K. Functional morphology of the human fetal pituitary. Pathol Ann 1984;19[pt 1]:275–315.

42. Asa SL, Kovacs K, Bilbao JM. The pars tuberalis of the human pituitary. A histologic, immunohistochemical, ultrastructural and immunoelectron microscopic analysis. Virchows Arch [A] 1983;399:49–59.

43. Asa SL, Kovacs K, Hammer GD, Liu B, Roos BA, Low MJ. Pituitary corticotroph hyperplasia in rats implanted with a medullary thyroid carcinoma cell line transfected with a corticotropin-releasing hormone complementary deoxyribonucleic acid expression vector. Endocrinology 1992;131:715–20.

44. Asa SL, Kovacs K, Horvath E, et al. Human fetal adenohypophysis. Electron microscopic and ultrastructural immunocytochemical analysis. Neuroendocrinology 1988;48:423–31.

45. Asa SL, Kovacs K, Laszlo FA, Domokos I, Ezrin C. Human fetal adenohypophysis. Histologic and immunocytochemical analysis. Neuroendocrinology 1986;43:308–16.

46. Asa SL, Kovacs K, Melmed S. The hypothalamic-pituitary axis. In: Melmed S, ed. The pituitary. Boston: Blackwell Scientific Publication, 1995:3–44.

47. Asa SL, Penz G, Kovacs K, Ezrin C. Prolactin cells in the human pituitary. A quantitative immunocytochemical analysis. Arch Pathol Lab Med 1982;106:360–3.

48. Asa SL, Puy LA, Lew AM, Sundmark VC, Elsholtz HP. Cell type-specific expression of the pituitary transcription activator Pit-1 in the human pituitary and pituitary adenomas. J Clin Endocrinol Metab 1993;77:1275–80.

49. Baes M, Allaerts W, Denef C. Evidence for functional communication between folliculo-stellate cells and hormone-secreting cells in perifused anterior pituitary aggregates. Endocrinology 1987;120:685–91.

50. Baker BL, Dermody WC, Reell JR. Localization of luteinizing hormone-releasing hormone in the mammalian hypothalamus. Am J Anat 1974;139:129–34.

51. Bergland RM, Torack RM. An electron microscopic study of the human infundibulum. Z Zellforsch Mikrosk Anat 1969;99:1–12.

52. Carey RM, Varma SK, Drake CR Jr, et al. Ectopic secretion of corticotropin-releasing factor as a cause of Cushing's syndrome. A clinical, morphologic, and biochemical study. N Engl J Med 1984;311:13–20.

53. Cezayirli RC, Robertson JT. Pharmacologic modulation of hypothalamic control of appetite. In: Givens JR, ed. The hypothalamus. Chicago: Year Book Medical Publishers, 1984:115–28.

54. Chaidarun SS, Klibanski A, Alexander JM. Tumor-specific expression of alternatively spliced estrogen receptor messenger ribonucleic acid variants in human pituitary adenomas. J Clin Endocrinol Metab 1997;82:1058–65.

55. Coates PJ, Doniach I. Development of folliculo-stellate cells in the human pituitary. Acta Endocrinol (Copenh) 1988;119:16–20.

56. Drolet DW, Scully KM, Simmons DM, et al. TEF, a transcription factor expressed specifically in the anterior pituitary during embryogenesis, defines a new class of leucine zipper proteins. Genes Dev 1991;5:1739–53.

57. Ezzat S, Melmed S. The role of growth factors in the pituitary. J Endocrinol Invest 1990;13:691–8.

58. Ferrara N, Schweigerer L, Neufeld G, Mitchell R, Gospodarowicz D. Pituitary follicular cells produce basic fibroblast growth factor. Proc Natl Acad Sci USA 1987;84:5773–7.

59. Frawley LS, Boockfor FR. Mammosomatotropes: presence and functions in normal and neoplastic pituitary tissue. Endocr Rev 1991;12:337–55.

60. Friend KE, Chiou YK, Laws ER Jr, Lopes MB, Shupnik MA. Pit-1 messenger ribonucleic acid is differentially expressed in human pituitary adenomas. J Clin Endocrinol Metab 1993;77:1281–6.

61. Friend KE, Chiou YK, Lopes MB, Laws ER Jr, Hughes KM, Shupnik MA. Estrogen receptor expression in human pituitary: correlation with immunohistochemistry in normal tissue, and immunohistochemistry and morphology in macroadenomas. J Clin Endocrinol Metab 1994;78:1497–04.

62. Girod C, Trouillas J. Hypophyse: embryologie, anatomie et histologie. Paris: Encycl Med Chir, 1993:1–24.

63. Girod C, Trouillas J, Dubois MP. Immunocytochemical localization of S-100 protein in stellate cells (folliculo-stellate cells) of the anterior lobe of the normal human pituitary. Cell Tissue Res 1985;241:505–11.

64. Gorski RA. Sexual differentiation of the brain. Hosp Pract 1978;13:55–62.

65. Hart MN. Hypertrophy of human subventricular hypothalamic nucleus in starvation. Arch Pathol 1971;91:493–6.

66. Hommes OR. Effects of hypophysectomy and age on the infundibular nucleus in man. J Endocrinol 1974;62: 479–88.

67. Honda SI, Morohashi KI, Nomura M, Takeya H, Kitajima M, Omura T. Ad4BP regulating steroidogenic P-450 gene is a member of steroid hormone receptor superfamily. J Biol Chem 1993;268:7494–502.

68. Horvath E, Ilse G, Kovacs K. Enigmatic bodies in human corticotroph cells. Acta Anat (Basel) 1977;98:427–33.

69. Horvath E, Kovacs K. Fine structural cytology of the adenohypophysis in rat and man. J Electron Microsc Tech 1988;8:401–32.

70. Horvath E, Kovacs K. The adenohypophysis. In: Kovacs K, Asa SL, eds. Functional endocrine pathology. Boston: Blackwell Scientific Publications, 1991:245–81.

71. Horvath E, Kovacs K, Penz G, Ezrin C. Origin, possible function and fate of "follicular cells" in the anterior lobe of the human pituitary. Am J Pathol 1974;77:199–212.

72. Horvath E, Lloyd RV, Kovacs K. Propylthiouracil-induced hypothyroidism results in reversible transdifferentiation of somatotrophs into thyroidectomy cells. A morphologic study of the rat pituitary including immunoelectron microscopy. Lab Invest 1990;63:511–20.

73. Höfler H, Walter GF, Denk H. Immunohistochemistry of folliculo-stellate cells in normal human adenohypophyses and in pituitary adenomas. Acta Neuropathol (Berl) 1984;65:35–40.

74. Ingraham HA, Lala DS, Ikeda Y, et al. The nuclear receptor steroidogenic factor 1 acts at multiple levels of the reproductive axis. Genes Dev 1994;8:2302–12.

75. Kovacs K, Horvath E. Tumors of the pituitary gland. Atlas of Tumor Pathology, 2nd Series, Fascicle 21. Washington, D.C.: Armed Forces Institute of Pathology, 1986.

76. Kovacs K, Horvath E, Bilbao JM. Oncocytes in the anterior lobe of the human pituitary gland. A light and electron microscopic study. Acta Neuropathol (Berl) 1974;27:43–54.

77. Kovacs K, Horvath E, Ryan N. Immunocytology of the human pituitary. In: DeLellis RA, ed. Diagnostic immunohistochemistry. New York: Masson Publishing, 1981:17–35.

78. Kovacs K, Sheehan HL. Pituitary changes in Kallman's syndrome: a histologic, immunocytologic, ultrastructural, and immunoelectronmicroscopic study. Fertil Steril 1982;37:83–9.

79. Lala DS, Rice DA, Parker KL. Steroidogenic factor I, a key regulator of steroidogenic enzyme expression, is the mouse homolog of fushi tarazu-factor I. Mol Endocrinol 1992;6:1249–58.

80. Lamonerie T, Tremblay JJ, Lanctot C, Therrien M, Gauthier Y, Drouin J. Ptx1, a bicoid-related homeo box transcription factor involved in transcription of the proopiomelanocortin gene. Genes Dev 1996;10:1284–95.

81. Lauriola L, Cocchia D, Sentinelli S, Maggiano N, Maira G, Michetti F. Immunohistochemical detection of folliculo-stellate cells in the human pituitary. Virchows Arch [B] 1984;47:189–97.

82. Li S, Crenshaw EB III, Rawson EJ, Simmons DM, Swanson LW, Rosenfeld MG. Dwarf locus mutants lacking three pituitary cell types result from mutations in the POU-domain gene pit-1. Nature 1990;347:528–33.

83. Liebelt RA, Perry JH. Handbook of physiology. Washington, D.C.: American Physiological Society 1967:271–85.

84. Lloyd RV, Anagnostou D, Cano M, Barkan AL, Chandler WF. Analysis of mammosomatotropic cells in normal and neoplastic human pituitary tissues by the reverse hemolytic plaque assay and immunocytochemistry. J Clin Endocrinol Metab 1988;66:1103–10.

85. Losinski NE, Horvath E, Kovacs K, Asa SL. Immunoelectron microscopic evidence of mammosomatotrophs in human adult and fetal adenohypophyses, rat adenohypophyses and human and rat pituitary adenomas. Anat Anz 1991;172:11–6.

86. Luo X, Ikeda Y, Parker KL. A cell-specific nuclear receptor is essential for adrenal and gonadal development and sexual differentiation. Cell 1994;77:481–90.

87. Marin F, Kovacs K, Stefaneanu L, Horvath E, Cheng Z. S-100 protein immunopositivity in human non-tumorous hypophyses and pituitary adenomas. Endocr Pathol 1992;3:28–38.

88. May V, Wilber JF, U'Prichard DC, Childs GV. Persistence of immunoreactive TRH and GnRH in long-term primary anterior pituitary cultures. Peptides 1987;8:543–58.

89. Moriarty GC, Garner LL. Immunocytochemical studies of cells in the rat adenohypophysis containing both ACTH and FSH. Nature 1977;265:356–8.

90. Neumann PE, Horoupian DS, Goldman JE, Hess MA. Cytoplasmic filaments of Crooke's hyaline change belong to the cytokeratin class. An immunocytochemical and ultrastructural study. Am J Pathol 1984;116:214–22.

91. Nishioka H, Llena JF, Hirano A. Immunohistochemical study of folliculostellate cells in pituitary lesions. Endocr Pathol 1991;2:155–60.

92. Pellegrini I, Barlier A, Gunz G, et al. Pit-1 gene expression in the human pituitary and pituitary adenomas. J Clin Endocrinol Metab 1994;79:189–96.

93. Pfäffle RW, DiMattia GE, Parks JS, et al. Mutation of the POU-specific domain of Pit-1 and hypopituitarism without pituitary hypoplasia. Science 1992;257:1118–21.

94. Radovick S, Nations M, Du Y, Berg LA, Weintraub BD, Wondisford FE. A mutation in the POU-homeodomain of Pit-1 responsible for combined pituitary hormone deficiency. Science 1992;257:1115–8.

95. Rance NE, McMullen NT, Smialek JE, Price DL, Young WS III. Postmenopausal hypertrophy of neurons expressing the estrogen receptor gene in the human hypothalamus. J Clin Endocrinol Metab 1990;71:79–85.

96. Rosenfeld MG. POU-domain transcription factors: powerful developmental regulators. Genes Dev 1991;5:897–907.

97. Scheithauer BW, Kovacs K, Randall RV. The pituitary gland in untreated Addison's disease. A histologic and immunocytologic study of 18 adenohypophyses. Arch Pathol Lab Med 1983;107:484–7.

98. Scheithauer BW, Kovacs K, Randall RV, Ryan N. Effects of estrogen on the human pituitary: a clinicopathologic study. Mayo Clin Proc 1989;64:1077–84.

99. Scheithauer BW, Sano T, Kovacs KT, Young WF Jr, Ryan N, Randall RV. The pituitary gland in pregnancy: a clinicopathologic and immunohistochemical study of 69 cases. Mayo Clin Proc 1990;65:461–74.

100. Seyama S, Pearl GS, Takei Y. Ultrastructural study of the human neurohypophysis. III. Vascular and perivascular structures. Cell Tissue Res 1980;206:291–302.

101. Seyama S, Pearl GS, Takei Y. Ultrastructural study of the human neurohypophysis. I. Neurosecretory axons and their dilations in the pars nervosa. Cell Tissue Res 1980;205:253–71.

102. Sheehan HL. Variations in the subventricular nucleus. J Pathol Bacteriol 1967;94:409–16.

103. Sheehan HL. Le noyau subventriculaire de l'hypothalamus. Rev Fr Endocrinol Clin 1975;16:111–4.

104. Sheehan HL, Kovacs K. The subventricular nucleus of the human hypothalamus. Brain 1966;89:589–614.

105. Sheehan HL, Kovacs K. Neurohypophysis and hypothalamus. In: Bloodworth JM Jr, ed. Endocrine pathology. General and surgical. 2nd ed. Baltimore: Williams & Wilkins, 1982:45–99.

106. Siperstein ER, Allison VF. Fine structure of the cells responsible for secretion of adrenocorticotrophin in the adrenalectomized rat. Endocrinology 1965;76:70–9.

107. Smith AI, Funder JW. Proopiomelanocortin processing in the pituitary, central nervous system, and peripheral tissues. Endocr Rev 1988;9:159–79.

108. Stefaneanu L, Kovacs K, Lloyd RV, et al. Pituitary lactotrophs and somatotrophs in pregnancy: a correlative in situ hybridization and immunocytochemical study. Virchows Arch [B] 1992;62:291–6.

109. Steinfelder HJ, Radovick S, Wondisford FE. Hormonal regulation of the thyrotropin α-subunit gene by phosphorylation of the pituitary-specific transcription factor Pit-1. Proc Natl Acad Sci USA 1992;89:5942–5.

110. Swaab DF, Fliers E. A sexually dimorphic nucleus in the human brain. Science 1985;228:1112–5.

111. Takei Y, Seyama S, Pearl GS, Tindall GT. Ultrastructural study of the human neurohypophysis. II. Cellular elements of neural parenchyma, the pituicytes. Cell Tissue Res 1980;205:273–87.

112. Therrien M, Drouin J. Cell-specific helix-loop-helix factor required for pituitary expression of the proopiomelanocortin gene. Mol Cell Biol 1993;13:2342–53.

113. Trouillas J, Loras B, Guigard MP, Girod C. α-subunit secretion by normal and tumoral growth hormone cells in humans [Abstract]. Endocr Pathol 1992;3:S53.

114. Ule G, Schwechheimer K, Tschahargane C. Morphological feedback effect on neurons of the nucl. arcuatus (sive infundibularis) and nucl. subventricularis hypothalami due to gonadal atrophy. Virchows Arch [A] 1983;400:297–308

115. Vankelecom H, Carmeliet P, van Damme J, Billiau A, Denef C. Production of interleukin-6 by folliculo-stellate cells of the anterior pituitary gland in a histiotypic cell aggregate culture system. Neuroendocrinology 1989;49:102–6.

116. Velkeniers B, Vergani P, Trouillas J, D'Haens J, Hooghe RJ, Hooghe-Peters EL. Expression of IL-6 mRNA in normal rat and human pituitaries and in human pituitary adenomas. J Histochem Cytochem 1994;42:67–76.

117. Webster J, Ham J, Bevan JS, Scanlon MF. Growth factors and pituitary tumors. Trends Endocrinol Metab 1989;1:95–8.

118. Whitehead R. The hypothalamus in postpartum hypopituitarism. J Pathol Bacteriol 1963;86:55–67.

119. Yang HJ, Ozawa H, Kurosumi K. Ultrastructural changes in growth hormone cells in the rat anterior pituitary after thyroidectomy as studied by immunoelectron microscopy and enzyme histochemistry. J Clin Electr Microsco 1989;22:269–83.

120. Zafar M, Ezzat S, Ramyar L, Pan N, Smyth HS, Asa SL. Cell-specific expression of estrogen receptor in the human pituitary and its adenomas. J Clin Endocrinol Metab 1995;80:3621–7.

❖❖❖

2

METHODS IN PITUITARY PATHOLOGY

INTRAOPERATIVE CONSULTATION

Intraoperative consultations are felt to be of value by some surgeons whereas in some institutions they are rarely requested. Some experienced surgeons suggest that the role of intraoperative consultation in the management of pituitary tumors is restricted to distinguishing pituitary adenomas from other lesions that occur in the region of the sella turcica, such as meningiomas, germinomas, and craniopharyngiomas, and metastatic tumors or inflammatory lesions such as lymphocytic hypophysitis. If there is a pituitary hormone hypersecretory state and radiologic evidence of pituitary tumor, there is little need for intraoperative consultation to confirm the diagnosis of pituitary adenoma; occasionally, however, the surgeon may encounter either another unexpected lesion or anatomic complications that require clarification. Since freezing results in disruption of tissue morphology that can interfere with the subsequent histologic and immunohistochemical examination, frozen sections should be performed only when necessary.

The accuracy of pituitary frozen section is lower than that at other sites. While most surgical pathologists achieve accuracy rates of greater than 90 percent at frozen section, the figures for pituitary frozen sections are closer to 80 percent (3,4). The reason for this low rate is largely technical, due to the small size of samples, freezing artefact, fibrosis, and other architectural distortions. Moreover, as will become apparent throughout this text, the use of standard staining techniques is not very helpful in pituitary pathology, and most special methods are not applicable to rapid intraoperative consultations.

When indicated, frozen sections or cytologic touch preparations are used. The former results in extensive artefact, but allows more accurate assessment of architecture, which may be necessary to identify an adenoma. Some authors have recommended the use of 16 μm rather than standard 4 to 8 μm sections, with various histochemical stains to identify secretory granules in cell cytoplasm (2). Rapid reticulin staining can distinguish adenoma from nontumorous ad-

enohypophysis (9), but this can be technically difficult. Stromal configuration, such as determined by the fluoresceinated lectin *Ricinus communis* agglutinin 120 (RCA 120); nuclear morphology after staining with propidium iodide; and cell-to-stroma ratios have also been suggested to diagnose pituitary adenoma by frozen section (8), but for these methods, a fluorescence microscope is required.

The use of cytologic smears has the advantage of being rapid, using little tissue, avoiding freezing artefact, and providing superb cellular detail (figs. 2-1, 2-2) (1,6,7). Although architectural detail is lost, a homogeneous cell population, binucleate cells, atypical or pleomorphic nuclei, or mitotic figures suggest the presence of an adenoma. This method, however, cannot be used to determine invasion by the tumor or to examine resection margins.

Some surgeons request frozen section examination of the margins of a specimen to establish complete tumor resection at the time of surgery. Experienced pathologists have found that this is extremely difficult and the expectation is often unrealistic. If there is a clear indication for this approach, it may be necessary.

In cases of hormone hypersecretion unaccompanied by detectable radiologic abnormality, such as occurs occasionally in patients with Cushing's disease, it may be necessary to determine the lateralization of a microadenoma biochemically using inferior petrosal sinus sampling (see chapter 3). The pathologist often cannot visualize a lesion grossly at the time of intraoperative consultation, and serial sectioning is not desirable for identifying a microadenoma on frozen section since it may be lost for permanent identification. In this situation, one can perform rapid intraoperative hormone measurements, such as for adrenocorticotropic hormone (ACTH) in the case of Cushing's disease, in peripituitary blood (5).

Perhaps the most important role of the pathologist at the time of pituitary surgery is to process the resected tissue for optimal handling that will result in the most accurate diagnosis. When a

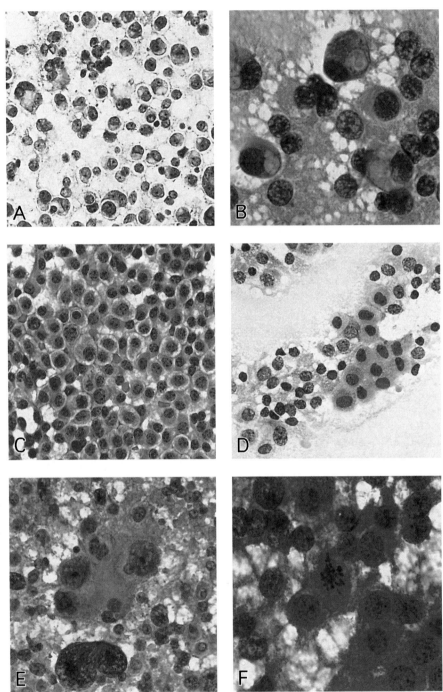

Figure 2-1
CYTOLOGIC SMEARS OF PITUITARY ADENOMAS AT INTRAOPERATIVE CONSULTATION

A: Sparsely granulated somatotroph adenoma. Note the eccentric distorted or lobulated nuclei that surround the clearing of fibrous bodies.

B: Corticotroph adenoma. Note the basophilic granules and "enigmatic bodies," cytoplasmic vacuoles corresponding to complex lysosomes.

C: Gonadotroph adenoma. The tumor is composed of a homogeneous population of small cells with chromophobic cytoplasm.

D: Gonadotroph adenoma with oncocytic change. This tumor is composed of small monotonous cells with chromophobic cytoplasm interspersed with cells that have abundant eosinophilic granular cytoplasm.

E: Somatotroph adenoma with giant cells and nuclear pleomorphism. These worrisome features confirm the presence of a neoplasm but are not indicative of malignancy.

F: Mitotic figures in a smear are not indicative of malignancy.

(Courtesy of Dr. J. M. Bilbao, Toronto, Canada.)

tumor is small, the tissue should be fixed for histologic and immunohistochemical analysis. If there is sufficient tissue, a small piece should be processed for electron microscopy. Depending on the interest of those involved in the investigation, sterile tissue can also be put in culture medium for in vitro analysis and some can be frozen for biochemical or molecular studies. Rapid handling of the tissue is essential, since delay of fixation and drying can damage the small fragments that are usually obtained by transsphenoidal surgery, the routine surgical approach for most pituitary tumors.

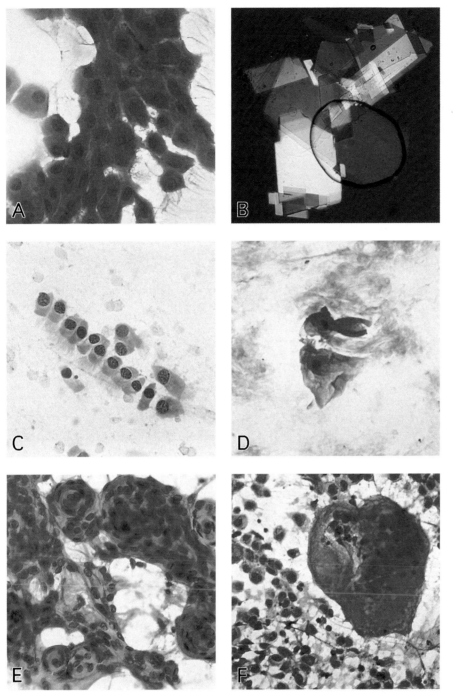

Figure 2-2
CYTOLOGIC SMEARS
OF PITUITARY TUMORS
OTHER THAN ADENOMAS
AT INTRAOPERATIVE
CONSULTATION

A: Craniopharyngioma can be diagnosed in a smear by identifying squamoid epithelial cells that adhere to form sheets.

B: Keratin in a craniopharyngioma forms crystalloid structures that have colorful birefringent patterns on polarized light.

C: A Rathke cleft cyst can be diagnosed at intraoperative consultation by the recognition of ciliated columnar epithelium that has bland nuclear features.

D: An epidermoid cyst contains desquamated epithelium and keratin debris.

E: A meningioma in the region of the sella turcica can be mistaken for a pituitary adenoma clinically, but is readily recognized by the characteristic meningotheliomatous whorls on a smear.

F: A germinoma is composed of epithelioid cells, infiltrating lymphocytes, and a multinucleate giant cell.

(Courtesy of Dr. J. M. Bilbao, Toronto, Canada.)

HISTOLOGY AND IMMUNOHISTOCHEMISTRY

The diagnosis of pituitary disorders, both neoplastic and non-neoplastic, relies mainly on histology and immunohistochemistry. Neutral buffered formalin is the best routine fixative for these studies. Some pathologists prefer Bouin's or Zamboni's fixatives because cytologic detail may be improved, but immunostaining for most pituitary antigens is better with formalin, so it is usually recommended that formalin be the primary fixative. If tissue is available, some may be fixed in the other preparations.

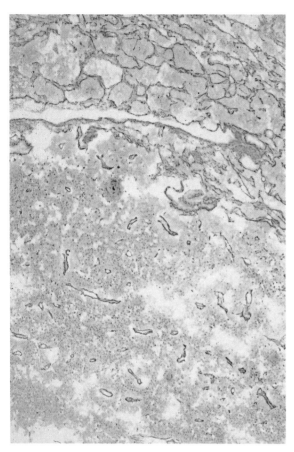

Figure 2-3
RETICULIN STAINING OF PITUITARY ADENOMA
The reticulin fiber network is completely disrupted in pituitary adenoma. The nontumorous adenohypophysis (top) retains normal acinar architecture.

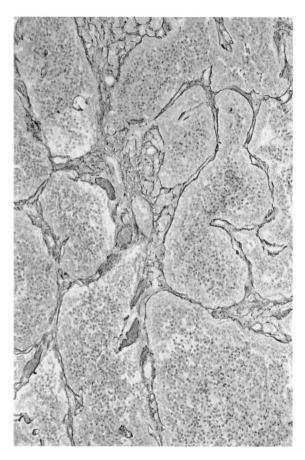

Figure 2-4
RETICULIN STAINING OF
ADENOHYPOPHYSIAL HYPERPLASIA
In adenohypophysial hyperplasia, the reticulin fiber network remains intact but the acini are expanded.

Routine histology relies on the conventional hematoxylin and eosin stain. A number of histochemical stains have been applied to the analysis of pituitary tissues, such as the periodic acid–Schiff (PAS) method, various trichrome stains, aldehyde fuchsin and aldehyde thionine techniques, orange G, Herlant's erythrosin, or Brookes' carmoisine. In the era of immunohistochemistry, these beautiful but relatively nonspecific stains have been relegated to the status of morphologic curiosities. The major exception is the reticulin stain which is essential for distinguishing normal adenohypophysial architecture, hyperplasia, and adenoma (figs. 2-3, 2-4) (22,23). Rare pituitary adenomas may contain amyloid material that stains with Congo red and has apple-green birefringence with polarized light (12,13,16,18,24).

Immunohistochemistry is perhaps the most valuable tool in the diagnosis of pituitary tumors (14,22). This technique, along with routine histology, is useful for determining cell differentiation and classifying a lesion into one of the numerous categories of pituitary tumors listed in the chapters that follow. In the case of pituitary adenoma, it is the most efficient and reliable means to characterize hormone production; other markers of adenohypophysial cell differentiation, such as transcription factors (10,11), chromogranins (17), and keratins (19–21), can also be determined by immunohistochemical staining. The same is true for proliferation markers, growth factor and receptor expression, and oncogene product expression which may have diagnostic, prognostic, or therapeutic implications in the future. Antigenic markers of other tumors, including meningiomas, germinomas, craniopharyngiomas, metastatic tumors, and sarcomas, allow the definite diagnosis of these lesions.

In the past pathologists were faced with problems of interpretation due to suboptimal tissue fixation, which caused artefactual immunonegativity, or crossreactivity of antisera, which gave rise to artefactual positivity; the latter was a particularly common problem with respect to hormone localization. Improvements in tissue fixation have been achieved in many laboratories as the role of immunohistochemistry has expanded in diagnostic pathology; this has resulted in far fewer artefactually immunonegative cases.

The problem of crossreactivity and artefactual positivity was addressed in 1991 by a collaborative study of the Pathologists of the Club Français de l'Hypophyse. These investigators evaluated 29 monoclonal antibodies and polyclonal antisera and recommended the use of highly specific and sensitive commercially available products that could be used to accurately determine the hormonal profile of pituitary adenomas (15). Although they did not evaluate antisera against ACTH or other proopiomelanocortin (POMC) derivatives, their analysis of other antisera and antibodies is of great value in the study of pituitary adenomas. The reader is referred to their important paper for the details; a list of the recommended antisera and antibodies is provided in Table 2-1.

ELECTRON MICROSCOPY

The role of electron microscopy in pituitary tumor diagnosis is controversial. Ultrastructural examination has played a pivotal role in shaping our understanding of adenohypophysial cytology and structure-function correlations (25,27). However, this knowledge as well as improved immunohistochemical methodology, has led to the development of light microscopic markers of tumor cell differentiation which obviate the need for this time-consuming and expensive examination for the usual forms of pituitary tumors. Nevertheless, electron microscopy remains an essential tool for rare or unusual tumors.

For this type of analysis, small fragments of fresh tumor tissue should be fixed in 2.5 percent glutaraldehyde. Retrieval of tissue from paraffin

Table 2-1

ANTIBODIES RECOMMENDED FOR HORMONE IMMUNOLOCALIZATION IN PITUITARY ADENOMAS

Hormone	Polyclonal vs Monoclonal	Source
GH	polyclonal	NIDDK*
		Miles
	monoclonal	Amersham
PRL	monoclonal	Miles
		Immunotech
α-subunit	polyclonal	NIDDK
	monoclonal	Serotec
		Immunotech
β-TSH	monoclonal	Miles
		Immunotech
β-FSH	monoclonal	Immunotech
β-LH	polyclonal	NIDDK
	monoclonal	Immunotech

*NIDDK - National Institute of Diabetes and Digestive and Kidney Disorders.

is of dubious value in those difficult cases in which electron microscopy is indicated, therefore it is recommended that a small fragment of tissue be fixed in every case in the event that it may be needed. Postfixation in osmium and embedding in an epoxy resin is suitable for conventional transmission electron microscopy to determine the ultrastructural characteristics of tumor cells.

Ultrastructural immunolocalization of some tumor cell antigens such as growth hormone (GH), prolactin, and ACTH is readily performed by application of postembedding immunocytochemical procedures (28); in some instances, omission of osmium postfixation improves the result. Other antigens, particularly the glycoprotein hormones, are significantly altered during routine processing and require either special fixation and embedding procedures or, alternatively, localization by preembedding staining (26,29).

TISSUE CULTURE

The role of tissue culture is primarily as a research tool but it can be applied to the diagnosis of unusual pituitary tumors. Numerous studies have documented hormone synthesis and secretion as well as their regulation in vitro; tissue culture is useful for the determination of response of tumors to various regulatory hormones and drugs. This subject has been reviewed in several publications (30,31).

The technical aspects of pituitary tumor cell culture can be challenging. Pituitary cells attach poorly to culture substrates and hormonal activity in vitro is highly dependent on cell-to-cell interactions as well as on the additives to culture media, such as hormones or growth factors found in serum or supplemented to serum-free media. The interested reader is referred to the work of investigators in the field for further information (32,37–39).

Cultured cells can be characterized by conventional histochemical techniques, immunocytochemical methods, electron microscopy, and in situ hybridization. Individual cells can be analyzed in vitro using the reverse hemolytic plaque assay which detects antigen release or surface presentation by single cells; it permits both qualitative assessment of mixed cell populations and quantitation of amounts of hormone released, since plaque size is proportional to the amount of hormone that diffuses around a given cell (41). The technique can be applied sequentially to measure temporal variations in hormonal activity or to identify cells that secrete more than one substance (33,35,36). It can be combined with immunocytochemistry (34,42), electron microscopy (40), autoradiography, or in situ hybridization.

FLOW CYTOMETRY

Flow cytometry has been used to examine DNA ploidy in pituitary adenomas (43–45). Studies indicate that pituitary adenomas have a low incidence of aneuploidy, which occurs primarily in GH- and prolactin-producing tumors. Both fresh tissue and fixed specimens have been used, however the latter yield lower aneuploidy figures and lower S-phase fractions.

The significance of these data remains to be established by follow-up of patients and more rigorous prospective studies. At this time, flow cytometry for DNA ploidy does not appear to be of major importance in the routine analysis of pituitary adenomas.

MOLECULAR ANALYSIS

Molecular analyses are rapidly becoming the most sophisticated tools of the investigative pathologist. For the moment, in situ hybridization,

Northern and Southern blot analyses, polymerase chain reaction (PCR), and other such tools are relegated to the realm of research. In rare cases, they are required for diagnosis; for example, occasional tumors may not store detectable hormone and the application of in situ hybridization can clarify the profile of hormone production by a pituitary adenoma (66,68–71,77). This technique is easily applicable to sections of formalin-fixed, paraffin-embedded tissue when the mRNA being examined is abundant, as it usually is for pituitary hormones. However, the cost and time involved limit this approach for routine diagnosis.

Northern blots and reverse transcription-PCR (RT-PCR) have been used to characterize gene expression in pituitary tumors. They identify not only hormone production (64), but also other substances, such as transcription factors (47,49,59,60,75,82) and growth factors (46,57,58, 61,67,79,81), that may be involved in tumor cell differentiation and proliferation.

Genetic analyses have also attempted to define the molecular basis of pituitary tumorigenesis (51,54–56,63,65,74,78,80,83). These studies are reviewed in chapter 3.

Transgenic models have been developed to examine pituitary cytodifferentiation (50,52) and tumorigenesis (48,53,62,72,73,76). Further applications of these sophisticated technologies will no doubt clarify the answers to many questions about pituitary tumor development.

A PRACTICAL APPROACH TO THE DIAGNOSIS OF A PITUITARY TUMOR

The first approach to a pituitary tumor is routine histology. This will usually allow classification of a lesion as an adenohypophysial proliferation, as another tumor type (see chapters 5 to 10), or as a tumor-like lesion (see chapter 11).

If the lesion is a proliferation of adenohypophysial cells, a reticulin stain is imperative to confirm neoplastic as opposed to hyperplastic disease. Immunostains are then used to classify the cells involved. A hyperplastic process will contain hormone-immunoreactive cells of all types with predominance of one type; the regional distribution of the various hormone-containing cells within the gland (see chapter 1) must be considered when assessing cell numbers. Neoplasms should be first classified, as reviewed in the following pages, based on hormone reactivity, transcription factors, or both, but subclassification entails the addition of other stains; for example, among growth hormone-producing adenomas, the pattern of low molecular weight cytokeratins (using the Cam 5.2 antibody) distinguishes sparsely from densely granulated adenomas without the need to resort to electron microscopy.

Electron microscopy is indicated for more precise evaluation of unusual tumors that are not readily classified on the basis of classic immunohistochemical profiles. This includes tumors that do not contain immunoreactive hormones, in which case other markers should also be used to exclude other tumors discussed in chapters 5 through 10. Tumors with unusual patterns of hormone reactivity also warrant ultrastructural investigation. The diagnosis of unusual adenomas, such as the aggressive silent subtype III adenomas (see pages 125 and 126) or acidophil stem cell adenomas (see pages 77–81) usually requires ultrastructural confirmation once the suspicion is raised by atypical immunohistochemical results. The results are not academic only; these diagnoses predict a worse prognosis and therefore indicate the need for closer clinical surveillance, and in some cases, prompt more aggressive postoperative management with early radiotherapy.

Tissue culture techniques, flow cytometry, and molecular analyses remain ancillary tools without direct diagnostic applications at this point in time.

Tumors not composed of adenohypophysial cells, such as craniopharyngiomas, neurogenic neoplasms, germ cell tumors, hematologic lesions, vascular and mesenchymal proliferations, and metastatic malignancies, are usually classified on the basis of histologic and immunohistochemical parameters described in the following chapters; ultrastructural examination should be performed when these techniques are not diagnostic.

REFERENCES

Intraoperative Consultation

1. Adams H, Graham DI, Doyle D. Brain biopsy. The smear technic for neurosurgical biopsies. Philadelphia: JB Lippincott, 1981.
2. Adelman LS, Post KD. Intraoperative frozen section technique for pituitary adenomas. Am J Surg Pathol 1979;3:173–5.
3. Lang HD, Saeger W, Lüdecke DK, Muller D. Rapid frozen section diagnosis of pituitary tumors. Endocr Pathol 1990;1:116–22.
4. Lloyd RV. Frozen sections in the diagnosis of pituitary lesions. In: Lloyd RV, ed. Surgical pathology of the pituitary gland. Philadelphia: WB Saunders, 1993:22–4.
5. Lüdecke DK. Intraoperative measurement of adrenocorticotropic hormone in peripituitary blood in Cushing's disease. Neurosurgery 1989;24:201–5.
6. Marshall LF, Adams H, Doyle D, Graham DI. The histological accuracy of the smear technique for neurosurgical biopsies. J Neurosurg 1973;39:82–8.
7. Martinez AJ, Moossy J. Cytological diagnosis of pituitary adenomas. J Neuropathol Exp Neurol 1983;412:307–11.
8. McKeever PE, Laverson S, Oldfield EH, Smith BH, Gadille D, Chandler WF. Stromal and nuclear markers for rapid identification of pituitary adenomas at biopsy. Arch Pathol Lab Med 1985;109:509–14.
9. Velasco ME, Sindely SO, Roessmann U. Reticulum stain for frozen-section diagnosis of pituitary adenomas. J Neurosurg 1977;46:548–50.

Histology and Immunohistochemistry

10. Asa SL, Bamberger AM, Cao B, Wong M, Parker KL, Ezzat S. The transcription activator steroidogenic factor-1 is preferentially expressed in the human pituitary gonadotroph. J Clin Endocrinol Metab 1996;81:2165–70.
11. Asa SL, Puy LA, Lew AM, Sundmark VC, Elsholtz HP. Cell type-specific expression of the pituitary transcription activator Pit-1 in the human pituitary and pituitary adenomas. J Clin Endocrinol Metab 1993;77:1275–80.
12. Bilbao JM, Horvath E, Hudson AR, Kovacs K. Pituitary adenoma producing amyloid-like substance. Arch Pathol Lab Med 1975;99:411–5.
13. Bilbao JM, Kovacs K, Horvath E, et al. Pituitary melanocorticotrophinoma with amyloid deposition. J Can Sci Neurol 1975;2:199–202.
14. Giannattasio G, Bassetti M. Human pituitary adenomas. Recent advances in morphological studies. J Endocrinol Invest 1990;13:435–54.

15. Labat-Moleur F, Trouillas J, Seret-Bregue D, Kujas M, Delisle M-B, Ronin C. Evaluation of 29 monoclonal and polyclonal antibodies used in the diagnosis of pituitary adenomas. A collaborative study from pathologists of the Club Français de l'Hypophyse. Pathol Res Pract 1991;187:534–8.

16. Landolt AM, Kleihues P, Heitz PU. Amyloid deposits in pituitary adenomas. Differentiation of two types. Arch Pathol Lab Med 1987;111:453–8.

17. Lloyd RV, Cano M, Rosa P, Hille A, Huttner WB. Distribution of chromogranin A and secretogranin I (chromogranin B) in neuroendocrine cells and tumors. Am J Pathol 1988;130:296–4.

18. Mori H, Mori S, Saitoh Y, Moriwaki K, Iida S, Matsumoto K. Growth hormone-producing pituitary adenoma with crystal-like amyloid immunohistochemically positive for growth hormone. Cancer 1985;55:96–102.

19. Neumann PE, Goldman JE, Horoupian DS, Hess MA. Fibrous bodies in growth hormone-secreting adenomas contain cytokeratin filaments. Arch Pathol Lab Med 1985;109:505–8.

20. Neumann PE, Horoupian DS, Goldman JE, Hess MA. Cytoplasmic filaments of Crooke's hyaline change belong to the cytokeratin class. An immunocytochemical and ultrastructural study. Am J Pathol 1984;116:214–22.

21. Sano T, Ohshima T, Yamada S. Expression of glycoprotein hormones and intracytoplasmic distribution of cytokeratin in growth hormone-producing pituitary adenomas. Pathol Res Pract 1991;187:530–3.

22. Stefaneanu L, Kovacs K. Light microscopic special stains and immunohistochemistry in the diagnosis of pituitary adenomas. In: Lloyd RV, ed. Surgical pathology of the pituitary gland. Philadelphia: WB Saunders, 1993:34–51.

23. Thorner MO, Perryman RL, Cronin MJ, et al. Somatotroph hyperplasia: successful treatment of acromegaly by removal of a pancreatic islet tumor secreting a growth hormone-releasing factor. J Clin Invest 1982;70:965–77.

24. Voigt C, Saeger W, Gerigk CH, Lüdecke DK. Amyloid in pituitary adenomas. Pathol Res Pract 1988;183:555–7.

Electron Microscopy

25. Horvath E, Kovacs K. Fine structural cytology of the adenohypophysis in rat and man. J Electron Microsc Tech 1988;8:401–32.

26. Horvath E, Lloyd RV, Kovacs K. Propylthiouracil-induced hypothyroidism results in reversible transdifferentiation of somatotrophs into thyroidectomy cells. A morphologic study of the rat pituitary including immunoelectron microscopy. Lab Invest 1990;63:511–20.

27. Kovacs K, Horvath E. Tumors of the pituitary gland. Atlas of Tumor Pathology, 2nd Series, Fascicle 21. Washington, D.C.: Armed Forces Institute of Pathology, 1986.

28. Losinski NE, Horvath E, Kovacs K, Asa SL. Immunoelectron microscopic evidence of mammosomatotrophs in human adult and fetal adenohypophyses, rat adenohypophyses and human and rat pituitary adenomas. Anat Anz 1991;172:11–6.

29. Osamura RY. Immunoelectron microscopic studies of GH and alpha subunit in GH secreting pituitary adenomas. Pathol Res Pract 1988;183:569–71.

Tissue Culture

30. Asa SL. In vitro culture techniques. In: Kovacs K, Asa SL, eds. Functional endocrine pathology. Boston: Blackwell Scientific Publications, 1991:109–23.

31. Asa SL. Tissue culture in the diagnosis and study of pituitary adenomas. In: Lloyd RV, ed. Surgical pathology of the pituitary gland. Philadelphia: WB Saunders, 1993:94–115.

32. Denef C. Paracrine interaction in anterior pituitary. In: MacLeod RM, Thorner MO, Scapagnini U, eds. Prolactin, basic and clinical correlates. Padova: Liviana Press, 1984:53–7.

33. Frawley LS, Boockfor FR, Hoeffler JP. Identification by plaque assays of a pituitary cell type that secretes both growth hormone and prolactin. Endocrinology 1985;116:734–7.

34. Lloyd RV, Anagnostou D, Cano M, Barkan AL, Chandler WF. Analysis of mammosomatotropic cells in normal and neoplastic human pituitary tissues by the reverse hemolytic plaque assay and immunocytochemistry. J Clin Endocrinol Metab 1988;66:1103–10.

35. Neill JD, Smith PF, Luque EH, Munoz de Toro M, Nagy G, Mulchahey JJ. Detection and measurement of hormone secretion from individual pituitary cells. Recent Prog Horm Res 1987;43:175–229.

36. Smith PF, Luque EH, Neill JD. Detection and measurement of secretion from individual neuroendocrine cells using a reverse hemolytic plaque assay. Methods Enzymol 1986;124:443–65.

37. Thodou E, Ramyar L, Cohen AI, Singer W, Asa SL. A serum-free system for primary cultures of human pituitary adenomas. Endocr Pathol 1995;6:289–99.

38. Vale W, Grant G, Amoss M, Blackwell R, Guillemin R. Culture of enzymatically dispersed anterior pituitary cells: functional validation of a method. Endocrinology 1972;91:562–72.

39. Weiner RI, Bethea CL, Jaquet P, Ramsdell JS, Gospodarowicz DJ. Culture of dispersed anterior pituitary cells on extracellular matrix. Methods Enzymol 1983;103:287–93.

40. Yamada S, Aiba T, Hattori A, Suzuki T, Asa SL, Kovacs K. Reverse hemolytic plaque assay. Electron microscopic observation of plaque-forming single adenoma cells in GH producing adenomas. Pathol Res Pract 1991;187:546–51.

41. Yamada S, Asa SL. Applications of the reverse hemolytic plaque assay in the study of human pituitary adenomas. Neuroprotocols 1994;5:209–15.

42. Yamada S, Asa SL, Kovacs K, Muller P, Smyth HS. Analysis of hormone secretion by clinically nonfunctioning human pituitary adenomas using the reverse hemolytic plaque assay. J Clin Endocrinol Metab 1989;68:73–80.

Flow Cytometry

43. Anniko M, Tribukait B, Wersäll J. DNA ploidy and cell phase in human pituitary tumors. Cancer 1984; 53:1708–13.
44. Camplejohn RS, Macartney JC. Comparison of DNA flow cytometry from fresh and paraffin-embedded samples of non-Hodgkin's lymphoma. J Clin Pathol 1985;38:1096–9.
45. Fitzgibbons PL, Appley AJ, Turner RR, et al. Flow cytometric analysis of pituitary tumors. Correlation of nuclear antigen p105 and DNA content with clinical behavior. Cancer 1988;62:1556–60.

Molecular Analysis

46. Alexander JM, Swearingen B, Tindall GT, Klibanski A. Human pituitary adenomas express endogenous inhibin subunit and follistatin messenger ribonucleic acids. J Clin Endocrinol Metab 1995;80:147–52.
47. Asa SL, Bamberger AM, Cao B, Wong M, Parker KL, Ezzat S. The transcription activator steroidogenic factor-1 is preferentially expressed in the human pituitary gonadotroph. J Clin Endocrinol Metab 1996;81:2165–70.
48. Asa SL, Kovacs K, Stefaneanu L, et al. Pituitary adenomas in mice transgenic for growth hormone-releasing hormone. Endocrinology 1992;131:2083–9.
49. Asa SL, Puy LA, Lew AM, Sundmark VC, Elsholtz HP. Cell type-specific expression of the pituitary transcription activator Pit-1 in the human pituitary and pituitary adenomas. J Clin Endocrinol Metab 1993;77:1275–80.
50. Behringer RR, Mathews LS, Palmiter RD, Brinster RL. Dwarf mice produced by genetic ablation of growth hormone-expressing cells. Genes Dev 1988;2:453–61.
51. Boggild MD, Jenkinson S, Pistorello M, et al. Molecular genetic studies of sporadic pituitary tumors. J Clin Endocrinol Metab 1994;78:387–92.
52. Borrelli E, Heyman RA, Arias C, Sawchenko PE, Evans RM. Transgenic mice with inducible dwarfism. Nature 1989;339:538–41.
53. Borrelli E, Sawchenko PE, Evans RM. Pituitary hyperplasia induced by ectopic expression of nerve growth factor. Proc Natl Acad Sci USA 1992;89:2764–8.
54. Brystom C, Larsson C, Blomberg C, et al. Localization of the MEN-1 gene to a small region within chromosome 11q13 by deletion mapping in tumors. Proc Natl Acad Sci USA 1990;87:1968–72.
55. Cai WY, Alexander JM, Hedley-Whyte ET, et al. Ras mutations in human prolactinomas and pituitary carcinomas. J Clin Endocrinol Metab 1994;78:89–93.
56. Cryns VL, Alexander JM, Klibanski A, Arnold A. The retinoblastoma gene in human pituitary tumors. J Clin Endocrinol Metab 1993;77:644–6.
57. Ezzat S, Melmed S. The role of growth factors in the pituitary. J Endocrinol Invest 1990;13:691–8.
58. Ezzat S, Smyth HS, Ramyar L, Asa SL. Heterogenous in vivo and in vitro expression of basic fibroblast growth factor by human pituitary adenomas. J Clin Endocrinol Metab 1995;80:878–84.
59. Friend KE, Chiou YK, Laws ER Jr, Lopes MB, Shupnik MA. Pit-1 messenger ribonucleic acid is differentially expressed in human pituitary adenomas. J Clin Endocrinol Metab 1993;77:1281–6.
60. Friend KE, Chiou YK, Lopes MB, Laws ER Jr, Hughes KM, Shupnik MA. Estrogen receptor expression in human pituitary: correlation with immunohistochemistry in normal tissue, and immunohistochemistry and morphology in macroadenomas. J Clin Endocrinol Metab 1994;78:1497–504.
61. Haddad G, Penabad JL, Bashey HM, et al. Expression of activin/inhibin subunit messenger ribonucleic acids by gonadotroph adenomas. J Clin Endocrinol Metab 1994;79:1399–403.
62. Helseth A, Siegal GP, Haug E, Bautch VL. Transgenic mice that develop pituitary tumors. A model for Cushing's disease. Am J Pathol 1992;140:1071–80.
63. Herman V, Drazin NZ, Gonsky R, Melmed S. Molecular screening of pituitary adenomas for gene mutations and rearrangements. J Clin Endocrinol Metab 1993;77:50–5.
64. Jameson JL, Klibanski A, Black PM, et al. Glycoprotein hormone genes are expressed in clinically nonfunctioning pituitary adenomas. J Clin Invest 1987;80:1472–8.
65. Karga HJ, Alexander JM, Hedley-Whyte ET, Klibanski A, Jameson JL. Ras mutations in human pituitary tumors. J Clin Endocrinol Metab 1992;74:914–9.
66. Kovacs K, Lloyd R, Horvath E, et al. Silent somatotroph adenomas of the human pituitary. A morphologic study of three cases including immunocytochemistry, electron microscopy, in vitro examination, and in situ hybridization. Am J Pathol 1989;134:345–53.
67. LeRiche VK, Asa SL, Ezzat S. Epidermal growth factor and its receptor (EGF-R) in human pituitary adenomas: EGF-R correlates with tumor aggressiveness. J Clin Endocrinol Metab 1996;81:656–62.
68. Li J, Stefaneanu L, Kovacs K, Horvath E, Smyth HS. Growth hormone (GH) and prolactin (PRL) gene expression and immunoreactivity in GH- and PRL-producing human pituitary adenomas. Virchows Arch [A] 1993;422:193–201.
69. Lloyd RV. Analysis of human pituitary tumors by in situ hybridization. Pathol Res Pract 1988;183:558–60.
70. Lloyd RV, Fields K, Jin L, Horvath E, Kovacs K. Analysis of endocrine active and clinically silent corticotropic adenomas by in situ hybridization. Am J Pathol 1990;137:479–88.
71. Lloyd RV, Jin L, Fields K, et al. Analysis of pituitary hormones and chromogranin A mRNAs in null cell adenomas, oncocytomas, and gonadotroph adenomas by in situ hybridization. Am J Pathol 1991;139:553–64.
72. McAndrew J, Paterson AJ, Asa SL, McCarthy KJ, Kudlow JE. Targeting of transforming growth factor-expression to pituitary lactotrophs in transgenic mice results in selective lactotroph proliferation and adenomas. Endocrinology 1995;136:4479–88.
73. Murphy D, Bishop A, Rindi G, et al. Mice transgenic for a vasopressin-SV40 hybrid oncogene develop tumors of the endocrine pancreas and the anterior pituitary. A possible model for human multiple endocrine neoplasia type 1. Am J Pathol 1987;129:552–66.

74. Pei L, Melmed S, Scheithauer B, Kovacs K, Prager D. H-ras mutations in human pituitary carcinoma metastases. J Clin Endocrinol Metab 1994;78:842–6.

75. Pellegrini I, Barlier A, Gunz G, et al. Pit-1 gene expression in the human pituitary and pituitary adenomas. J Clin Endocrinol Metab 1994;79:189–96.

76. Schechter J, Windle JJ, Stauber C, Mellon PL. Neural tissue within anterior pituitary tumors generated by oncogene expression in transgenic mice. Neuroendocrinology 1992;56:330–11.

77. Stefaneanu L, Kovacs K, Lloyd RV, et al. Pituitary lactotrophs and somatotrophs in pregnancy: a correlative in situ hybridization and immunocytochemical study. Virchows Arch [Cell Pathol] 1992;62:291–6.

78. Vallar L, Spada A, Giannattasio G. Altered Gs and adenylate cyclase activity in human GH-secreting pituitary adenomas. Nature 1987;330:566–8.

79. Webster J, Ham J, Bevan JS, Scanlon MF. Growth factors and pituitary tumors. Trends Endocrinol Metab 1989;1:95–8.

80. Woloschak M, Roberts JL, Post KD. Loss of heterozygosity at the retinoblastoma locus in human pituitary tumors. Cancer 1994;74:693–6.

81. Yamashita S, Weiss M, Melmed S. Insulin-like growth factor I regulates growth hormone secretion and messenger ribonucleic acid levels in human pituitary tumor cells. J Clin Endocrinol Metab 1986;63:730–5.

82. Zafar M, Ezzat S, Ramyar L, Pan N, Smyth HS, Asa SL. Cell-specific expression of estrogen receptor in the human pituitary and its adenomas. J Clin Endocrinol Metab 1995;80:3621–7.

83. Zhu J, Leon SP, Beggs AH, Busque L, Gilliland DG, Black PM. Human pituitary adenomas show no loss of heterozygosity at the retinoblastoma gene locus. J Clin Endocrinol Metab 1994;78:922–7.

3
PITUITARY ADENOMAS

Pituitary adenomas are benign neoplasms composed of adenohypophysial cells. These tumors are clonal proliferations and exhibit a wide range of behavior, both functional and proliferative. Although they usually arise in the sella turcica, they may occasionally be ectopic.

 Some pituitary adenomas are small, with a slow rate of growth. When hormonally inactive, such tumors are not usually detected clinically and therefore represent either radiologic "incidentalomas" or incidental findings at postmortem examination. When they produce hormones in excess, however, they can give rise to a severe clinical syndrome, such as acromegaly or Cushing's disease, that can be lethal despite the relative paucity of tumor growth.

Other adenomas are rapidly growing tumors that give rise to symptoms of an intracranial mass or cause visual field disturbances. They may invade locally downwards into the paranasal sinuses, laterally into the cavernous sinuses, and upwards into the parenchyma of the brain. These more aggressive tumors are either hormonally active, secreting any number of hormones in excess, or clinically nonfunctional.

This chapter reviews the epidemiology and classification of these lesions and discusses the clinical, biochemical, radiologic, and morphologic features as well as the prognosis and therapy of each tumor type. A comprehensive discussion of the pathogenesis of these intriguing neoplasms follows.

EPIDEMIOLOGY OF
PITUITARY ADENOMAS

The true incidence of pituitary tumors is difficult to establish with certainty. The recognized incidence of tumors of any type in a given population is determined by the limitations of diagnostic techniques. With modern methods of imaging and biochemical analysis of hormonal activity, the most recent data, reviewed below, suggest that pituitary adenomas are common, occurring in approximately 20 percent of the general population.

Various studies have examined the incidence of such lesions at autopsy (fig. 3-1) or at routine radiologic evaluation of asymptomatic patients, yielding data on the development of incidental, slowly growing tumors that do not give rise to clinical symptoms of either a sellar mass or hormonal excess. While one study found incidental pituitary adenomas in only 2.7 percent of the population (6), careful histologic assessment yields higher numbers (16) and some have shown prevalences of 22.5 (3) and 27 percent (2). Using high resolution computed tomography (CT) or magnetic resonance imaging (MRI), approximately 20 percent of "normal" pituitary glands are shown to harbor an incidental lesion measuring 3 mm or more in diameter (4). Most asymptomatic patients have clinically nonfunctioning tumors that are now recognized to be of gonadotroph differentiation, or prolactinomas that have not caused symptoms recognized by the patient (12,13). The sex incidence is equal in these studies and the incidence increases with age in autopsy analyses so that the more than 30 percent of patients 50 to 60 years of age have clinically undetected tumors.

Clinically diagnosed pituitary adenomas (figs. 3-2–3-4) traditionally were said to represent 10 percent of intracranial neoplasms, however, improvements in radiographic imaging, biochemical detection of hormonal abnormalities, and

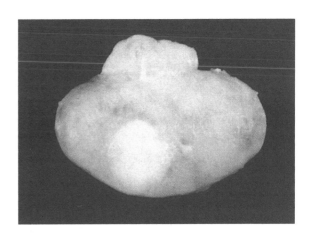

Figure 3-1
INCIDENTAL PITUITARY ADENOMA
This small microadenoma was identified incidentally at autopsy. The patient had no evidence of hormone excess and no symptoms of a sellar mass.

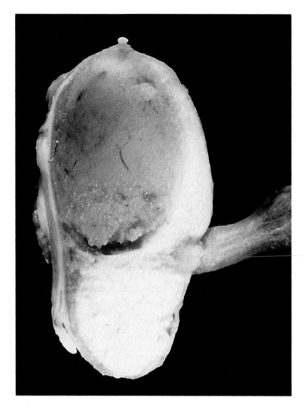

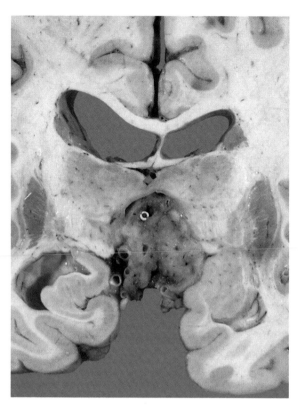

Figure 3-2
INTRASELLAR PITUITARY ADENOMA
This intrasellar adenoma, occupying one of the lateral wings, was found incidentally at the autopsy of a 65-year-old man who died of coronary heart disease. The tumor caused no obvious endocrine symptoms and contained no immunoreactive hormones. (Plate IVC from Fascicle 21, 2nd Series.)

Figure 3-3
INVASIVE PITUITARY ADENOMA
This large pituitary adenoma intrudes into the brain of a 74-year-old woman who had a 2-year history of dementia and visual impairment. Obstruction of the third ventricle resulted in hydrocephalus, requiring a ventriculo-peritoneal shunt. (Courtesy of Dr. J.M. Bilbao, Toronto, Canada.)

microsurgical techniques have increased diagnostic accuracy, such that pituitary adenomas now represent approximately 25 percent of surgically resected intracranial neoplasms in some series (17). Epidemiologic data obtained prior to 1969 indicated annual incidence rates of up to 1.85 per 100,000 population (5) with geographic and racial variation; again these figures may be low and the diagnosis appears to be more frequent today because of increased awareness and improved diagnostic techniques.

Prolactinomas are the most common type of adenoma. About one third of pituitary adenomas are not associated with clinical hypersecretory syndromes but present with symptoms of an intracranial mass, such as headaches, nausea, vomiting, or visual field disturbances. Growth hormone- or adrenocorticotropic (ACTH)-producing adenomas each account for 10 to 15 percent of pituitary adenomas while thyroid-stimulating hormone (TSH)-producing adenomas are rare (14,20).

The relative frequency of the various adenoma types encountered by the surgical pathologist varies with several factors, including geography and the therapeutic approach involved. For example, in some centers, prolactinomas are rare in surgical material because the endocrinologists prefer a medical approach to management (8,11,18,20). There is usually a female preponderance in tumor occurrence. In women, adenomas usually present at a younger age and there is a higher incidence of prolactin (PRL)- and ACTH-secreting tumors whereas in men they tend to present in middle or older age as clinically nonfunctioning tumors (18).

Pituitary adenomas are infrequent in childhood: only about 3.5 to 8.5 percent are diagnosed before the age of 20 years (7,15). Childhood tumors exhibit a female preponderance and some have

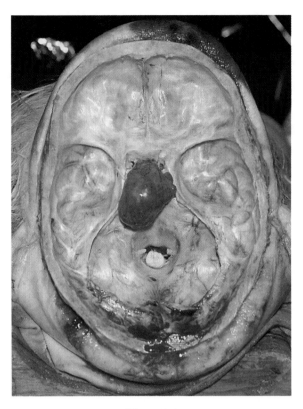

Figure 3-4
GIANT PITUITARY ADENOMA
This very large pituitary adenoma grew upwards to compress the hypothalamus but exhibited no invasive properties and still maintains a capsule.

suggested that they are smaller, less invasive, and less aggressive than tumors of adults (7). Hormone excess is common and only a few are clinically nonfunctioning tumors that present with mass effects. Tissue destruction results in a decreased secretion of growth hormone (GH), with resultant growth retardation. Patients with GH-secreting adenomas have an almost uniform incidence of PRL production by the tumor and pure GH adenomas are rare in children (7).

In random autopsies, 0.9 percent of pituitary adenomas identified were multiple (9). As expected of incidental adenomas encountered at postmortem, most were small and clinically silent. In another review of more than 3000 surgically resected pituitary adenomas, 11 were defined as "double adenomas" (10) and in 2 of these cases, hormone excess attributable to both tumors was manifest. In surgical series, multiple adenomas are rarely reported; synchronous de-

tection of more than one tumor has been reported (1,9,10) and metachronous double adenomas have occurred in the same patient (19).

CLASSIFICATIONS OF PITUITARY ADENOMAS

Pituitary adenomas have been classified by various groups of investigators in different ways.

Functional Classification

A functional classification characterizes a pituitary adenoma based on its hormonal activity in vivo. This is the common clinical approach, and places adenomas into the categories of GH-producing adenomas associated with acromegaly and/or gigantism, adenomas causing hyperprolactinemia and its clinical sequelae, ACTH-producing adenomas associated with Cushing's or Nelson's syndromes, TSH-producing tumors, the rare clinically detectable gonadotroph adenomas, and the large group of clinically nonfunctioning adenomas.

Anatomic or Radiologic Classification

Neuroradiologic examination provides a method of classification of pituitary adenomas based on tumor size and degree of local invasion. These data are of critical importance to the surgeon when planning for tumor resection. The most widely used classification, proposed by Hardy in the 1970s (24), was based primarily on skull X rays, pneumoencephalography, polytomography, and carotid angiography (fig. 3-5). It remains valid with the application of CT and MRI scanning which are more accurate (fig. 3-6).

This classification places adenomas into one of four grades: 1) grade I adenomas, or microadenomas, are intrapituitary lesions that measure less than 1 cm in diameter. While these lesions may be detected with sophisticated imaging techniques, by definition they do not cause bony changes to the sella turcica that can be identified by conventional X rays (fig. 3-6A; compare with fig. 3-1); 2) grade II adenomas are larger than 1 cm in diameter but still remain intrasellar or exhibit suprasellar expansion without invasion. Sellar enlargement is usually identified but these tumors do not cause bony destruction (fig. 3-6B; compare with fig. 3-2); 3) grade III adenomas are small or large locally invasive tumors that may be associated with diffuse sellar

SUPRA SELLAR EXPANSION

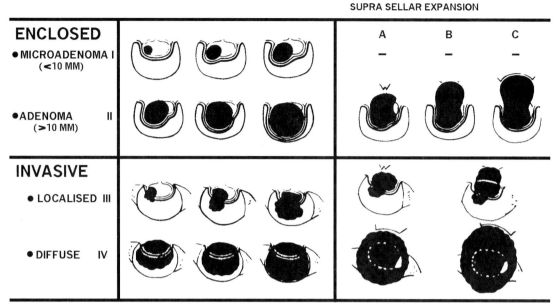

Figure 3-5
RADIOLOGIC CLASSIFICATION OF PITUITARY ADENOMAS
(Fig. 43 from Fascicle 21, 2nd Series.)

enlargement or may have suprasellar extension, but in either case cause bony erosion of the sella turcica (fig. 3-6C; compare with fig. 3-7); and 4) grade IV adenomas are large invasive tumors that involve extrasellar structures including bone, hypothalamus, and the cavernous sinus (fig. 3-6D; compare with figs. 3-3, 3-4, 3-8).

A subclassification of grade I, II, and III tumors identifies the degree of suprasellar invasion as small (A), moderate (B), or large (C).

Invasive adenomas are a subject of controversy. Some have suggested that significant local invasion should be considered a sign of malignant potential (see chapter 4). However, infiltrative pituitary tumors that invade dura, bone, and the cavernous sinus are relatively common (32–34), yet they do not metastasize; these are generally classified as benign but aggressive adenomas. Large invasive pituitary adenomas can invade the sphenoid bone and further downward to present as nasopharyngeal masses (36) or may invade posteriorly to involve or destroy the clivus (37), creating significant diagnostic dilemmas.

The incidence of invasion varies depending on whether the lesion is examined grossly or microscopically. Invasive lesions are less frequently identified by imaging techniques or by the sur-

geon than by the pathologist examining dural biopsies microscopically (34).

Invasiveness appears to correlate to some extent with tumor type and size. The most invasive groups include thyrotroph adenomas and silent corticotroph adenomas (32,33); in addition, the unusual plurihormonal silent subtype III adenomas are generally invasive (25). Macroadenomas are more often invasive than are microadenomas. Grossly invasive adenomas are recognized by the surgeon and are usually not amenable to complete resection; for smaller lesions, however, there are no well accepted markers to predict invasive behavior and possible recurrence. Cytologic features are not valid, since they do not differ in recurrent and non-recurrent tumors. Ploidy analyses have not shown aneuploidy to correlate with hormone profile or recurrence (21,22). Some authors have suggested that the proliferation markers Ki-67, proliferating cell nuclear antigen (PCNA) or p105 (22,23,26,27,30,31), or the purine-binding factor nm23 (35) may be useful in this regard.

Histologic Classification

The histologic diagnosis of pituitary adenomas prior to the era of immunohistochemistry and electron microscopy was a frustrating and

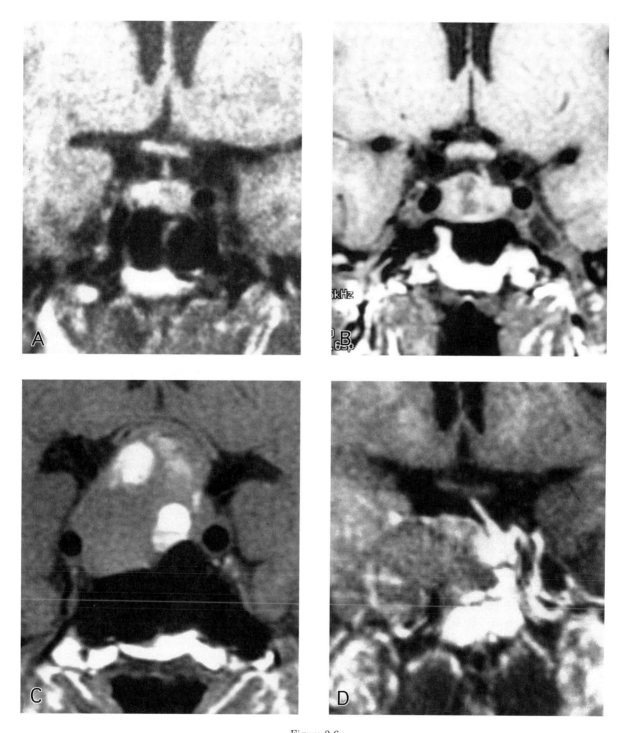

Figure 3-6
RADIOLOGIC CLASSIFICATION OF PITUITARY ADENOMAS (MRI, T1-WEIGHTED IMAGES)

A: A grade I microadenoma is a small intrapituitary lesion that measures less than 1 cm in diameter. This left-sided microadenoma is slightly hypointense.

B: A grade II adenoma is intrasellar but larger than 1 cm in diameter. This tumor exhibits mild suprasellar extension.

C: A grade III adenoma is locally invasive with suprasellar extension and chiasmal stretching. The tumor also exhibits focal areas of hyperintensity consistent with recent hemorrhage.

D: A grade IV adenoma is large and invasive, involving extrasellar structures including the right cavernous sinus and extending into the right temporal lobe. (Courtesy of Dr. S. Ezzat, Toronto, Ontario.)

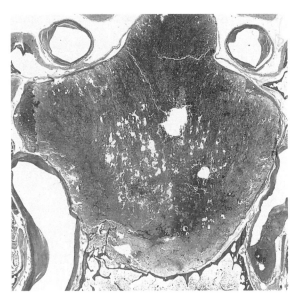

Figure 3-7
GRADE III PITUITARY ADENOMA

This clinically nonfunctioning adenoma is a grade III tumor with suprasellar extension and focal bony erosion of the sella turcica. (Courtesy of Dr. J.M. Bilbao, Toronto, Ontario.)

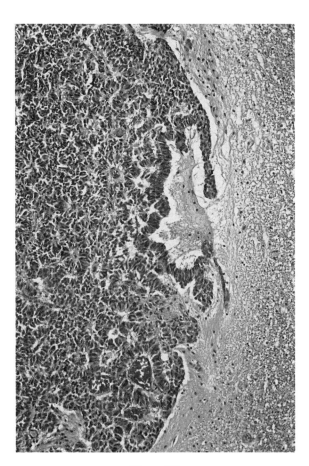

Figure 3-8
GRADE IV INVASIVE PITUITARY ADENOMA

This invasive tumor is the same as illustrated in figure 3-3. The tumor invades the brain parenchyma of the hypothalamus.

unsuccessful exercise. These tumors were classified by microscopists as acidophilic, basophilic, and chromophobic using conventional stains; acidophilic adenomas were said to be associated with acromegaly or gigantism, basophilic adenomas were thought to be the cause of Cushing's disease, and chromophobic tumors were considered to be nonfunctioning from the endocrine perspective. However, the value of such classification was questioned when it became obvious that some chromophobic adenomas were associated with the florid clinical symptomatology of hormone excess, and some acidophilic or basophilic adenomas were clinically hormonally inactive.

The application of more sophisticated histochemical stains led to an enhanced classification of these adenomas, but still proved to be relatively insensitive, nonspecific, and therefore unreliable.

Immunohistochemical Classification

The development of techniques for the immunologic detection of antigens in tissue revolutionized the classification of pituitary adenomas. Since hormones are well recognized as antigenic substances by other species, this technology allowed the development of highly specific anti-

sera to adenohypophysial hormones and precipitated the morphologist's ability to accurately determine hormone content of tumor cells.

The classification of pituitary adenomas currently relies most heavily on the use of the immunohistochemical characteristics of tumor cells. However, there is still controversy concerning the most important reactivities of these adenomas. From the clinical perspective, hormonal activity is the basis for diagnosis and therapy. Biologically, however, it remains to be established whether other characteristics, such as proliferation markers, growth factor and receptor expression, or oncogene product expression, will prove to be the most important predictors of tumor behavior, reflecting invasive growth, recurrence, or metastasis. If these markers are found to be useful in the

Table 3-1

IMMUNOHISTOCHEMICAL CLASSIFICATION OF PITUITARY ADENOMAS

Major Component	Other Reactivities
GH-PRL-TSH family	**Pit-1**
GH-cell adenomas	α-subunit
GH-cell adenomas with fibrous bodies	keratin whorls
GH- and PRL-cell (mammo-somatotroph) adenomas	α-subunit, ER
PRL-cell adenomas	ER
PRL-cell adenomas with GH reactivity	ER
TSH-cell adenomas (β-TSH and α-subunit)	
GH-, PRL-, and TSH-producing adenomas	ER
ACTH family	**?**
ACTH-cell adenomas	keratins
Gonadotropin family	**SF-1, ER**
FSH/LH-cell adenomas (β-subunits and α-subunit)	
Unclassified adenomas	
Unusual plurihormonal adenomas	
Hormone-negative adenomas	

guidance of therapeutic management, the classification of these tumors will undergo a revolution. Nevertheless, the application of immunohistochemical staining methods to determine tumor cytogenesis and pathogenesis will likely remain a mainstay of morphologic classification.

Currently, pituitary adenomas are classified by hormone content. This functional approach most closely correlates with the clinical presentation of the patient. The outline for this system is provided in Table 3-1. Other markers of cell differentiation, such as the transcription factors that regulate hormone expression and keratins, can also be used to classify and subclassify pituitary adenomas immunohistochemically. Some of these obviate the need for ultrastructural examination except in unusual situations. Other predictive indicators, such as proliferation markers, can be incorporated into this type of classification.

Ultrastructural Classification

Electron microscopy is useful to characterize the cytologic differentiation of tumor cells. The applications of this technology, combined with immunolocalization of hormones, at both the light and electron microscopic levels, allow structure-function correlations that provide the basis for a morphologic classification (28). This type of analysis allows recognition of specific subcellular characteristics of somatotrophs, mammosomatotrophs, lactotrophs, thyrotrophs, corticotrophs, and gonadotrophs. In most tumors, immunolocalization of hormones can achieve these objectives.

Careful examination by electron microscopy permitted the subclassification of tumors that produce GH and PRL. This led to the recognition of densely and sparsely granulated somatotroph adenomas as well as lactotroph adenomas. Now that the variants are known, they can be distinguished by immunostaining and light microscopy. Densely granulated lactotroph adenomas are exceedingly rare, and the variants of somatotroph adenomas are conveniently recognized with the application of keratin stains, since sparsely granulated somatotroph adenomas are characterized by the presence of conspicuous fibrous bodies that are readily decorated by the Cam 5.2 antibody. Subclassification of GH- and PRL-producing adenomas as densely granulated somatotroph adenomas with PRL content, mammosomatotroph adenomas, or mixed somatotroph-lactotroph adenomas is difficult without ultrastructural analysis; the significance of these subtleties for clinical management remains unclear.

In the family of glycoprotein-producing adenomas, there has been some controversy concerning the diagnosis of gonadotroph adenomas without ultrastructural confirmation of cytodifferentiation. Previously, immunolocalization of glycoprotein hormones was unreliable; there was significant crossreactivity, particularly because of the common α-subunit, and fixation led to artefactual negativity in some cases. These problems have been reduced by the development of more sensitive and specific antisera and improvements in tissue fixation for antigen recognition. It now appears that the gonadotropic hormones, as detected by antisera to β-follicle-stimulating hormone (FSH) and β-luteinizing hormone (LH) are present in many clinically

Table 3-2

CLINICOPATHOLOGIC CLASSIFICATION OF PITUITARY ADENOMAS

Functioning Adenomas	Nonfunctioning Adenomas
GH-PRL-TSH family	
Adenomas causing GH excess	
Densely granulated somatotroph adenomas	
Sparsely granulated somatotroph adenomas with fibrous bodies	Silent somatotroph adenomas
Mammosomatotroph adenomas	
Adenomas causing hyperprolactinemia	
Lactotroph adenomas	Silent lactotroph adenomas
Lactotroph adenomas with GH reactivity (Acidophil stem cell	
adenomas)	
Adenomas causing TSH excess	
Thyrotroph adenomas (β-TSH and α-subunit)	Silent thyrotroph adenomas
ACTH family	
Adenomas causing ACTH excess	
Corticotroph adenomas	Silent corticotroph adenomas
Gonadotropin family	
Adenomas causing gonadotropin excess	
Gonadotroph adenomas	Silent gonadotroph adenomas
	Null cell adenomas, oncocytomas
Unclassified adenomas	
Unusual plurihormonal adenomas	Hormone-negative adenomas

nonfunctioning adenomas. Some of these are recognized by electron microscopy as having gonadotropic differentiation, but some have less well-differentiated cells, resembling the "null" cells that were initially thought to be undifferentiated precursors of adenohypophysial cells (29). The role of electron microscopy in the classification of these tumors remains controversial, but since there is little clinical impact, the need for this expensive and time-consuming exercise remains academic.

For unusual plurihormonal adenomas, electron microscopy continues to play an important role in determining cytodifferentiation and structure-function correlations.

Clinicopathologic Classification

The ideal classification of any group of tumors is one which maximizes the ability to reflect clinical and morphologic features. The endocrine manifestations and aggressivity of pituitary adenomas are usually correlated with specific morphologic phenotypes. Table 3-2 summarizes a scheme that permits maximal structure-function identification. Generally, aggressive behav-

ior is a phenomenon of silent adenomas and unusual plurihormonal adenomas as well as the rare lactotroph adenoma with GH immunoreactivity, known as the "acidophil stem cell adenoma." Additional information, such as tumor size; radiologic, gross, or microscopic evidence of invasion; and the proliferative activity level of a tumor as identified by flow cytometry or immunohistochemical proliferation markers, can be incorporated in a multidisciplinary fashion to determine the optimal therapeutic approach to management of the individual patient.

PITUITARY ADENOMAS CAUSING GROWTH HORMONE EXCESS

Clinical Features. GH excess causes acromegaly, gigantism, or both. The clinical syndrome of acromegaly, characterized by prognathism, thickening of the soft tissues of the face and lip (fig. 3-9), and acral enlargement (fig. 3-10), was first described by Pierre Marie in 1886 (103); its association with pituitary tumor was noted by Minkowski in 1887 (106). The chronic hypersecretion of GH as the cause of acromegaly and gigantism was confirmed by the experiments of Evans and Long (59). Gigantism is the result of GH excess prior to epiphyseal closure and is frequently accompanied by the soft tissue thickening characteristic of acromegaly.

Of historic interest, the first case of acromegaly was probably documented in 1365 BCE: the Egyptian king Akhenaton displayed the classic clinical features of acromegaly including prognathism, enlargement of the nose and upper jaw, and thickening of the soft tissues of the face and lip. Speculation may lead one to attribute major historic significance to the visual field defects that may be caused by large pituitary somatotroph tumors; it is likely that the giant Goliath had a pituitary adenoma with GH excess, and his defeat by David may be attributed to these complications.

Acromegaly is insidious in onset and may not be noted by the patient, friends, or family. This often results in delay in diagnosis, which may be made at the time of investigation of an unrelated problem or of symptoms of complications such as headache, carpal tunnel syndrome, diabetes mellitus, hypertension, hypogonadism, or other manifestations of hypopituitarism (48,107). The chronic hypertension can lead to cerebrovascular disease, coronary artery disease, congestive heart failure, and early death. Patients with acromegaly also have a higher incidence of malignancy, including colonic polyps and carcinomas and breast carcinomas, than the general population.

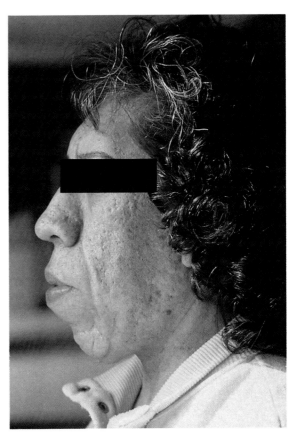

Figure 3-9
CLINICAL MANIFESTATIONS OF ACROMEGALY
This patient with a longstanding growth hormone–producing adenoma exhibits the characteristic facies of acromegaly, with prognathism and thickening of soft tissues of the face and lip. (Courtesy of Dr. S. Ezzat, Toronto, Canada.)

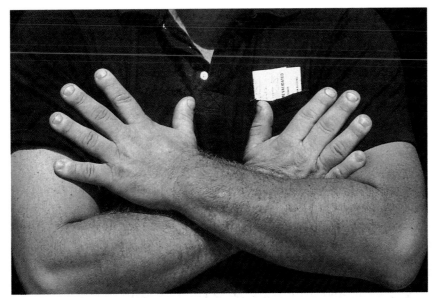

Figure 3-10
CLINICAL MANIFESTATIONS OF ACROMEGALY
Chronic growth hormone excess in acromegaly results in significant acral enlargement as shown in this illustration. (Courtesy of Dr. S. Ezzat, Toronto, Canada.)

Biochemical Findings. The dominant chemical abnormality in acromegaly and gigantism is GH excess. The hormone exists in a number of different forms as a result of alternative mRNA processing and post-translational modifications (127). The heterogeneity involves both molecular size and molecular charge. Size heterogeneity is due to the existence of oligomeric forms as well as to differential binding of GH to carrier proteins in plasma. Charge isomerism is the expression of several monomeric molecular forms: 22K, 20K, acetylated and deamidated GH. The various molecular forms can be demonstrated in the normal pituitary gland and in tumors, in tissue extracts, in culture media, and in the blood of normal and acromegalic patients. The relative proportions of the monomeric GH forms are the same in tumors and nontumorous pituitary.

GH is thought to exert many of its biologic functions through stimulation of somatomedins, a family of peptides also known as insulin-like growth factors (IGF) (48,50,113). IGF-1 and IGF-2 are single chain polypeptide hormones of 70 and 67 amino acids, respectively. They show more than 60 percent homology to each other and have over 40 percent homology to insulin. Somatomedins are synthesized in a number of sites; liver is thought to be the major source of circulating IGF-1 but a variety of other tissues have also been shown to express IGF mRNA (113).

The diagnosis of acromegaly relies upon documentation of elevated serum GH levels as well as elevated IGF-1 (somatomedin-C) (79,105). Although random GH levels are occasionally not elevated, the 24-hour GH profile, in which serum GH is measured at frequent intervals throughout the day and night, may be of diagnostic significance; normals generally show very low serum GH values, less than 1 to 2 ng/ml, at some time during the day or night whereas acromegalics almost never achieve such low values. Administration of glucose suppresses serum GH in normals but not in acromegalics. This maneuver is now routinely used as a diagnostic tool; failure to observe suppression of GH following an oral glucose load is considered to be the single most useful and definitive diagnostic test for acromegaly. Some acromegalics actually show a "paradoxical" stimulation of GH in response to glucose loading. Ancillary tests of GH secretion include administration of thyrotropin-releasing hormone

(TRH): normals rarely show GH stimulation in response to this substance but a significant proportion of acromegalics have at least a 50 percent rise in serum GH. L-DOPA testing is used by some endocrinologists: in normals, GH is stimulated but in 50 to 100 percent of acromegalics GH is suppressed by L-DOPA. GH responses to insulin-induced hypoglycemia, arginine, and GH-releasing hormone (GRH) are nondiscriminating and have not proven useful for diagnosis.

Some acromegalic patients and many with gigantism have hyperprolactinemia in the absence of a macroadenoma that could explain the phenomenon as "stalk section effect" (123). It is now recognized that many GH-producing tumors secrete PRL (55,67,81,82). Clinical studies have also documented elevated blood levels of the α-subunit of glycoprotein hormones in some acromegalic patients (109). GH-producing adenomas are often immunopositive for α-subunit (86) and coexistence of GH and α-subunit in the same cell and colocalization in the same secretory granule have been demonstrated by immunoelectron microscopy (49,111). Release of α-subunit in association with GH has been documented in vitro (86).

Elevated levels of plasma GRH have been found in cases of acromegaly secondary to extrahypothalamic GRH-producing neoplasms (see chapter 11), but plasma GRH has been generally undetectable in patients with primary pituitary disease (129).

Radiologic Findings. Pituitary and sellar enlargement found on skull roentgenography is useful in the diagnosis of acromegaly; sellar enlargement is found in 75 to 95 percent of patients (85,105,107). A pituitary tumor is nearly always demonstrable on CT scanning or with MRI (fig. 3-11). Tumor size can also be estimated by the addition of lateral polytomography, air encephalography, or carotid angiography; in the case of microadenomas, these techniques are unnecessary. Recently, the demonstration of somatostatin receptors in pituitary tumors has led to the use of scintigraphic visualization of radiolabeled somatostatin analogs to localize some adenomas (fig. 3-12) (91). However, in addition to identifying tumors that produce GH or TSH as well as functionally inactive pituitary adenomas, this imaging technique has localized other lesions, such as metastatic deposits (133), and therefore it is not as specific as originally postulated.

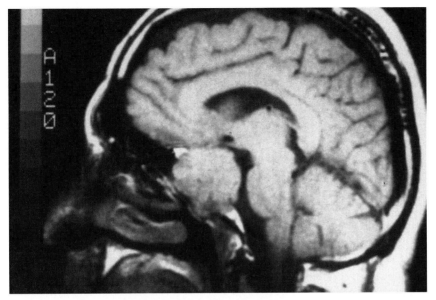

Figure 3-11
RADIOGRAPHIC FEATURES
OF ACROMEGALY
A T1-weighted MRI image of a patient with a pituitary adenoma causing growth hormone excess reveals a large adenoma causing marked destruction of the sella turcica. The image also shows the thickening of soft tissues around the orbit and skull, correlating with the clinical appearance of the patient.

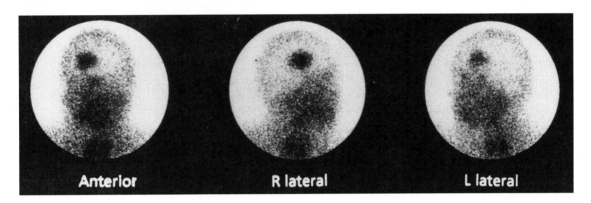

Figure 3-12
OCTREOSCAN LOCALIZATION OF GROWTH HORMONE–PRODUCING PITUITARY ADENOMA
Octreotide scintigraphy in a patient with acromegaly localizes a suprasellar pituitary adenoma that shows selective uptake of the radiolabelled somatostatin analogue.

Considerable attention is also paid to extracranial radiographic findings. Of these, measurement of heel pad thickness has been proposed as a useful diagnostic test. There is, however, considerable overlap of normal values and those of acromegalic patients, and the technique has found its greatest use in monitoring the effects of therapy.

Gross Findings. Unlike tumors that are not detected until they have grown beyond the sella turcica, these adenomas are often diagnosed early because of the striking clinical syndrome they create. The most characteristic finding in acromegaly is, therefore, a well-demarcated adenoma, often confined to the anterior lobe of the pituitary gland (122). Microadenomas are usually located in one of the lateral wings, the principle site of GH-producing cells in the normal adenohypophysis (88). Larger tumors may distort the sella, spread into the suprasellar area, and occasionally invade neighboring tissues. GH levels are thought to correlate with pituitary tumor size, and the presence of suprasellar extension also correlates with increased circulating GH levels (85,131).

Microscopic Findings. The morphologic appearance of GH-producing adenomas has led to their division into several categories. These categories are based on the immunohistochemical profile of the tumor cells and ultrastructural parameters. GH production is dependent on the presence of the transcription factor Pit-1, and most of these tumors contain nuclear immunoreactivity for this protein as well as for GH (42). In general, GH-producing tumors also contain immunoreactive α-subunit, as do nontumorous somatotrophs (87,112,120,132). Pure *somatotroph adenomas* have been subclassified into densely and sparsely granulated variants (81,88). However, many GH-producing adenomas are also immunoreactive for prolactin; this phenomenon is being recognized with increasing frequency, probably due to improved methodologies. In the normal gland, bihormonal cells that produce GH and PRL as well as α-subunit are known as mammosomatotrophs. The mammosomatotroph is a cell type that has been recognized to fluctuate: it is thought to be capable of altering its behavior and hormonal activity to become a monohormonal somatotroph or lactotroph and probably can revert to a plurihormonal state (68). The fluidity of this cell type explains why many GH-producing pituitary adenomas are immunoreactive for PRL. Initially, such tumors were classified as *mammosomatotroph adenomas* and were described as being composed of a single population of plurihormonal cells capable of producing GH, PRL, and α-subunit. Other tumors were identified by electron microscopy as containing individual tumor cell populations with distinct features of differentiated somatotrophs and lactotrophs and were classified as mixed somatotroph-lactotroph adenomas. However, sophisticated techniques, such as ultrastructural immunocytochemistry, in situ hybridization, tissue culture, and molecular analysis (41,95,101,136) have shown extensive overlap between densely granulated somatotroph adenomas, mammosomatotroph adenomas, and mixed somatotroph-lactotroph adenomas. Therefore, the distinction between these different tumor types is becoming more difficult. Since there is no known clinical or pathogenetic significance in distinguishing these various tumors that produce GH and PRL, a more simplistic approach based on light microscopy and immunohistochemistry alone, as detailed below, is recommended as the most useful.

Densely Granulated Somatotroph Adenoma. This is the classic acidophilic tumor associated with acromegaly. The tumors are relatively slow growing and cause gradual ballooning of the

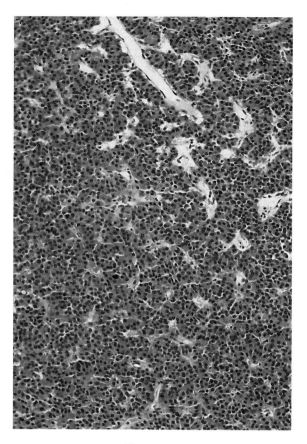

Figure 3-13
HISTOLOGY OF DENSELY GRANULATED
SOMATOTROPH ADENOMA
This eosinophilic adenoma has a sinusoidal architectural pattern. Focal nuclear pleomorphism is identified and occasional binucleate cells are seen. The stroma is highly vascular.

sella turcica. They have a trabecular, sinusoidal, or diffuse histologic pattern (figs. 3-13, 3-14). Immunohistochemistry shows densely granulated somatotroph cells with relatively strong uniform immunoreactivity for GH distributed throughout the cell cytoplasm (fig. 3-15). These tumors often contain α-subunit of the glycoprotein hormones (fig. 3-16). They are moderately positive for low molecular weight cytokeratins in a perinuclear distribution (fig. 3-17), and characteristically have strong nuclear immunoreactivity for Pit-1 (fig. 3-18) (42).

Ultrastructural examination of densely granulated somatotroph adenomas reveals cells that strongly resemble nontumorous somatotrophs (figs. 3-19, 3-20). The cells are polyhedral or elongated with spherical euchromatic nuclei containing conspicuous nucleoli. The cytoplasm

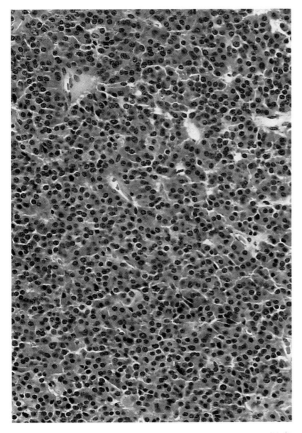

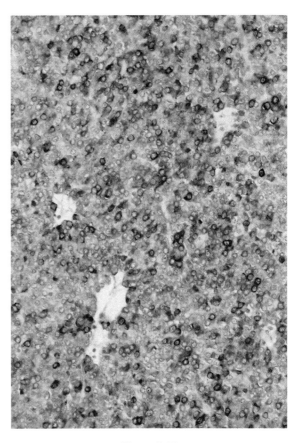

Figure 3-14
HISTOLOGY OF DENSELY GRANULATED
SOMATOTROPH ADENOMA
The tumor cells have abundant eosinophilic granular
cytoplasm. Nuclear pleomorphism is only moderate.

Figure 3-15
IMMUNOHISTOCHEMICAL LOCALIZATION OF
GROWTH HORMONE IN DENSELY GRANULATED
SOMATOTROPH ADENOMA
The majority of tumor cells have abundant immunoreactive growth hormone in their cytoplasm.

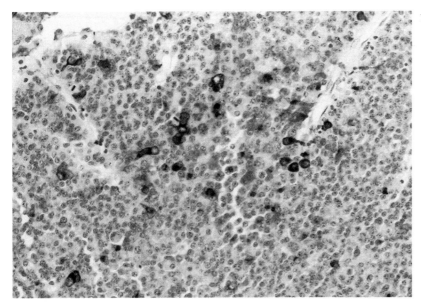

Figure 3-16
IMMUNOHISTOCHEMICAL
LOCALIZATION OF α-SUBUNIT
IN DENSELY GRANULATED
SOMATOTROPH ADENOMA
These tumors often contain α-subunit of glycoprotein hormones in scattered tumor cells; the immunoreactivity is variable but can be very intense throughout the cytoplasm.

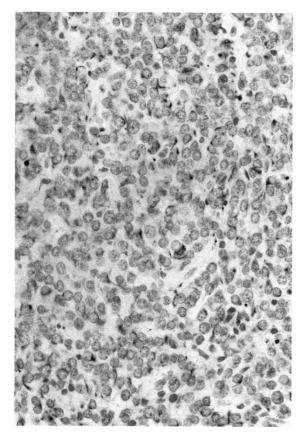

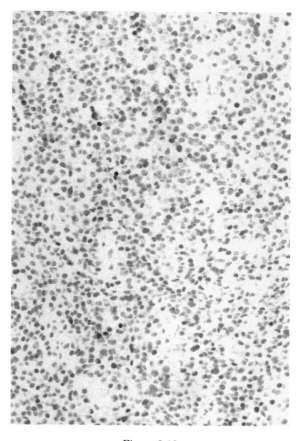

Figure 3-17

IMMUNOHISTOCHEMICAL LOCALIZATION OF
CYTOKERATINS IN DENSELY GRANULATED
SOMATOTROPH ADENOMA

The tumor cells are moderately positive for low molecular
weight cytokeratins using the Cam 5.2 antibody; the staining pattern is characteristically perinuclear.

Figure 3-18

IMMUNOHISTOCHEMICAL LOCALIZATION
OF PIT-1 IN DENSELY GRANULATED
SOMATOTROPH ADENOMA

The tumor cells have a strong and monotonous nuclear
immunoreactivity for Pit-1.

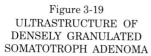

Figure 3-19

ULTRASTRUCTURE OF
DENSELY GRANULATED
SOMATOTROPH ADENOMA

The tumor cells resemble nontumorous somatotrophs. They have
well-developed rough endoplasmic
reticulum, juxtanuclear Golgi complexes, and numerous round, electron
dense secretory granules.

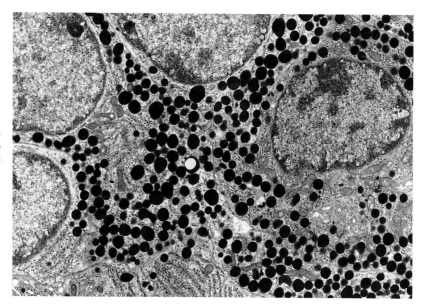

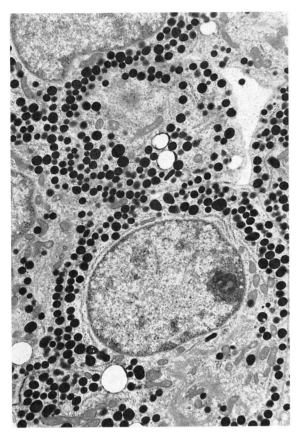

Figure 3-20
ULTRASTRUCTURE OF DENSELY GRANULATED
SOMATOTROPH ADENOMA
The juxtanuclear Golgi region is highly developed and
harbors pleomorphic secretory granules.

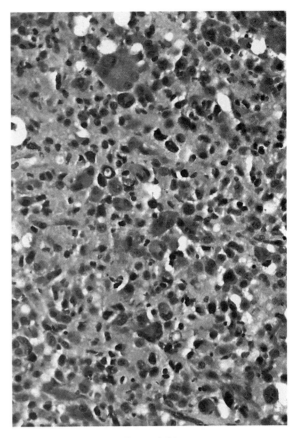

Figure 3-21
HISTOLOGY OF SPARSELY GRANULATED
SOMATOTROPH ADENOMA
The sparsely granulated somatotroph adenoma is characterized by marked cellular pleomorphism. The tumor cells have a diffuse architecture and multinucleated cells are conspicuous. The nuclei tend to be eccentric, pushed to the periphery of the cell by the fibrous body. The significant nuclear atypia often raises the question of malignancy but is not reflective of malignant potential.

is abundant and contains well-developed organelles. The rough endoplasmic reticulum is arranged in parallel stacks, usually at the periphery of the cell. The Golgi complex, composed of slightly dilated sacculi, is globular and often harbors forming secretory granules. The cytoplasm is almost filled with numerous large spherical or ovoid, electron dense secretory granules which usually measure 400 to 500 nm in diameter (range, 150 to 600 nm).

Sparsely Granulated Somatotroph Adenoma with Fibrous Bodies. These chromophobic tumors are slightly more common than the acidophilic form and are thought to be more aggressive, with a faster growth rate than their densely granulated counterpart (81). They are generally large at the time of diagnosis and the histologic pattern is almost always diffuse. Tumor cells

display considerable nuclear and cellular pleomorphism (figs. 3-21, 3-22) which may raise the question of malignancy; sometimes the atypia is suggestive of a metastatic carcinoma. The nuclear features, although worrisome, are not predictive of malignant potential. Immunoreactivity for GH is variable but is usually faint and focal (figs. 3-23, 3-24) because positivity in the sparse secretory granules is not readily detectable by light microscopy; strong staining is generally limited to a juxtanuclear location that corresponds to the Golgi area. These tumors are rarely significantly positive for α-subunit. The most characteristic immunohistochemical

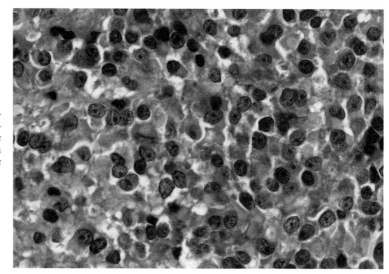

Figure 3-22
HISTOLOGY OF SPARSELY
GRANULATED
SOMATOTROPH ADENOMA

Sparsely granulated somatotroph adenomas are composed of cells with chromophobic cytoplasm and only focal eosinophilic granularity. The tumor cell cytoplasm often harbors juxtanuclear, pale, eosinophilic globules that represent fibrous bodies.

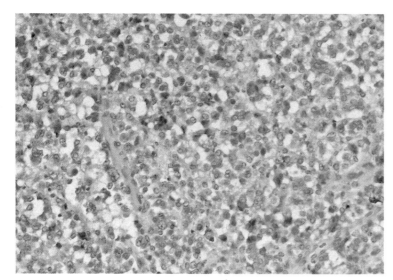

Figure 3-23
IMMUNOHISTOCHEMICAL
LOCALIZATION OF GROWTH
HORMONE IN SPARSELY
GRANULATED SOMATOTROPH
ADENOMA

Growth hormone is identified in the majority of cells in a sparsely granulated somatotroph adenoma, however, the immunoreactivity is variable in amount and intensity. The scattered cells contain strong juxtanuclear staining patterns corresponding to the Golgi complex.

Figure 3-24
IMMUNOHISTOCHEMICAL
LOCALIZATION OF GROWTH
HORMONE IN SPARSELY
GRANULATED
SOMATOTROPH ADENOMA

In this sparsely granulated somatotroph adenoma, the majority of tumor cells are immunonegative but scattered cells are immunoreactive for growth hormone in the sparse secretory granules or a juxtanuclear Golgi complex.

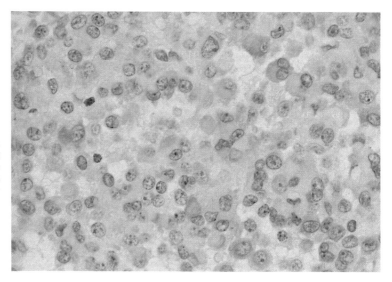

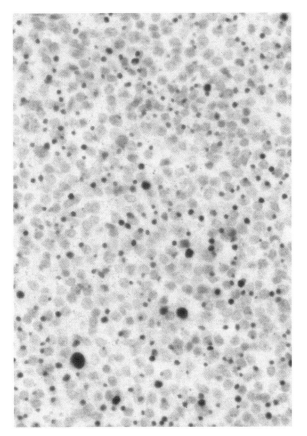

Figure 3-25
IMMUNOHISTOCHEMICAL LOCALIZATION
OF CYTOKERATINS IN SPARSELY
GRANULATED SOMATOTROPH ADENOMA
Immunostaining with the Cam 5.2 antibody identifies the characteristic juxtanuclear globular positivity that decorates fibrous bodies in this tumor. This characteristic immunohistochemical pattern allows recognition of this tumor type.

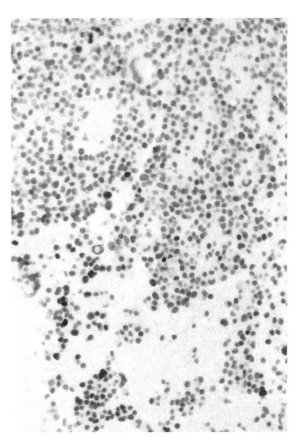

Figure 3-26
IMMUNOHISTOCHEMICAL LOCALIZATION OF
PIT-1 IN SPARSELY GRANULATED
SOMATOTROPH ADENOMA
Immunostaining for Pit-1 decorates the nuclei of tumor cells in a sparsely granulated somatotroph adenoma. This stain allows recognition of the nuclear pleomorphism. In this photograph, a nucleus is indented by a fibrous body, giving it a "halo" appearance.

marker of this tumor is the globular juxtanuclear positivity for low molecular weight cytokeratins (fig. 3-25) in the "fibrous body" that was initially recognized by electron microscopy (see below). These lesions usually exhibit nuclear immunoreactivity for the transcription factor Pit-1 (fig. 3-26).

Sparsely granulated somatotroph adenomas have a highly characteristic ultrastructure distinctly different from that of normal somatotrophs or the densely granulated somatotroph adenoma (fig. 3-27). The irregular cells show marked variability in size and shape. They have eccentric nuclei which are frequently pleomorphic and concave or multilobed. The rough endoplasmic reticulum varies from small, scattered, short profiles

to well-developed parallel stacks and arrays. The area of the Golgi usually contains the highly characteristic fibrous body (fig. 3-28), a spherical accumulation of intermediate filaments known to be keratin (108,120) and associated with variable amounts of smooth endoplasmic reticulum. The filamentous aggregates may trap sacculi of the Golgi complex as well as other cytoplasmic organelles including centrioles. Secretory granules are sparse and small, ranging from 100 to 250 nm.

Mammosomatotroph Adenoma. Bihormonal adenomas producing GH and PRL are often associated with acromegaly and are the most frequent cause of gigantism (81). These adenomas are usually acidophilic tumors with a diffuse or

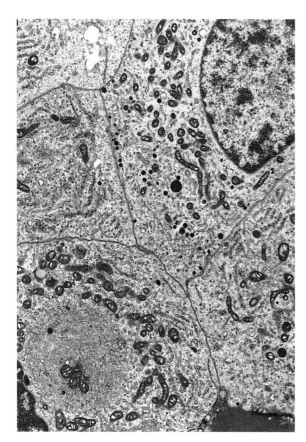

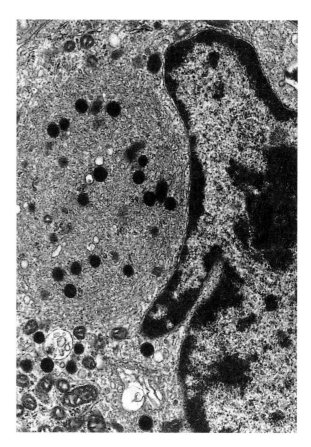

Figure 3-27

ULTRASTRUCTURE OF SPARSELY GRANULATED
SOMATOTROPH ADENOMA

The tumor is composed of round to polygonal cells that contain abundant cytoplasm. There are short profiles of rough endoplasmic reticulum and some tumor cells have prominent juxtanuclear Golgi complexes. The hallmark of this tumor is the fibrous body, a juxtanuclear accumulation of intermediate filaments associated with rough endoplasmic reticulum that traps cytoplasmic organelles. Secretory granules are sparse and small but electron dense.

Figure 3-28

ULTRASTRUCTURE OF SPARSELY GRANULATED
SOMATOTROPH ADENOMA

The fibrous body can indent the nucleus of a sparsely granulated somatotroph adenoma cell, creating marked nuclear pleomorphism. The filamentous aggregate is associated with smooth endoplasmic reticulum and trapped cytoplasmic organelles, including secretory granules.

solid growth pattern (fig. 3-29). Occasional interspersed chromophobic cells may be seen. The tumor cells exhibit intense cytoplasmic immunopositivity for GH (fig. 3-30) and variable immunoreactivity for PRL (fig. 3-31). Most adenomas also contain the α-subunit of glycoprotein hormones. The pattern of staining for low molecular weight cytokeratins resembles that of the densely granulated somatotroph adenoma (fig. 3-32), but occasional fibrous bodies, similar to those of the sparsely granulated somatotroph adenoma, can be recognized. Nuclear staining for Pit-1 is usually strong (fig. 3-33) and some tumor cells are reactive for estrogen receptor (ER) (136). Occa-

sionally they produce β-TSH and can be associated with hyperthyroidism and goiter.

The diagnosis may be readily confirmed by electron microscopy (81,88): the mammosomatotrophs resemble densely granulated somatotrophs but have differences in secretory granule size and morphology (figs. 3-34, 3-35). Secretory granules vary from ovoid to pleomorphic in shape and may be very large, up to 1000 nm in maximum dimension. They frequently have asymmetric mottled cores and demonstrate the hallmark of PRL secretion, the misplaced exocytosis. Ultrastructural immunocytochemistry localizes both GH and PRL within the same cell and within the same secretory granules (fig. 3-36); size and morphology of secretory granules do not correlate with hormone content.

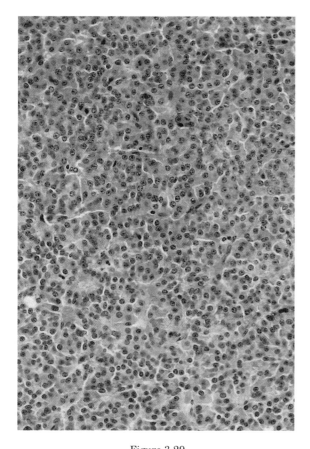

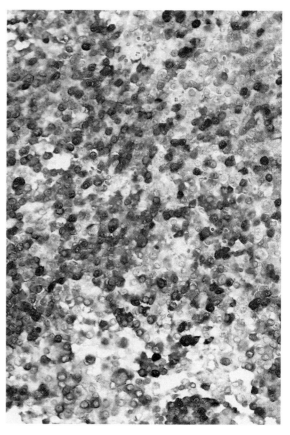

Figure 3-29
HISTOLOGY OF MAMMOSOMATOTROPH ADENOMA
This pituitary tumor has a solid or sinusoidal growth pattern and is composed predominantly of acidophilic cells with interspersed chromophobes.

Figure 3-30
IMMUNOHISTOCHEMICAL LOCALIZATION OF GROWTH HORMONE IN MAMMOSOMATOTROPH ADENOMA
The majority of tumor cells have very strong diffuse cytoplasmic reactivity for growth hormone.

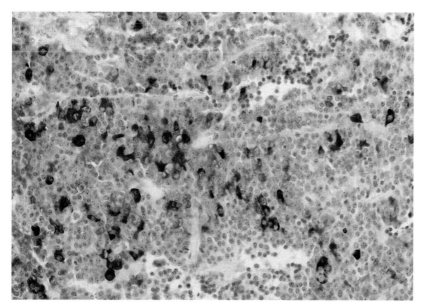

Figure 3-31
IMMUNOHISTOCHEMICAL LOCALIZATION OF PROLACTIN IN MAMMOSOMATOTROPH ADENOMA
A smaller population of tumor cells stains for prolactin; the pattern is usually strong and diffuse throughout the cytoplasm.

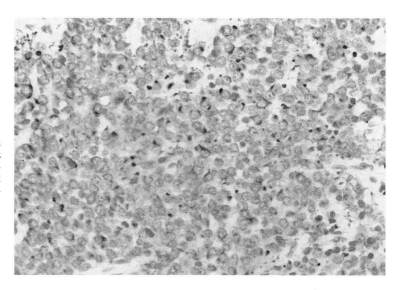

Figure 3-32
IMMUNOHISTOCHEMICAL
LOCALIZATION OF CYTOKERATINS
IN MAMMOSOMATOTROPH ADENOMA

The cells of a mammosomatotroph adenoma are immunoreactive for low molecular weight cytokeratins using the Cam 5.2 antibody. Usually the pattern is perinuclear, but occasional round juxtanuclear globules suggest the presence of fibrous bodies in some tumor cells.

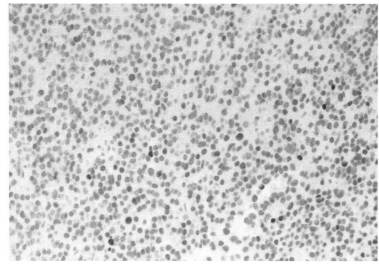

Figure 3-33
IMMUNOHISTOCHEMICAL
LOCALIZATION OF PIT-1 IN
MAMMOSOMATOTROPH ADENOMA

The nuclei of tumor cells in a mammosomatotroph adenoma stain strongly for Pit-1.

Figure 3-34
ULTRASTRUCTURE OF
MAMMOSOMATOTROPH ADENOMA

The tumor cells resemble densely granulated somatotrophs but have more pleomorphic secretory granules. They also exhibit misplaced exocytosis (arrows), extrusion of secretory material along the lateral cell borders, a feature that is indicative of prolactin secretion.

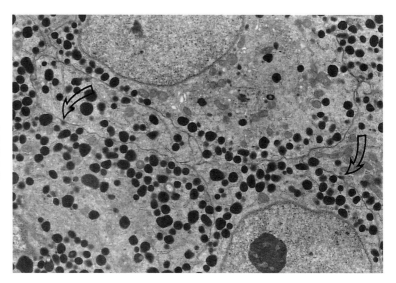

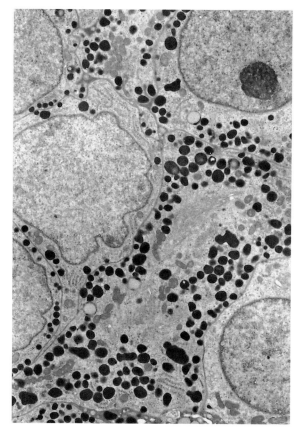

Figure 3-35
ULTRASTRUCTURE OF
MAMMOSOMATOTROPH ADENOMA
The striking pleomorphism of secretory granules in this
tumor distinguishes it from the densely granulated
somatotroph adenoma.

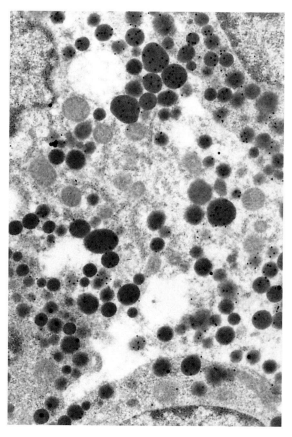

Figure 3-36
ULTRASTRUCTURAL IMMUNOLOCALIZATION
OF GROWTH HORMONE AND PROLACTIN IN
MAMMOSOMATOTROPH ADENOMA
These bihormonal tumor cells contain growth hormone
(small gold particles) as well as prolactin (large gold particles)
within the same cell and even within the same secretory granule.

In some of these tumors, mature somatotrophs and lactotrophs may be recognized. These mixed somatotroph-lactotroph adenomas are most commonly composed of a densely granulated somatotroph component and a sparsely granulated lactotroph component (81,88) that can only be verified by electron microscopy.

In vitro, these adenomas usually release GH, PRL, and α-subunit; the bihormonal nature of individual tumor cells is demonstrated with the reverse hemolytic plaque assay (98). Parallel responses of hormone release to GRH or TRH stimulation and to bromocriptine or somatostatin inhibition indicate co-regulation of the three hormones (41). The inverse relationship between GH and PRL secretion in long-term cultures of human pituitary adenomas from acromegalic pa-

tients suggests that low cortisol levels may induce a shift in secretion to PRL (100).

Morphologic Effects of Drugs and Hormones. The morphologic alterations induced by various hormonal substances have been reported in GH-producing adenomas of all types. Short-term exposure to GRH in vitro causes rapid degranulation of densely granulated adenomas (99); after chronic exposure to GRH, the cytoplasmic volume densities of the synthetic organelles, rough endoplasmic reticulum, and Golgi complex are increased, reflecting increased hormone synthesis, and that of secretory granules is reduced, reflecting rapid release of GH (84). In contrast, there are no consistent morphologic alterations induced by somatostatin or its long-acting analogue SMS 201-995 (octreotide) (62). No alteration of synthetic

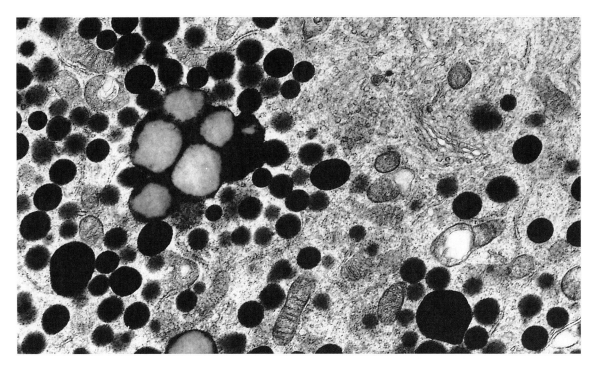

Figure 3-37
SOMATOSTATIN-TREATED SOMATOTROPH ADENOMA
This densely granulated somatotroph adenoma was exposed to octreotide therapy preoperatively. The tumor exhibits a marked prominence of lysosomes and there is crinophagy, uptake of secretory granules by complex lysosomes. This feature has been suggested to reflect intracellular degradation of stored hormone due to inhibition of hormone release by the drug.

organelles is seen; this supports the finding that somatostatin does not reduce GH mRNA levels (78). There have been reports of increases in lysosomes in some cases both in vivo (71) and in vitro (40), suggesting intracellular degradation of stored hormone that may result from reduced GH release (fig. 3-37). Octreotide has not been reported to reduce tumor cell size in a consistent fashion, but in some cases it causes preoperative tumor mass reduction that eases surgical resection (fig. 3-38) (63); there seems to be an increase in perivascular and interstitial fibrosis in adenomas preoperatively exposed to somatostatin analogue (62).

Differential Diagnosis. The diagnosis of pituitary adenoma is generally confirmed clinically, biochemically, and radiologically prior to surgical exploration of the sella and resection of adenohypophysial tissue. However, there are patients with clinical evidence of GH excess who do not have detectable adenohypophysial pathology radiologically or who have evidence of diffuse sellar enlargement without a focal tumor. This clinical scenario raises the possibility of an ectopic source of hormone excess: either ectopic production of growth hormone or production of hormones that can stimulate pituitary growth hormone secretion, with or without associated adenohypophysial hyperplasia.

Ectopic secretion of GH is rare, and has been convincingly associated with acromegaly in only a single pancreatic endocrine carcinoma (61). However, the clinical syndrome of acromegaly is now recognized to be caused by ectopic secretion of GH-releasing hormone (GRH). Whereas the presence of immunoreactive GRH is not uncommon in endocrine tumors, frank acromegaly due to ectopic GRH production is rare and only approximately 40 cases of acromegaly secondary to ectopic GRH hypersecretion have been described (66,119); the majority of these neoplasms have been pancreatic, pulmonary, or gastrointestinal endocrine tumors, with the rare pheochromocytoma (119). The diagnosis of acromegaly caused by a GRH-producing tumor is based on biochemical findings because

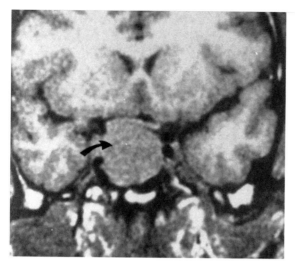 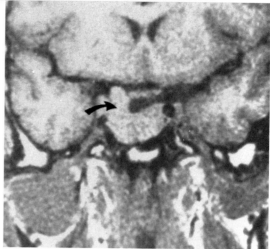

Figure 3-38
RADIOGRAPHIC APPEARANCE OF A DENSELY GRANULATED SOMATOTROPH ADENOMA
BEFORE AND FOLLOWING OCTREOTIDE THERAPY (MRI, T1 WEIGHTED)
There is asymmetric involution of the tumor with reduction in overall size and relief of pressure on the optic chiasm.
(Courtesy of Dr. S. Ezzat, Toronto, Canada.)

the clinical phenotype is usually indistinguishable from acromegaly of pituitary origin. The diagnosis is particularly complex because sellar radiography is abnormal in both situations. However, the adenohypophysial pathology in primary pituitary acromegaly is usually that of a discrete adenoma unassociated with hyperplasia. In contrast, patients with ectopic GRH secretion display the full spectrum from somatotroph hyperplasia (130) to adenomatous transformation arising in the background of hyperplasia (119) (see chapter 11). The duration and intensity of exposure to GRH may be responsible for the presentation. The acromegaly may be associated with hyperprolactinemia, consistent with the stimulation of PRL secretion by GRH and the presence of lactotroph hyperplasia noted in the pituitaries of these patients. A paradoxical GH response to thyrotropin-releasing hormone (TRH) may be observed in patients with tumoral GRH production as it is in those with GH-producing pituitary adenomas (66). These patients usually do not exhibit an in vivo GH response to GRH provocation (73,121); this is not surprising, since the small dose of exogenous GRH would not significantly increase an already high level of circulating GRH. Elevation of circulating GRH levels is diagnostic of the condition. A reduced GH response to GRH has been reported in patients

harboring adenomas with Gs mutations (124) but may also reflect GRH receptor down-regulation which has been documented in vitro in pituitary somatotroph adenomas (84,126) and nontumorous somatotrophs (60).

Hypothalamic neuronal tumors producing GRH may be associated with acromegaly (see chapter 5). These rare lesions present as a sellar mass that mimics a simple pituitary GH-producing pituitary adenoma or may involve the hypothalamus; microscopic examination reveals a gangliocytoma associated with a pituitary adenoma in most cases (43,51,96,115).

Prognosis and Therapy. The local effects of tumor growth may cause adenohypophysial insufficiency resulting in headache, nausea and vomiting, and cranial nerve lesions. The insulin-antagonistic effects of GH lead to diabetes mellitus in patients with somatotroph adenoma. Patients with chronic GH excess develop hypertension that leads to cerebrovascular disease, cardiomyopathy, severe coronary artery disease, congestive heart failure, and early death. They also have a higher incidence of malignancy, including colonic polyps and carcinomas, and breast carcinomas, than the general population (105,107).

Although there have been occasional reports of spontaneous remission of acromegaly due to hemorrhage and infarction of the tumor (69), these are rare occurrences and most patients require therapy. The primary objectives in treating acromegaly are to relieve the hypersomatotropic state and its complications, and to remove or relieve the compressive effects of the mass without compromising other pituitary function. Three major therapeutic modalities are available: surgery (118), drug therapy (69), and irradiation (58,69,135). Regardless of the approach it is important to recognize that cure is often difficult to achieve. Partial fulfillment represents control of the disease.

Surgery constitutes the primary form of treatment for most patients with acromegaly. Transsphenoidal adenomectomy is preferred but a subfrontal approach is sometimes necessary for patients with tumors demonstrating extensive suprasellar or parasellar extension. In several clinical studies, rapid normalization of blood GH level was accomplished in more than 60 percent of patients and in more than 90 percent with small to medium-sized tumors (70,94,102,117,122). The frequency of surgical success, however, is closely correlated to the size and degree of invasiveness of the tumor, as well as to surgical expertise. The results with large tumors are worse and tumors with evidence of invasion also have poor long-term results (72,94). In a worldwide review of 1366 cases of acromegaly managed by transsphenoidal surgery, a modest criterion of cure (GH level <10 µg/L) was achieved in only 50 percent of patients (118). Significant complications, including diabetes insipidus and cerebrospinal fluid leakage, occurred in approximately 5 percent of patients. Delayed relapse has been reported in patients who retain abnormal GH dynamics on provocative testing postoperatively (38,39,122).

The relatively low surgical correction rate in patients with large or invasive tumors suggests that treatment to decrease tumor size prior to surgery would be appropriate. Approximately 20 percent of subjects respond to dopaminergic drugs, such as bromocriptine or lisuride, which lower blood GH levels and reduce signs and symptoms of active disease (110); however, IGF-1 levels are normalized in only 10 percent of patients. Many patients report subjective improvement in clinical symptoms with dopaminergic treatment (76,83,89,92,125) yet do not demonstrate objective reduction in GH/IGF-1 levels. An elevated serum PRL level portends a favorable GH response to bromocriptine, consistent with the in vitro response of bihormonal tumors (41). Nevertheless, tumor shrinkage during therapy is not a constant feature of this treatment (83).

Results have been more encouraging with octreotide (Sandostatin), a synthetic octapeptide analogue of somatostatin which resists enzymatic degradation and has an extended half life (47,64,65,74,104,134). A number of reports have shown that this substance is capable of reducing blood GH levels in the majority of acromegalic patients (45,46,53,80,90,93). Mean GH levels decline significantly (by more than 25 percent) in 70 percent of subjects, usually within 30 minutes of subcutaneous octreotide administration and maximal suppression is reached within 2 hours (65). However, GH levels often begin to rise by the 7th hour of drug administration, necessitating frequent injections or continuous subcutaneous infusion by pump (54,77). Rapid and significant improvement in most clinical features is noted; excessive perspiration, soft tissue swelling, fatigue, arthralgias, acne, and headaches improve in 50 to 75 percent of octreotide-treated patients with acromegaly (128). Headaches are frequently reported to improve within minutes of analog administration while other symptoms resolve within weeks (64,65,75,116). Cardiovascular function may improve within 3 months of treatment (52,97). The use of this analog is of particular benefit to those patients with persistently nonsuppressible GH levels and elevated IGF-1 levels following pituitary surgery or after radiotherapy until radiation effects are noticeable. It may also constitute primary therapy for those who decline or cannot tolerate surgery or irradiation.

Despite the rapid response of headaches to this medical therapy, tumor shrinkage is a controversial issue; a few authors have indicated that some tumors do reduce in size and therefore preoperative therapy may improve the results of surgery (45,46), however, in the majority of reports tumor shrinkage is not a prominent feature (80,93). When it occurs, it is rapid (within weeks) and may be reversible after drug withdrawal (44,65). The degree of size reduction is usually modest. While some earlier reports have suggested that this effect may facilitate surgical removal and improve outcome (46,63), this question remains to be resolved.

The importance of morphologic diagnosis in predicting response to therapy is emphasized in this area. The variable morphologic appearance of GH-producing pituitary adenomas correlates with their response to octreotide: densely granulated adenomas exhibit an enhanced reduction of GH levels compared to sparsely granulated somatotroph adenomas (63). Interestingly, the densely granulated tumors are also thought to be the group of adenomas with activating mutations of Gsα and high basal adenylyl cyclase levels (124) (see Pathogenesis of Pituitary Adenomas).

Radiation with either conventional X-ray high voltage photons or heavy particles has been used to treat acromegaly (56,58,135). Pituitary implantation of radioactive yttrium (90Y) is a procedure that has been used in Europe with variable success (114). These procedures generally result in decreased plasma GH levels but frequently have more severe side effects including late hypopituitarism, empty sella syndrome, visual impairment due to optic pathway damage, and temporal lobe epilepsy. GH hypersecretion may continue due to extension of the tumor into areas that are difficult to reach with a sufficient dose of radiation. These therapies are generally suitable for elderly patients and those who are poor candidates for surgery or anesthesia; they are also used for patients who have had unsuccessful pituitary surgery or medical therapy (57,58). The results achieved by all forms of irradiation are highly comparable and are mainly limited by their slow onset of action.

PITUITARY ADENOMAS CAUSING PROLACTIN EXCESS

Clinical Features. Although PRL was not discovered as a human hormone until 1971 (151, 167), the association of amenorrhea and galactorrhea dates back to 1855 when Chiari and colleagues reported two cases of puerperal atrophy of the uterus with amenorrhea and persistent lactation (140). The syndrome was redescribed in 1882 by Frommel (147), in 1932 by Ahumada and del Castillo (137), and in 1953 by Argonz and del Castillo (137a). Forbes and her associates (146) were the first to suggest that the syndrome characterized by galactorrhea, amenorrhea, and low levels of urinary follicle-stimulating hormone (FSH) might be associated with a pituitary tumor,

however, only 25 percent of patients were recognized to have such tumors at the time. After the discovery of PRL, the use of radioimmunoassay confirmed that serum levels were elevated in many patients who were thought to harbor "functionless" pituitary tumors (150,171). It is now recognized that prolactinomas represent approximately 25 percent of surgically removed pituitary adenomas (163) and nearly 50 percent of pituitary tumors in autopsy series (141,164,169,174); the lower prevalence in surgical material is likely due to successful nonsurgical management with dopaminergic agonists.

Lactotroph adenomas present most frequently with galactorrhea and ovulatory disorders in women (140,150,153,173,182). The galactorrhea may be unilateral or bilateral, continuous or intermittent, free flowing or expressible. A significant number of patients with striking hyperprolactinemia present only with amenorrhea (140). Some patients have less severe ovulatory disorders such as luteal phase defects and disorders of folliculogenesis. Although most lactotroph adenomas occur in adults, occasionally primary amenorrhea and delayed puberty may be attributed to the development of a lactotroph adenoma in youth.

In surgical material, lactotroph adenomas are less common in men, in whom hyperprolactinemia results in decreased libido and impotence (163). Interestingly, there is no sex-related difference in autopsy series, and the prevalence in women in surgical series probably reflects their greater awareness of the sequela. Women generally present at a younger age and tend to have microadenomas; men present at older ages with larger tumors that cause visual field abnormalities and hypopituitarism due to pituitary tissue destruction (149); rarely they may have galactorrhea (182). The serum concentration of PRL correlates with tumor size (153); because women generally present with smaller tumors, their serum PRL levels are not as high as those of men (171).

Some lactotroph microadenomas do not grow and cause only mild symptoms. Some experts advocate clinical surveillance of these patients and suggest therapy only if the symptoms are bothersome. However, many patients require treatment of amenorrhea, infertility, and persistent galactorrhea, and prolonged estrogen deficiency may result in vaginal complications and osteopenia. Large invasive tumors can cause the complications of a parasellar mass.

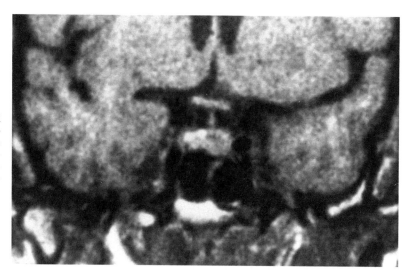

Figure 3-39
RADIOGRAPHIC APPEARANCE
OF PROLACTINOMA
(MRI, T1 WEIGHTED)
This patient with amenorrhea and galactorrhea has a microadenoma detectable as a small hypointense mass on the left, resulting in asymmetry of the pituitary. Notice the normally enhancing pituitary gland on the right after gadolinium administration.

Occasional patients with a lactotroph adenoma have subtle acromegalic features, however, elevation of blood GH may not be documented. Nevertheless, their tumors produce PRL and GH. Clinicopathologic correlations have implicated the unusual and aggressive tumor known as acidophil stem cell adenoma as the cause of hyperprolactinemia with "fugitive acromegaly" (157, 158,163). These adenomas must be distinguished from the usual lactotroph adenomas because of their propensity grow aggressively and recur.

Biochemical Findings. The dominant chemical abnormality in patients with lactotroph adenomas is the marked elevation of serum PRL levels. On a single measurement, elevated serum PRL levels that are not over 250 ng/ml are not diagnostic. PRL has a sleep-entrained secretory pattern with elevated levels in the early morning. Many physiologic events can trigger the release of this hormone including stress, food intake, physical activity, pregnancy, lactation, nipple stimulation, and female orgasm. Pharmacologic agents including dopamine receptor agonists (phenothiazines, metoclopramide), tricyclic antidepressants, reserpine, estrogens, opiates, and cimetidine can elevate serum PRL (153).

Other pathologic causes of hyperprolactinemia include hypothalamic diseases and interruption of the pituitary stalk which prevent the tonic dopamineric inhibition of pituitary lactotrophs. Systemic disorders, such as hypothyroidism and chronic renal failure, cause hyperprolactinemia; determination of thyroid and renal function are

therefore indicated in the evaluation of persistent hyperprolactinemia. In compensated hypothyroidism, thyroxine levels may be low to normal but blood TSH and PRL levels are elevated. This may be accompanied by pituitary hyperplasia which can mimic a lactotroph adenoma. These abnormalities usually all regress with thyroid hormone replacement. Idiopathic lactotroph hyperplasia is a rare cause of hyperprolactinemia; it is difficult to distinguish from prolactinoma clinically (160,175) and may even be associated with suprasellar extension of the gland (175).

The most commonly used diagnostic test to distinguish hyperprolactinemia due to a lactotroph adenoma from hyperprolactinemia of other causes is the TRH stimulation test (171). In normal persons, TRH induces an elevation of serum PRL to at least double basal values. Approximately 80 percent of patients with lactotroph adenoma have either no rise or a blunted increase in PRL levels with this test. Patients with hyperprolactinemia due to other causes, however, may also have an abnormal result on provocative testing.

Radiologic Findings. Because lactotroph adenomas in women are frequently microadenomas, they may be associated with normal skull X rays or with only subtle asymmetry of the pituitary fossa. High resolution CT with or without contrast or MRI reveals small tumors in most patients with hyperprolactinemia and normal skull X rays (fig. 3-39). Although it has been suggested that some of the small abnormalities found on scans may represent only artefact, in patients with a blood

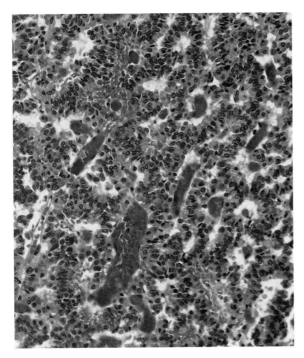

Figure 3-40
HISTOLOGY OF SPARSELY GRANULATED
LACTOTROPH ADENOMA
This sparsely granulated lactotroph adenoma has a characteristic papillary architecture, forming pseudorosettes around vascular channels. The tumor cells are crowded and have pale eosinophilic to chromophobic cytoplasm. The nuclear morphology is relatively monotonous.

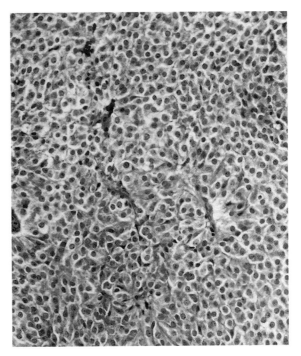

Figure 3-41
HISTOLOGY OF SPARSELY GRANULATED
LACTOTROPH ADENOMA
This sparsely granulated lactotroph adenoma has a more solid architectural pattern. The tumor cells are generally chromophobic with relatively bland nuclear morphology and occasional pseudorosettes around vascular channels.

PRL level greater than 200 ng/mL, they provide strong evidence of a pituitary adenoma. Patients with blood levels lower than that value who have radiographic evidence of a sizeable pituitary tumor likely have adenomas that are nonfunctional or produce other substances and the hyperprolactinemia is attributable to the "stalk section effect" (150,153,171).

Tumors generally present later in men than women because the symptoms are more subtle. The tumors are generally larger and there may be radiologic evidence of suprasellar extension as well as compression or invasion of adjacent structures.

Gross Findings. Microadenomas are frequently found in young women and are usually located in the lateral portions of the gland where lactotrophs are most numerous (163). Some of the tumors are expansile, compressive lesions; many have a microinvasive pattern without a well-defined capsule. Macroadenomas can be widely invasive of local structures, extending into dura,

sinuses, and bone; they can present as nasal masses or undetected large tumors that result in death due to destruction of hypothalamic structures or obstruction of the third ventricle.

These pituitary adenomas vary from soft, red, friable lesions to firm grayish white tumors that have abundant fibrous or amyloid stroma. Occasionally they contain gritty calcifications that represent psammoma bodies.

Microscopic Findings. Lactotroph adenomas are recognized to have two variants, analogous to the two types of somatotroph adenomas (156,163), however, sparsely granulated tumors comprise the overwhelming majority.

Sparsely Granulated Lactotroph Adenomas. These common adenomas are usually chromophobic with conventional histologic techniques. They exhibit a wide variation in architecture: some tumors are trabecular or papillary (fig. 3-40), others are composed of solid sheets (fig. 3-41). There may be a slight cytoplasmic basophilia

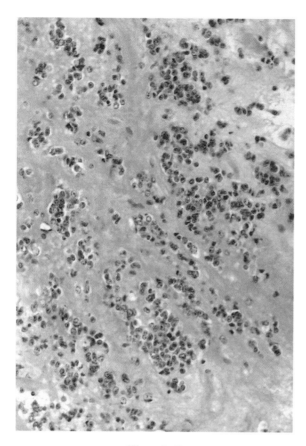

Figure 3-42
HISTOLOGY OF SPARSELY GRANULATED
LACTOTROPH ADENOMA: FIBROSIS
Sparsely granulated lactotroph adenomas often exhibit fibrous stroma.

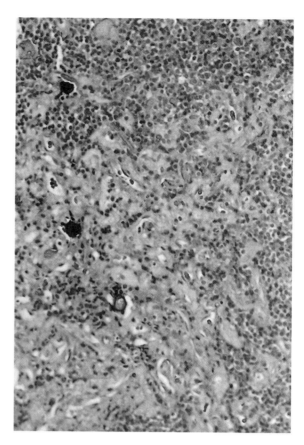

Figure 3-43
HISTOLOGY OF SPARSELY GRANULATED
LACTOTROPH ADENOMA: PSAMMOMA BODIES
Sparsely granulated lactotroph adenomas may form psammoma bodies, adding meningioma to the differential diagnosis. This tumor also exhibits a fibrous stroma.

attributable to abundant rough endoplasmic reticulum rich in RNA. Occasionally, the stroma is fibrous (figs. 3-42, 3-43). Calcification may take the form of psammoma bodies (fig. 3-43) or may be so extensive as to form a "pituitary stone" (fig. 3-44). The reason for this phenomenon and its preferential occurrence in lactotroph adenomas is not certain (168), however, it is important to distinguish these tumors from other parasellar tumors that calcify, such as meningiomas. Occasionally, lactotroph adenomas produce endocrine amyloid that stains with Congo red (fig. 3-45) and has apple green birefringence with polarized light (fig. 3-46).

By immunohistochemistry, positivity for PRL is intense in a juxtanuclear globular structure which corresponds to the Golgi complex (fig. 3-47). The tumor cells may exhibit nuclear positivity for Pit-1 (fig. 3-48) and for the estrogen

receptor (ER) (139,184). They almost never stain for other adenohypophysial hormones; rarely, they may contain α-subunit (152).

The ultrastructural features of sparsely granulated lactotroph adenomas are distinctive. The cells resemble stimulated nontumorous lactotrophs (figs. 3-49, 3-50). They have large, euchromatic nuclei with prominent nucleoli. The cytoplasm is almost totally occupied by parallel arrays of rough endoplasmic reticulum; Nebenkern formations, concentric whorls of rough endoplasmic reticulum membranes, are common. The Golgi complex is well developed and frequently contains immature granules which may be very pleomorphic in shape and electron density. Storage granules, which are sparse, vary from 150 to 300 nm in diameter and are generally spherical. One of the characteristics of PRL secretion in these

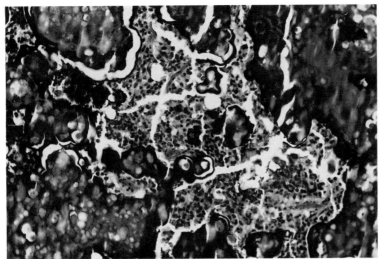

Figure 3-44
HISTOLOGY OF SPARSELY
GRANULATED LACTOTROPH
ADENOMA: PITUITARY STONE
This sparsely granulated lactotroph adenoma has undergone extensive calcification. Residual psammoma bodies are recognized but the calcification has become so extensive as to form an almost solid, calcified, stone-like tumor. The residual tumor cells have chromophobic cytoplasm.

Figure 3-45
HISTOLOGY OF SPARSELY
GRANULATED LACTOTROPH
ADENOMA: AMYLOID
This sparsely granulated lactotroph adenoma forms endocrine amyloid which stains with Congo red. Solid deposits of amyloid are recognized and individual tumor cells have ballooned cytoplasm filled with amyloid.

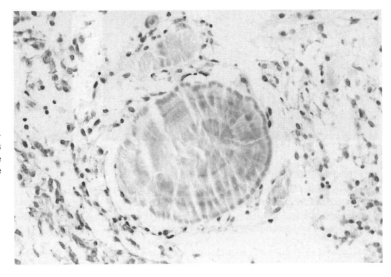

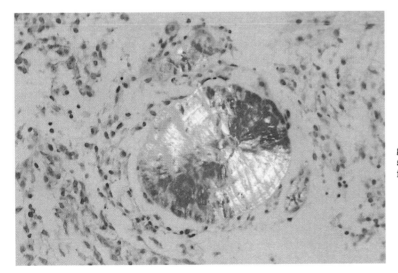

Figure 3-46
HISTOLOGY OF SPARSELY
GRANULATED LACTOTROPH
ADENOMA: AMYLOID
Polarized light reveals the characteristic green birefringence of amyloid in this section stained with Congo red, corresponding to figure 3-45.

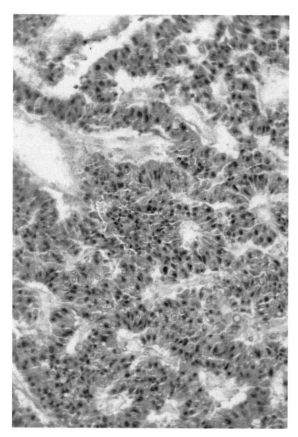

Figure 3-47
IMMUNOHISTOCHEMICAL LOCALIZATION
OF PROLACTIN IN SPARSELY
GRANULATED LACTOTROPH ADENOMA

The immunohistochemical pattern of staining for prolactin in sparsely granulated lactotroph adenomas is diagnostic. These tumors have juxtanuclear dot-like positivity corresponding to the Golgi complex. Stored secretory granules are sparse, therefore cytoplasmic staining is not diffuse.

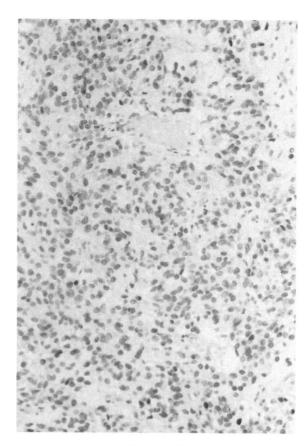

Figure 3-48
IMMUNOHISTOCHEMICAL LOCALIZATION
OF PIT-1 IN SPARSELY
GRANULATED LACTOTROPH ADENOMA

Prolactin-producing adenomas exhibit nuclear positivity for Pit-1.

and other PRL-producing tumors is the presence of granule extrusions along the lateral cell borders into the extracellular space; this diagnostic feature is known as "misplaced exocytosis."

Densely Granulated Lactotroph Adenoma. This very rare adenoma is a more acidophilic tumor (fig. 3-51), with intense diffuse positivity for PRL throughout the cell cytoplasm (fig. 3-52). The cells strongly resemble resting nontumorous lactotrophs. Their ultrastructure is that of a densely granulated cell with less abundant rough endoplasmic reticulum than in the sparsely granulated counterpart. The cells also contain well-developed Golgi complexes that often harbor pleomorphic, highly electron dense

forming granules. The numerous secretory granules within the cytoplasm are spherical and electron dense, measuring up to 700 nm in diameter. The largest granules frequently have a mottled appearance. Misplaced exocytosis may be recognized in this tumor type as well.

Acidophil Stem Cell Adenoma. Rarely, patients with hyperprolactinemia have minor symptoms or biochemical evidence of GH excess. This clinical phenomenon is associated with an unusual PRL-immunoreactive adenoma containing faint or focal GH immunoreactivity, and peculiar mitochondrial changes. The acidophil stem cell adenoma is a chromophobic or slightly acidophilic tumor with diffuse histologic architecture (fig. 3-53); the acidophilia is attributable to mitochondrial accumulation, considered to be a form of oncocytic change (fig.

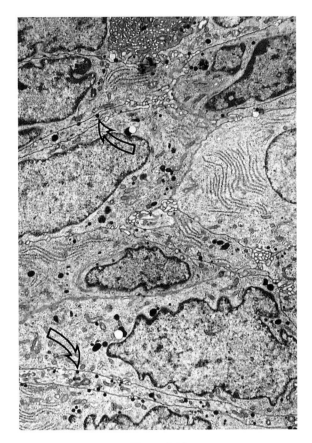

Figure 3-49
ULTRASTRUCTURE OF SPARSELY
GRANULATED LACTOTROPH ADENOMA

The cells of a sparsely granulated lactotroph adenoma are elongated and exhibit some degree of polarity. At one pole of the cell, rough endoplasmic reticulum is well formed. Juxtanuclear Golgi complexes are large and extremely well developed. Secretory granules are sparse and these tumors exhibit a characteristic feature, "misplaced exocytosis," which is extrusion of secretory material at the lateral cell borders (arrows).

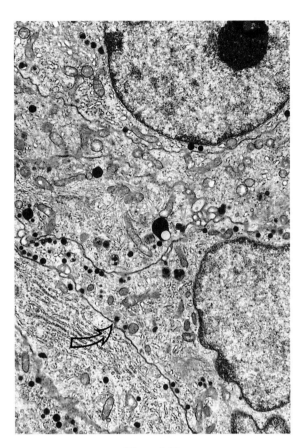

Figure 3-50
ULTRASTRUCTURE OF SPARSELY
GRANULATED LACTOTROPH ADENOMA

Sparsely granulated lactotroph adenoma cells have parallel arrays of well-developed rough endoplasmic reticulum, highly developed Golgi complexes, and sparse secretory granules that are highly variable in size and shape. Misplaced exocytosis is conspicuous (arrow).

3-54). Even in the absence of clinical evidence of GH production by a prolactinoma, the presence of oxyphilia should raise suspicion of this aggressive tumor. Clear cytoplasmic vacuoles may be recognized on histologic examination (fig. 3-55); these correspond to giant mitochondria. Immunohistochemistry documents predominant positivity for PRL (fig. 3-56), but not in the usual juxtanuclear dot-like pattern of the common sparsely granulated lactotroph adenoma (contrast with fig. 3-47), and occasionally there is scant positivity for GH (fig. 3-57). In some tumors, GH immunoreactivity cannot be demonstrated by light microscopy. These tumors contain scattered fibrous bodies,

identified as juxtanuclear whorls of low molecular weight cytokeratins (fig. 3-58).

This rare tumor has a distinctive and diagnostic ultrastructure (figs. 3-59, 3-60) and electron microscopy is usually required to confirm the diagnosis when it is suspected by light microscopy. Within irregular elongated cells that have ovoid or irregular nuclei, the mitochondria are numerous and often enlarged, forming unique giant mitochondria with loss of cristae and harboring electron dense tubular structures. Rough endoplasmic reticulum and Golgi complexes are moderately developed. The tumor cells contain fibrous bodies in a juxtanuclear location, identical to those of sparsely granulated somatotroph adenomas. In addition, they display the misplaced exocytosis seen in

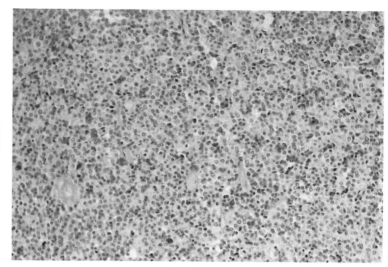

Figure 3-51
HISTOLOGY OF DENSELY
GRANULATED
LACTOTROPH ADENOMA
The densely granulated lactotroph ade-
noma is a rare tumor that resembles
sparsely granulated tumors but has more
cytoplasmic acidophilia.

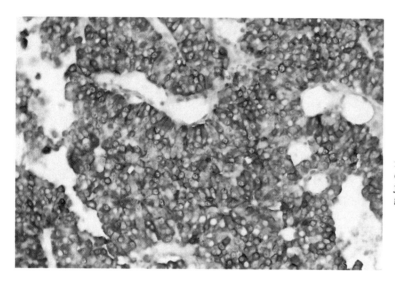

Figure 3-52
IMMUNOHISTOCHEMICAL
LOCALIZATION OF PROLACTIN
IN DENSELY GRANULATED
LACTOTROPH ADENOMA
This tumor has diffuse and intense immu-
noreactivity for prolactin throughout the tumor
cell cytoplasm, in contrast to the characteristic
juxtanuclear staining pattern of the sparsely
granulated variant of lactotroph adenoma.

lactotrophs. The secretory granules are sparse
and small, measuring 150 to 200 nm.

Tissue culture studies have documented release of small quantities of GH as well as PRL
by these tumors (138).

Morphologic Effects of Drugs and Hormones.
The administration of dopamine agonists such as
bromocriptine results in striking morphologic
changes accompanied by a dramatic clinical response (165). Most patients with lactotroph adenomas have striking and rapid reduction of serum
PRL levels when therapy is initiated, and within
days to weeks, there is symptomatic and radiologic
evidence of tumor shrinkage. Histologically, the
changes can evoke diagnostic problems. The tu-

mors become more cellular due to marked
shrinkage in cell size, predominantly affecting the
tumor cell cytoplasm (figs. 3-61, 3-62); ultrastructural analysis has confirmed a marked reduction
in the density of the cytoplasmic volume of rough
endoplasmic reticulum and Golgi complexes (fig.
3-63) (180). The nuclei become markedly irregular and heterochromatic. In some cases, the
number of secretory granules increases, but the
size and number of secretory granules are not
usually significantly altered and granule extrusions may still be recognized. There is often
associated perivascular and interstitial fibrosis
(figs. 3-61, 3-64); occasionally there is evidence
of hemorrhage (fig. 3-64). These changes can

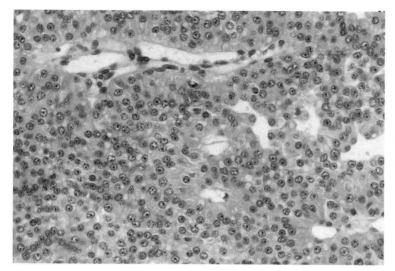

Figure 3-53
HISTOLOGY OF ACIDOPHIL
STEM CELL ADENOMA
This slightly acidophilic tumor generally exhibits a diffuse solid architectural pattern and, like the lactotroph adenoma, may form pseudorosettes around vascular channels.

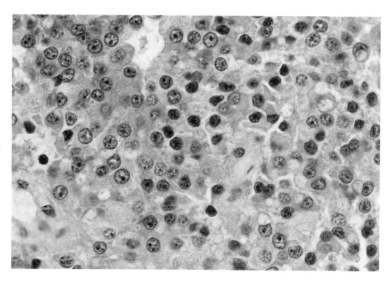

Figure 3-54
HISTOLOGY OF ACIDOPHIL
STEM CELL ADENOMA
The tumor cells have pale acidophilic cytoplasm with granularity, attributable to oncocytic change. The nuclear morphology of this tumor type is more pleomorphic than in well-differentiated lactotroph adenoma.

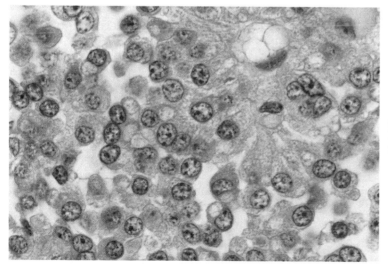

Figure 3-55
HISTOLOGY OF ACIDOPHIL
STEM CELL ADENOMA
The acidophilic granular cytoplasm due to mitochondrial accumulation often exhibits a large clear vacuole that corresponds to a giant mitochondrion seen by electron microscopy.

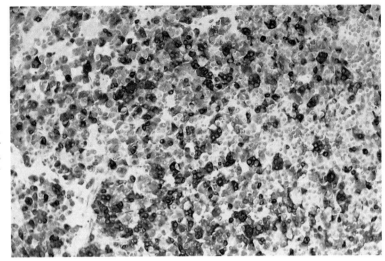

Figure 3-56
IMMUNOHISTOCHEMICAL
LOCALIZATION OF PROLACTIN IN
ACIDOPHIL STEM CELL ADENOMA

Immunostaining reveals prolactin positivity in these tumors. The pattern is variable: there may be juxtanuclear staining similar to that seen in lactotroph adenomas or, as in this case, diffuse cytoplasmic reactivity may be more prominent.

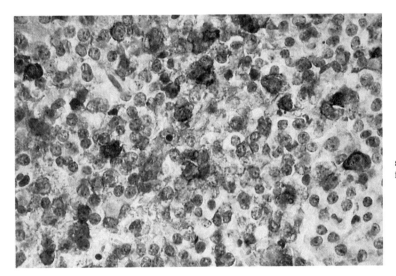

Figure 3-57
IMMUNOHISTOCHEMICAL
LOCALIZATION OF GROWTH
HORMONE IN ACIDOPHIL
STEM CELL ADENOMA

Occasionally, scattered cells in an acidophil stem cell adenoma exhibit immunoreactivity for growth hormone. This is generally weak.

Figure 3-58
IMMUNOHISTOCHEMICAL
LOCALIZATION OF CYTOKERATINS
IN ACIDOPHIL STEM CELL ADENOMA

Immunostaining for low molecular weight cytokeratins with the Cam 5.2 antibody reveals scattered juxtanuclear cytoplasmic globules (arrows) that correspond to fibrous bodies, similar to those seen in sparsely granulated somatotroph adenomas. These are much fewer in the acidophil stem cell adenoma and careful examination is required to identify them.

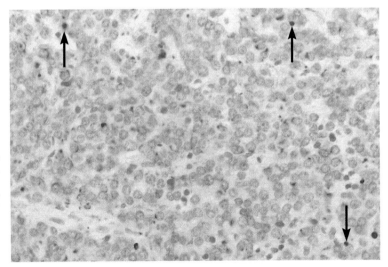

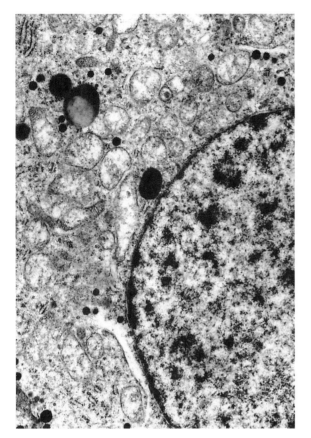

Figure 3-59
ULTRASTRUCTURE OF ACIDOPHIL
STEM CELL ADENOMA
The cells of this tumor have short profiles of rough endoplasmic reticulum, sparse small secretory granules, and numerous swollen mitochondria, creating an oncocytic appearance.

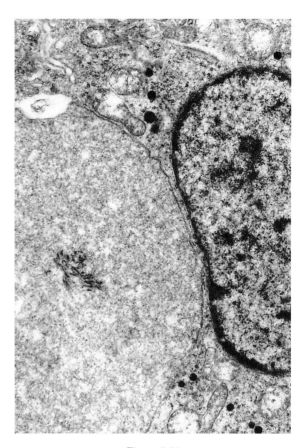

Figure 3-60
ULTRASTRUCTURE OF ACIDOPHIL
STEM CELL ADENOMA
The tumor cells in an acidophil stem cell adenoma have numerous dilated mitochondria. Scattered cells form unusual giant mitochondria with double membranes and loss of cristae and electron dense tubular inclusions.

result in a histologic picture that resembles lymphoma and immunohistochemical staining is required to address this differential diagnosis. Lack of staining for leukocyte common antigen (LCA) and the presence of PRL immunoreactivity (fig. 3-65), albeit focal or faint, provide guidance when facing this problem.

The morphologic alterations are usually rapidly reversible on termination of the therapy. Occasionally, a subpopulation of tumor cells may continue to demonstrate the "bromocriptine effect" (fig. 3-66), suggesting irreversible inhibition; the reason for this is not known.

Protracted exposure of these tumors to dopaminergic agonists may also result in extensive fibrosis which may adversely influence the outcome of subsequent surgery. Tissue culture stud-

ies suggest that acidophil stem cell adenomas may be unresponsive to bromocriptine inhibition (138).

Differential Diagnosis. The numerous physiologic and pathologic causes of hyperprolactinemia are discussed above. Many of these are unassociated with a pituitary tumor, or may be coincidentally associated with an unrelated pituitary tumor; it is therefore critical to prove that a surgically resected pituitary tumor is responsible for PRL production. First, the pathologist must establish the presence of an adenoma with the reticulin stain in dubious cases. Lactotroph and thyrotroph hyperplasia are often mistaken for prolactinoma (see Hyperplasias, chapter 11), and other tumor-like lesions such as inflammatory processes (see Inflammatory Lesions, chapter 11) can

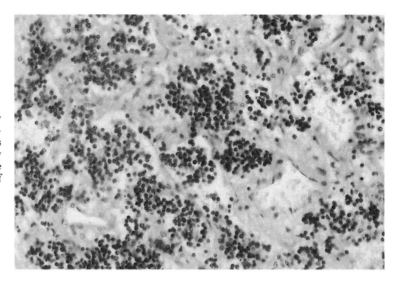

Figure 3-61
HISTOLOGY OF BROMOCRIPTINE-TREATED LACTOTROPH ADENOMA

Following bromocriptine therapy, sparsely granulated lactotroph adenomas undergo a remarkable change. The tumor cell cytoplasm is markedly reduced and the tumor cells are very small. The nuclei exhibit hyperchromasia. The stroma is fibrotic. The histologic appearance of this tumor resembles lymphoma.

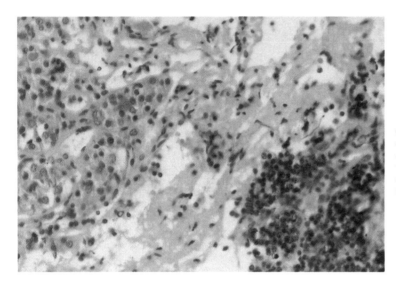

Figure 3-62
HISTOLOGY OF BROMOCRIPTINE-TREATED LACTOTROPH ADENOMA

The bromocriptine-treated prolactinoma (right) is strikingly different than the adjacent nontumorous pituitary (left) that is composed of cells of the usual size. The treated tumor cells are smaller and markedly increased in density with almost total reduction of tumor cell cytoplasm.

Figure 3-63
ULTRASTRUCTURE OF BROMOCRIPTINE-TREATED LACTOTROPH ADENOMA

Electron microscopy of a bromocriptine-treated lactotroph adenoma reveals a reduced cell size with irregular heterochromatic nuclei and a striking loss of rough endoplasmic reticulum and Golgi complexes. The scattered secretory granules appear more dense but this is attributable to a reduction in cytoplasmic area of other subcellular organelles.

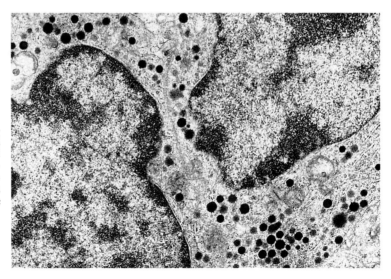

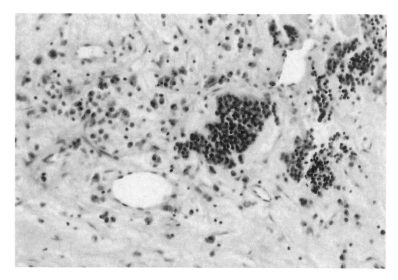

Figure 3-64
HISTOLOGY OF BROMOCRIPTINE-
TREATED LACTOTROPH ADENOMA:
FIBROSIS AND HEMORRHAGE

This lactotroph adenoma was treated with bromocriptine prior to surgery. In addition to cellular involution, there is stromal fibrosis, and hemosiderin-laden macrophages provide evidence of hemorrhage.

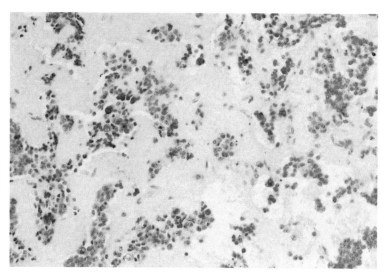

Figure 3-65
IMMUNOHISTOCHEMICAL
LOCALIZATION OF
PROLACTIN IN
BROMOCRIPTINE-TREATED
LACTOTROPH ADENOMA

Although this involuted adenoma can histologically resemble lymphoma, the scattered immunoreactivity for prolactin proves its true nature.

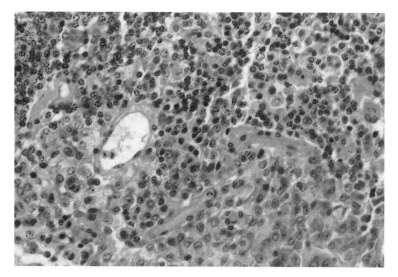

Figure 3-66
HISTOLOGY OF
BROMOCRIPTINE-TREATED
LACTOTROPH ADENOMA:
IRREVERSIBLE INHIBITION

This lactotroph adenoma was treated with bromocriptine but the medication was stopped more than a year prior to surgery. Although much of the tumor has resumed the typical appearance of a sparsely granulated lactotroph adenoma, there is focal residual cellular involution.

mimic this disorder, but careful histologic examination and a reticulin stain will identify these possibilities. Several plurihormonal pituitary adenomas produce PRL; these include GH-producing tumors (see Adenomas Causing Growth Hormone Excess) and unusual plurihormonal tumors (see Plurihormonal Pituitary Adenomas). Clinically nonfunctioning pituitary adenomas and any of the other mass lesions described in the various chapters of this text can cause stalk compression and hyperprolactinemia; the clue to these diagnoses is the relatively low serum PRL levels that do not correlate with tumor size.

Ectopic secretion of PRL has not been of clinical significance to date. PRL expression has been detected in endometrium, lymphocytes, and breast as well as sporadically in other tumors (145, 148,178), however, only rarely has the secretion given rise to a clinical diagnostic dilemma (154).

Prognosis and Therapy. Some lactotroph microadenomas do not grow and cause only mild symptoms (140). Investigators have advocated only clinical surveillance in these patients and suggest therapy only if the symptoms are bothersome. However, many tumors, especially macroadenomas, are a serious clinical problem. Untreated, they result, in women, in amenorrhea, infertility, persistent galactorrhea, and estrogen deficiency which may cause decreased vaginal secretion leading to dyspareunia and severe osteopenia with significant debilitation (161,162). Some women with PRL-secreting tumors have clinical evidence of androgen excess with hirsutism and acne (171). Tumor growth may extend suprasellar, giving rise to visual field defects and even blindness, or extend to the hypothalamus, resulting in disturbances of temperature regulation, food intake, fluid balance, sleep cycle, behavior, and autonomic nervous system function. Diabetes insipidus, somnolence, and hyperphagia with obesity may be manifestations of extensive hypothalamic involvement (171). Cranial nerves may be involved by tumor extension, particularly the third, fourth, and sixth cranial nerves. Involvement of the ophthalmic nerve and maxillary divisions of the fifth cranial nerve lead to ptosis, diplopia, ophthalmoplegia, and reduced facial sensation. Extension into the cavernous sinus can be lethal. Involvement of the temporal lobe may cause seizures. The frontal lobes may be infiltrated by tumor, resulting in alterations of personality and defects in smell. Acute hemorrhagic necrosis of the tumor (pituitary apoplexy) may lead to rapid tumor expansion, severe headache, lethargy, coma, or other signs of increased intracranial pressure. Without therapy, the tumors may lead to death.

Surgical resection can be undertaken by either the transsphenoidal or, in the case of large tumors, the transfrontal approach (142,143,177). The results of surgery indicate cure rates as high as 70 to 75 percent. The success of surgery in general and its relative merits compared to a medical approach are controversial. The variable response to transsphenoidal adenomectomies appears to be influenced by the biologic behavior of the tumor and the skill of the neurosurgeon. While most centers report postoperative normalization of serum prolactin in 60 to 80 percent of patients with microprolactinomas (181), the response rate for those with macroprolactinomas is considerably lower and ranges from 0 to 40 percent (176). The second problem with surgical adenomectomy for prolactinoma is long-term recurrence. Available data suggest that while surgery is effective in rapidly debulking large tumors, it is curative in only a small minority of patients with macroadenomas (177). Therefore, in patients with macroprolactinomas, the relative risks and complications from surgery must be carefully weighed against the anticipated benefits. Moreover, after initial surgical failure, the risk of repeat surgery is considerably higher (166) and medical management is recommended.

Most lactotroph adenomas respond to dopamine agonists such as the ergot alkaloid, 2-bromo-alpha-ergocryptine mesylate (bromocriptine), with a rapid fall in serum PRL levels and tumor shrinkage (179,180). This has revolutionized the therapeutic approach to patients with prolactinomas. Reduction of serum PRL ameliorates the endocrine symptoms; fertility is rapidly restored and conception can be achieved. The drug suppresses PRL gene transcription and causes cellular involution; shrinkage of tumor is well documented (fig. 3-67) and the morphologic correlates have been described above. The extent of shrinkage does not correlate with changes in blood hormone levels and the resolution of visual field defects can occur prior to radiologic evidence of tumor shrinkage (172). There appears to be no difference in response rate between

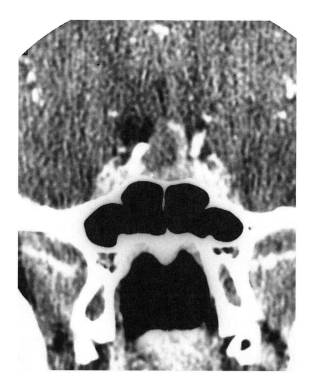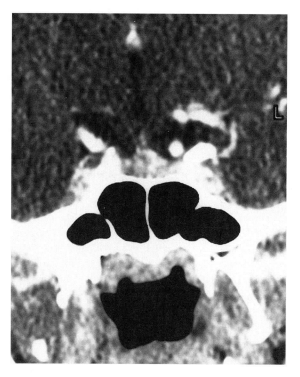

Figure 3-67

RADIOLOGIC APPEARANCE OF BROMOCRIPTINE-INDUCED TUMOR SHRINKAGE

Left: This prolactin-producing tumor was a macroadenoma with suprasellar extension documented by CT scan with contrast enhancement at the time of diagnosis.

Right: After 3 months of bromocriptine therapy, it has significantly reduced in size as shown in this corresponding CT image. (Courtesy of Dr. S. Ezzat, Toronto, Canada.)

patients with microadenomas and those with macroprolactinomas; the time taken to achieve normalization of PRL, however, may be longer in the latter group. This drug is now recommended as a primary treatment modality by some endocrinologists who reserve neurosurgery for refractory situations (172). However, the hormonal effects and tumor shrinkage are reversible following withdrawal of the medication which is therefore generally continuous and should be maintained at the lowest effective dose. New long-acting dopamine agonists such as bromocriptine-LAR (179) or CV 205-502 (155) provide alternatives for patients who do not tolerate bromocriptine or are refractory.

Macroadenomas may show only partial response to bromocriptine and may require surgery. Some investigators have found no difference in the frequency or extent of fibrosis, calcification, PRL immunoreactivity, or ultimate surgical outcome in patients pretreated with bromocriptine and those not so treated (159). Others have found that a

short (2- to 6-week) preoperative course of bromocriptine increased the efficacy of surgery in patients with larger adenomas (144,183). However, prolonged exposure to dopamine agonists may increase fibrous tissue which may adversely affect the outcome of subsequent surgery.

The acidophil stem cell adenoma appears not to be suppressible by bromocriptine (138) and failure of dopamine agonist therapy in vivo may suggest that the patient harbors this tumor type. In general, patients with this aggressive and infiltrative tumor require surgical resection and recurrence is not uncommon. Careful surveillance is warranted for early detection of recurrence and radiation therapy is usually indicated for recurrent tumors.

Small doses of radiation were administered in past years to patients with lactotroph adenoma. In general, this therapy has been relegated to small series of patients who do not respond to medical and surgical treatments (140). Assessment of the results is difficult, since these are clearly biased series including only patients with the most aggressive tumors. As sole treatment, it is rarely effective. A response is often not seen for months to years (170). The complications of radiation include optic nerve and chiasmatic injury, brain necrosis, hypopituitarism, and sarcoma formation. Proton radiosurgery using open or stereotactic techniques has also been used, particularly for older, surgically unfit patients; morbidity has been lower and cure rates better than those with low-dose radiation (140).

PITUITARY ADENOMAS CAUSING THYROTROPIN EXCESS

Clinical Features. The most common cause of hyperthyroidism is Graves' disease, diffuse thyroid hyperplasia caused by the autoimmune production of thyroid-stimulating immunoglobulins. Rarely, hyperthyroid patients have elevated levels of TSH due to a pituitary thyrotroph adenoma; these neoplasms represent less than 1 percent of pituitary tumors (192). The differential diagnosis includes patients who have pituitary resistance to thyroid hormone without an overt pituitary tumor (189), as well as the rare patient with ectopic TSH production. Clearly the management of these entities differs significantly and detailed biochemical and radiologic investigation is indicated to establish the cause of the TSH excess. In the investigation of patients with hyperthyroidism, primary thyroid disease causing hyperthyroidism should result in undetectable TSH levels; any elevation of TSH into the measurable range is inappropriate.

Pituitary-dependent TSH excess may also be associated with hypothyroidism (192,195). These patients most frequently have longstanding primary hypothyroidism which induces hypersecretion of TSH, secondary hyperplasia of pituitary thyrotrophs and even thyrotroph adenoma (199). In some patients, the TSH excess is associated with galactorrhea and hyperprolactinemia due to lactotroph hyperplasia; in these instances, the disorder may mimic a lactotroph adenoma (193). The sella turcica is usually enlarged and there may be signs of compression of the optic chiasm.

Patients with thyrotroph adenoma may present with symptoms of a mass lesion which appears to be nonfunctioning (200). Most patients have diffuse goiters although some have normal-sized glands (200,201). They generally do not have proptosis which is usually associated with Graves' disease.

Biochemical Findings. The TSH level is usually elevated and not suppressible in patients with this neoplasm, however, some patients have no evidence of TSH hypersecretion. Elevation of the α-subunit is frequently found in patients with TSH-secreting tumors. It has been suggested that calculation of the molar ratio of α-subunit to TSH may distinguish tumorous from nontumorous conditions with inappropriate TSH secretion (194).

The regulation of thyrotroph function is also useful for establishing TSH excess due to adenoma. TSH should be stimulated by dopamine antagonists and suppressed by administration of thyroid hormone, dopamine agonists, α-adrenergic antagonists, somatostatin, and glucocorticoids. Inappropriate responses to these substances may help in the differential diagnosis.

Adenomas causing hyperthyroidism may be plurihormonal and associated with acromegaly or hyperprolactinemia; in larger tumors the hyperprolactinemia may be attributed to stalk section effect.

Radiologic Findings. An important diagnostic study required in the evaluation of TSH excess is roentgenographic examination to establish a pituitary tumor. Most patients have macroadenomas that are evident on skull X rays. Microadenomas may require more sophisticated radiologic procedures such as CT or MRI. However, these tumors are usually large and invasive neoplasms that infiltrate parasellar structures.

Gross Findings. The tumors are usually large and invasive at the time of diagnosis. Reported cases are few and the gross appearance of these lesions is not noted to be characteristic. Microadenomas show no particular predilection for anatomic sites in the adenohypophysis. Occasionally the tumors are densely fibrotic.

Microscopic Findings. Thyrotroph adenomas are generally chromophobic and exhibit a solid or sinusoidal pattern (figs. 3-68, 3-69). They often have stromal fibrosis and occasionally form psammoma bodies (fig. 3-70). The tumor cells have chromophobic cytoplasm with indistinct cell borders and pleomorphic nuclei. In patients with primary hypothyroidism it is important to exclude the possibility of hyperplasia; reticulin staining provides a clear answer in this differential diagnosis (fig. 3-71).

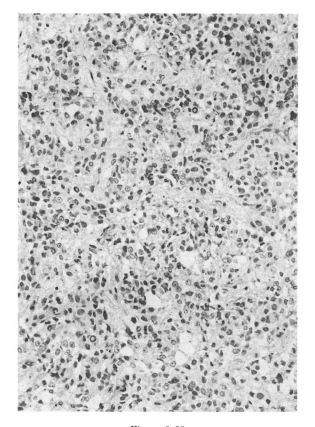

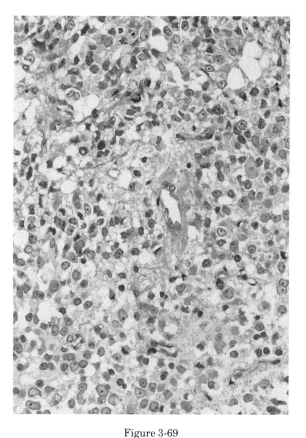

Figure 3-68
HISTOLOGY OF THYROTROPH ADENOMA
This thyrotroph adenoma has a solid architectural pattern with relatively abundant stromal fibrosis, a feature that is not uncommon in these tumors.

Figure 3-69
HISTOLOGY OF THYROTROPH ADENOMA
The tumor cells of a thyrotroph adenoma have indistinct cell borders and pale eosinophilic cytoplasm in which basophilic granules are rarely identified. The nuclei are quite pleomorphic and mitotic figures are often seen.

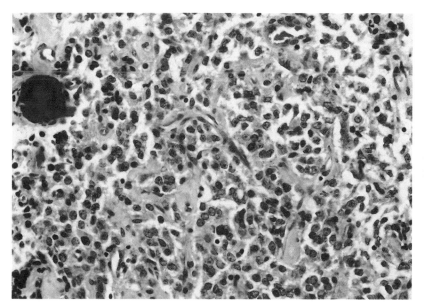

Figure 3-70
HISTOLOGY OF
THYROTROPH ADENOMA
Thyrotroph adenomas exhibit stromal fibrosis and occasionally harbor calcifications which may take the form of psammoma bodies.

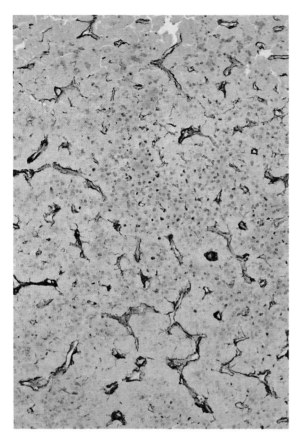

Figure 3-71
RETICULIN STAINING OF THYROTROPH ADENOMA
It is important to exclude thyrotroph hyperplasia in patients with hypothyroidism and TSH excess. The acinar reticulin pattern is totally disrupted in an adenoma whereas it is retained in hyperplasia.

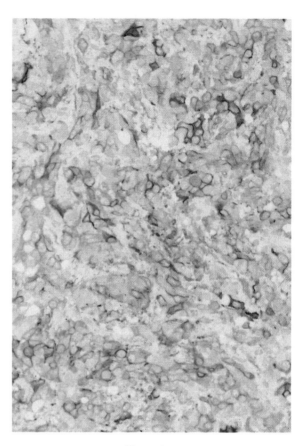

Figure 3-72
IMMUNOHISTOCHEMICAL LOCALIZATION OF α-SUBUNIT IN THYROTROPH ADENOMA
The cells of a thyrotroph adenoma are immunoreactive for α-subunit. The staining pattern is variable from cell to cell but clearly highlights the polygonal nature of these cells and decorates elongated cell processes.

Conventional histology and even immunohistochemistry can be disappointing in characterizing these lesions. In the past, tumors have been reported to lack positivity for TSH; the reason for this is not understood but may be attributed to artefact, since tissue fixation is known to alter the antigenicity of glycoprotein hormones (192). Improvements in tissue processing and the availability of highly specific and more sensitive antibodies have improved diagnosis. When properly handled, these lesions are usually positive for α-subunit (fig. 3-72) and β-TSH (fig. 3-73). The immunoreactivity usually varies from cell to cell; the staining pattern allows recognition of the angular morphology of the tumor cells.

Despite some variability in the ultrastructural appearance of thyrotrophs, electron microscopy can be rewarding for the diagnosis of these tumors. Most thyrotroph adenomas are well differentiated, composed of elongated cells which resemble nontumorous thyrotrophs (figs. 3-74–3-76). The cells have distinct polarity with spherical or oval euchromatic nuclei at one end. They contain abundant rough endoplasmic reticulum which may take the form of slightly dilated cisternae and may contain flocculent electron lucent contents. The Golgi apparatus is generally spherical and prominent. Secretory granules are variable in number but have a distinctive distribution, accumulating at the plasmalemma and in cytoplasmic processes. They are usually small and spherical, ranging from 150 to 250 nm in diameter; they exhibit variable electron density. Occasionally, densely granulated tumors contain

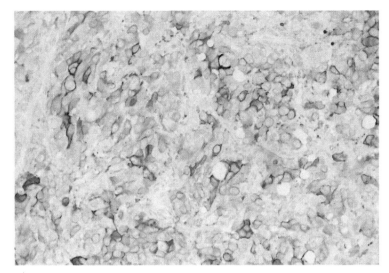

Figure 3-73
IMMUNOHISTOCHEMICAL
LOCALIZATION OF β-TSH
IN THYROTROPH ADENOMA

The cells of a thyrotroph adenoma are immunoreactive for β-TSH. The variable staining intensity allows clear delineation of the polygonal cell morphology and recognition of cell processes that store hormone.

Figure 3-74
ULTRASTRUCTURE OF
THYROTROPH ADENOMA

A thyrotroph adenoma is composed of cells that have angular morphology and elongated cell processes. The rough endoplasmic reticulum is well developed and Golgi complexes are found in a juxtanuclear location. Secretory granules are very small and tend to accumulate along the plasmalemma; some have peripheral electron lucent halos and the cores have highly variable electron density.

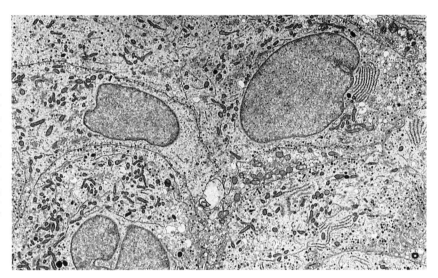

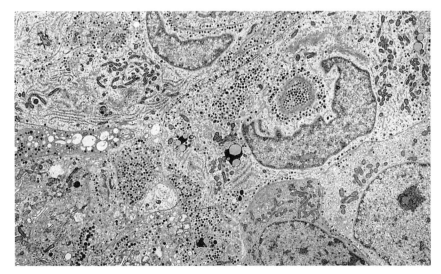

Figure 3-75
ULTRASTRUCTURE OF
THYROTROPH ADENOMA

Some cells in a thyrotroph adenoma have more abundant secretory granules and harbor prominent lysosomes which can produce PAS positivity focally in these tumors.

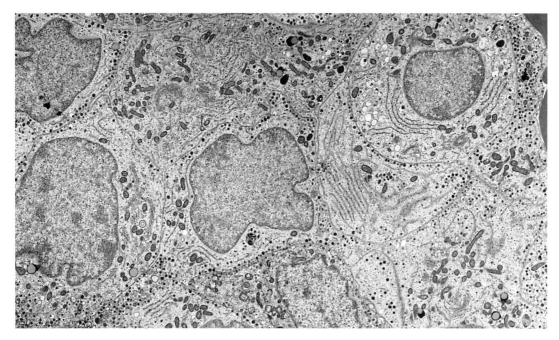

Figure 3-76
ULTRASTRUCTURE OF THYROTROPH ADENOMA
A less well-differentiated thyrotroph adenoma is composed of round to oval cells that do not exhibit the striking angularity of normal thyrotrophs and do not have prominent cell processes. Nevertheless, the subcellular organelles resemble those in a differentiated thyrotroph. Rough endoplasmic reticulum is well developed, Golgi complexes are conspicuous, and secretory granules are numerous, small, and displayed preferentially at the cell border. This tumor can resemble a null cell adenoma but the immunoreactivity for ß-TSH confirms the diagnosis.

larger secretory granules that may measure up to 350 nm in diameter. However, some tumors associated with TSH production are composed of less well-differentiated cells which resemble those of null cell adenomas.

In cases difficult to diagnose by morphology, tissue culture studies have documented release of TSH by adenoma cells in vitro (185,188,197,203,204).

Thyrotroph adenomas usually are associated with TSH excess, however, they can be associated with hyperthyroidism, hypothyroidism, or euthyroidism; usually, preexisting primary hypothyroidism masks clinical symptoms of TSH excess whereas a previously normal thyroid status allows the patient to develop hyperthyroidism. The various clinical presentations and settings cannot be distinguished morphologically, unless there is evidence of underlying thyrotroph hyperplasia indicative of primary hypothyroidism; the nontumorous thyrotrophs may have features of "thyroidectomy" or "thyroid deficiency" cells, with extreme cytoplasmic vacuolation due to dilation of rough endoplasmic reticulum cisternae (see chapter 1).

The cells may be almost totally devoid of secretory granules and, therefore, immunoreactivity. Thyrotroph hyperplasia may also be associated with lactotroph hyperplasia.

Differential Diagnosis. There are three substances that stimulate thyroid hormone synthesis and secretion: pituitary TSH, placental chorionic thyrotropin, and the thyroid-stimulating immunoglobulins that cause Graves' disease. Ectopic TSH secretion is exceedingly unusual. Rare cases of choriocarcinoma have been associated with hyperthyroidism and an ectopic TSH-like syndrome, presumably due to overproduction of a chorionic thyrotropin-like hormone (190).

Prognosis and Therapy. Several therapeutic approaches have been used to manage patients with thyrotroph adenoma. Surgery has had moderate success (201); the invasive behavior commonly found in these lesions often precludes a surgical cure (191). Only a few patients who have had radiation therapy as the initial treatment have been cured. Combined surgery and radiation has also been advocated.

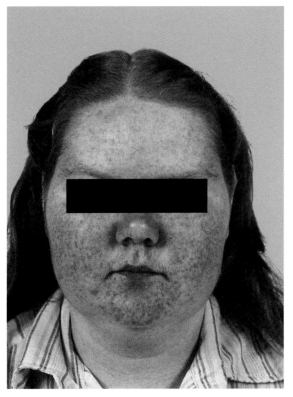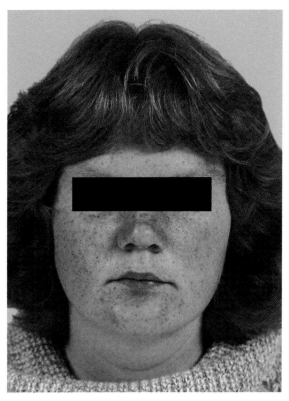

Figure 3-77
CLINICAL FEATURES OF CUSHING'S DISEASE
Left: This young woman presented with obesity, hirsutism, and acne. She had a plethoric, moon-shaped face and manifested other features of cortisol excess as detailed in the text. She was found to have a pituitary microadenoma which was resected.
Right: Postoperatively, the return to normal is striking. (Courtesy of Dr. H.S. Smyth, Toronto, Canada.)

Recently, medical therapy has been suggested for patients with this disorder. Bromocriptine was used by some investigators (202), however, the abnormal response to bromocriptine documented in vitro in some cases suggests that this therapy may be ineffective (186). The poor prognosis of these aggressive and invasive tumors led some authors to advocate octreotide therapy (187); reduction of TSH or α-subunit levels in most patients suggests the possibility of control of hypersecretion, but to date, only a single patient has had tumor shrinkage as a result of this treatment (196,198).

PITUITARY ADENOMAS
CAUSING ACTH EXCESS

Clinical Features. The syndrome recognized and described by Harvey Cushing is characterized by a number of clinical features that are attributable to prolonged overproduction of cortisol and other adrenocorticoids: centripetal obesity, plethoric moon-shaped facies, hirsutism, acne (fig. 3-77), hypertension, muscle weakness, bruisability, mental disorders, menstrual irregularities, and osteoporosis. The glucocorticoid excess leading to these manifestations can result from diverse secretory lesions of the adrenal cortex (adrenal Cushing's syndrome), or to ACTH-induced adrenocortical hyperplasia caused by ACTH-producing extrapituitary neoplasms (ectopic ACTH syndrome), excess corticotropin-releasing hormone (CRH) production by tumors, or pituitary-dependant ACTH excess. Overproduction of proopiomelanocortin (POMC) may also be associated with excess secretion of melatonin-stimulating hormone (MSH), resulting in hyperpigmentation in patients with ectopic ACTH production or with severe pituitary-dependent ACTH excess.

Pituitary-dependent hypercortisolism, known as Cushing's disease, is responsible for approximately

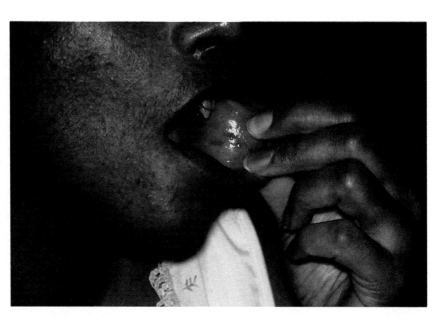

Figure 3-78
CLINICAL FEATURES OF
NELSON'S SYNDROME
This Caucasian patient had cortisol excess and no pituitary lesion was identified. She underwent bilateral adrenalectomy. Subsequently she developed a large, rapidly growing, ACTH-producing pituitary tumor. The excess MSH production by this lesion resulted in severe hyperpigmentation which even involved buccal mucosa. (Courtesy of Dr. H.P. Higgins, Toronto, Canada.)

two thirds of cases of Cushing's syndrome. Cushing recognized the pituitary basis for this disorder as published in his 1932 monograph entitled "Pituitary Basophilism" (211). He described the pituitary tumor or hyperplasia, adrenal tumor or hyperplasia, as "so many and varied as to baffle analysis." Today, despite the discovery of ACTH and cortisol, both unknown to Cushing, the diversity of Cushing's syndrome remains a diagnostic challenge and the pathogenesis of Cushing's disease remains enigmatic.

Prior to the development of sophisticated imaging techniques, patients with cortisol excess and no pituitary lesion detectable on routine X ray were treated with bilateral adrenalectomy; some subsequently manifested ACTH-producing pituitary tumors (234). This phenomenon is known as Nelson's syndrome: the patients have rapidly growing tumors that are unassociated with the classic features of cortisol excess because they lack adrenal tissue and are generally strikingly hyperpigmented (fig. 3-78). The iatrogenic basis of Nelson's syndrome emphasizes the need for careful imaging with nuclear MRI in patients with the clinical features of Cushing's disease. Inferior petrosal sinus sampling to measure basal and CRH-stimulated ACTH levels increases the accuracy of the diagnosis (239).

Untreated Cushing's disease results in severe complications that can be fatal. The need for rapid therapy cannot be overemphasized. If sur-

gery is contraindicated, several less successful medical therapies can be attempted.

Biochemical Findings. The diagnosis of Cushing' disease can be difficult and frequently requires multiple biochemical investigations (241). Cortisol excess is documented by measurement of elevated urinary free cortisol levels, loss of the diurnal variation of plasma cortisol, and lack of normal suppression of cortisol or its metabolites by dexamethasone administration. In patients with adrenal tumors or ectopic ACTH-producing tumors, administration of this potent synthetic glucocorticoid usually does not suppress adrenal function whereas in patients with pituitary-dependent disease, overnight administration of 8 mg of dexamethasone usually suppresses the pituitary and results in reduced cortisol secretion (205,236). Metyrapone, which inhibits 11-β hydroxylation in cortisol biosynthesis, causes a rapid fall in circulating cortisol and a compensatory elevation of ACTH levels in patients with pituitary-dependent ACTH excess, in contrast to patients with the ectopic ACTH syndrome whose suppressed pituitary glands are incapable of response (218).

In patients with Cushing's disease, the plasma ACTH level is usually elevated, but less so than in those with the ectopic ACTH syndrome. The ACTH level may, in fact, not be higher than the upper limit of normal, but even a high normal value is inappropriate in the face of cortisol excess. The ACTH response to stimulation by CRH, vasopressin, thyrotropin-releasing hormone (TRH) or insulin-induced hypoglycemia is abnormal in patients with Cushing's disease and Nelson's syndrome (229). TRH administration may cause a rise in ACTH derived from pituitary tumors but not in normal individuals. The increment in ACTH concentration in response to vasopressin administration is greater in patients with Cushing's disease or Nelson's syndrome than in normals, and in contrast, the increment in plasma cortisol or ACTH concentration following insulin-induced hypoglycemia is significantly less in patients with these diseases. The use of CRH has become one of the most useful diagnostic tools (237). Plasma ACTH responds significantly to stimulation by this hypophysiotropic hormone, despite basal hypercortisolism; this readily distinguishes patients with Cushing's disease from depressed patients who may also have basal hypercortisolism but have blunted responses to CRH stimulation (219,236,242).

Some patients with Cushing's disease have hyperprolactinemia in the absence of a macroadenoma that could cause a stalk section effect (252), and those with normal basal PRL levels may have blunted PRL responses to insulin-induced hypoglycemia, suggesting that either the tumor or hypercortisolism may interfere with the regulation of PRL at a suprahypophysial level (230). Several derivatives of POMC, such as β-endorphin, have been implicated as the stimulus for PRL release in these patients.

It should be remembered that hypercortisolism may have other causes including obesity and alcoholism as well as several drugs. Exogenous estrogens and pregnancy increase the hepatic synthesis of cortisol-binding globulin, resulting in an increased total plasma cortisol level, occasionally into the range seen in Cushing's syndrome. Diphenylhydantoin can interfere with dexamethasone, resulting in an apparent failure to suppress this steroid. The cortisol dynamics of patients with depression often mimic those of Cushing's syndrome and may require elaborate dynamic testing to clarify the diagnosis. Obesity also can result in a state of relative hypercortisolemia and the distinction from Cushing's syndrome can be confounding.

Radiologic Findings. The use of skull X rays in the diagnosis of Cushing's disease is unreli-

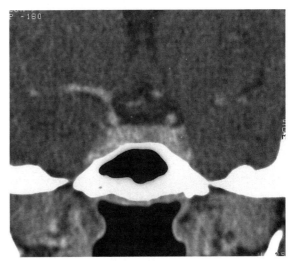

Figure 3-79
COMPUTED TOMOGRAPHY OF
THE PITUITARY IN CUSHING'S DISEASE
This CT scan with contrast enhancement shows an equivocal lesion in the left pituitary which is slightly hypodense. This turned out to be a microadenoma composed of corticotrophs.

able since only a minority of patients have evidence of sellar enlargement (205). This has led to the erroneous diagnosis of primary adrenal disease in some patients with pituitary-dependent Cushing's disease and the development of Nelson's syndrome following bilateral adrenalectomy.

The addition of CT scanning improved the radiologic detection of pituitary microadenomas in patients with Cushing's disease (205). Nevertheless, less than 60 percent have sellar abnormalities using this technique (fig. 3-79) (233). MRI has also improved diagnostic sensitivity (figs. 3-80, 3-81).

The localization of pituitary tumors in Cushing's disease can be difficult, yet is necessary for appropriate transsphenoidal microsurgical resection. The use of selective venous sampling from the inferior petrosal sinus has been reported to be a reliable and useful method for establishing the presence and laterality of ACTH-secreting microadenomas (205,215,238). Because of the possibility of episodic release of ACTH, inferior petrosal sinus sampling may lead to erroneous results; however, the addition of CRH stimulation in combination with inferior petrosal sinus sampling has been proposed as a useful adjunctive diagnostic tool (232).

Large tumors, including those associated with Nelson's syndrome and the more aggressive silent

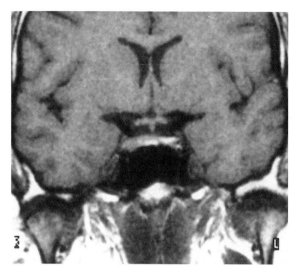

Figure 3-80
MAGNETIC RESONANCE IMAGING OF
THE PITUITARY IN CUSHING'S DISEASE

Even high resolution MRI scanning with gadolinium enhancement sometimes only reveals suspicious areas. The right side of the pituitary is slightly enlarged and the hypointense area is suspicious for a pituitary adenoma.

corticotroph adenomas, are usually demonstrable with CT scanning. Tumor size can be further estimated by other techniques such as polytomography, air encephalography, or angiography.

Gross Findings. The most common cause of pituitary-dependent Cushing's disease is a basophilic microadenoma (222,227). Corticotrophs are most numerous in the median wedge of the adenohypophysis, and some adenomas are found in this central location, however, they may also be present in a lateral wing and usually show lateralization of blood flow, as discussed above.

In contrast to Cushing's disease, patients with Nelson's syndrome usually have a large, invasive adenoma. Macroadenomas are also characteristic in patients with less severe ACTH excess who harbor chromophobic or sparsely granulated adenomas.

Microscopic Findings. *Densely Granulated Corticotroph Adenoma.* This is the usual tumor type in patients with ACTH excess. These basophilic adenomas have a sinusoidal architecture (fig. 3-82) and stain with periodic acid–Schiff

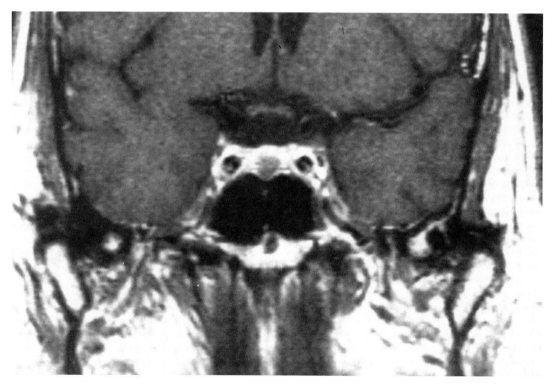

Figure 3-81
MAGNETIC RESONANCE IMAGING OF THE PITUITARY IN CUSHING'S DISEASE

This patient with Cushing's disease has an unequivocal midline hypointense lesion on T2-weighted imaging with gadolinium enhancement, corresponding to a corticotroph adenoma.

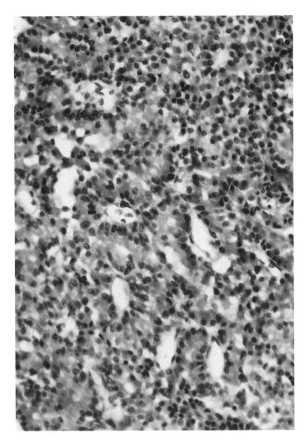

Figure 3-82
HISTOLOGY OF DENSELY GRANULATED
CORTICOTROPH ADENOMA
These tumors have sinusoidal architecture and are composed of relatively large cells with abundant cytoplasm that contains basophilic secretory granules.

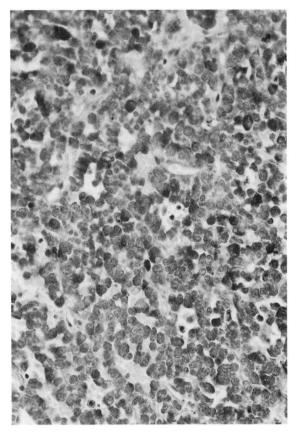

Figure 3-83
HISTOLOGY OF DENSELY GRANULATED
CORTICOTROPH ADENOMA: PAS STAIN
The PAS stain documents positivity in the vast majority of cells of this densely granulated corticotroph adenoma.

(PAS) (fig. 3-83). They have varying degrees of immunoreactivity for ACTH (fig. 3-84) and other derivatives of POMC, including β-endorphin. Positivity for low molecular weight cytokeratins is strong and diffuse in the cytoplasm of tumors that cause Cushing's syndrome (fig. 3-85) but not in tumors associated with Nelson's syndrome, reflecting the lack of cortisol feedback on the pituitary.

The typical corticotroph adenoma has a characteristic ultrastructure (fig. 3-86). It is composed of medium-sized corticotroph cells which are angular and contain ovoid or irregular nuclei; nucleoli are usually attached to the inner nuclear membrane. The cytoplasm contains well-developed rough endoplasmic reticulum and numerous free ribosomes. The Golgi complex is spherical and the majority of cells are densely granulated. The secretory granules vary from 150 to 450 nm in diameter and are distinguished from other secretory granules by the marked variability in electron density and shape; they may be tear-drop shaped, indented, or heart shaped. Another distinguishing feature of the corticotroph is the presence of bundles of intermediate filaments, located predominantly around the nucleus; these filaments correspond to immunoreactive low molecular weight cytokeratin proteins (235). They are helpful diagnostic markers, but are absent in patients with Nelson's syndrome (fig. 3-87).

Sparsely Granulated Corticotroph Adenoma. Occasionally, tumors producing ACTH excess are histologically chromophobic (fig. 3-88). They are likely to be macroadenomas associated with Cushing's disease and may, in fact, be associated with a less florid endocrine presentation, suggesting that they have lower hormonal activity. This

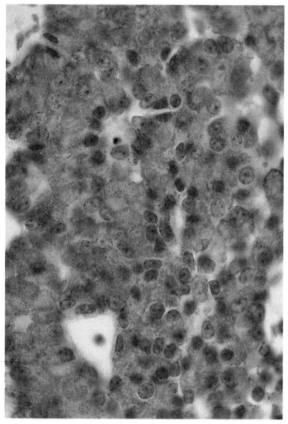

Figure 3-84
IMMUNOHISTOCHEMICAL LOCALIZATION
OF ACTH IN DENSELY GRANULATED
CORTICOTROPH ADENOMA

The tumor cells have abundant cytoplasmic positivity for ACTH. A similar picture is obtained with immunostaining for ß-endorphin and other derivatives of proopiomelanocortin.

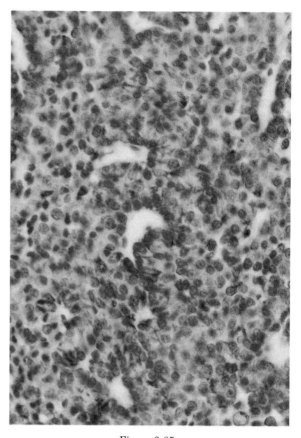

Figure 3-85
IMMUNOHISTOCHEMICAL LOCALIZATION
OF CYTOKERATINS IN DENSELY GRANULATED
CORTICOTROPH ADENOMA

This corticotroph adenoma from a patient with Cushing's disease has abundant immunoreactivity for cytokeratins in the perinuclear cytoplasm. Patients with Nelson's syndrome do not exhibit this feature.

Figure 3-86
ULTRASTRUCTURE OF
DENSELY GRANULATED
CORTICOTROPH ADENOMA

Most corticotroph adenomas are composed of cells resembling nontumorous corticotrophs. These cells have well-developed rough endoplasmic reticulum, prominent Golgi complexes, and numerous secretory granules that are extremely variable in size, shape, and electron density. In addition, tumor cells harbor numerous perinuclear intermediate filaments that form bundles; these correspond to cytokeratins. Lysosomes are complex and prominent in this tumor type. Some secretory granules are irregular in shape with indentations or tear-drop shapes (arrows).

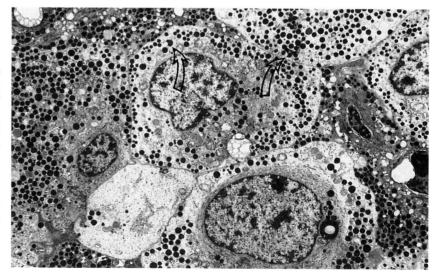

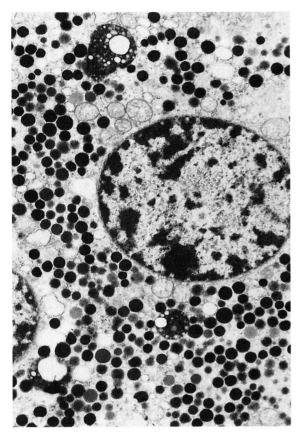

Figure 3-87
ULTRASTRUCTURE OF DENSELY
GRANULATED CORTICOTROPH ADENOMA
IN NELSON'S SYNDROME

The tumor cells in a corticotroph adenoma from a patient with Nelson's syndrome resemble the tumor cells of a densely granulated corticotroph adenoma from a patient with Cushing's syndrome (fig. 3-86) with the exception of a conspicuous absence of intermediate filaments that represent cytokeratins. Note the complex lysosomes and the marked variability in size, shape, and electron density of secretory granules.

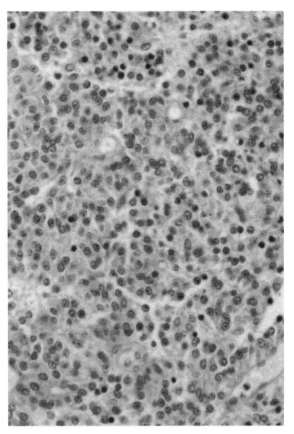

Figure 3-88
HISTOLOGY OF SPARSELY GRANULATED
CORTICOTROPH ADENOMA

These tumors usually have a diffuse architecture and are composed of cells with chromophobic cytoplasm.

rare variant of corticotroph adenoma usually has a diffuse architecture, is PAS negative or has only slight PAS positivity (fig. 3-89), and has only faint immunoreactivity for ACTH (fig. 3-90) but still contains strong keratin immunoreactivity (fig. 3-91).

The chromophobic tumors have an unusual ultrastructure (fig. 3-92): the cells generally have less well-developed membranous organelles and small, scanty secretory granules which measure 200 to 250 nm in diameter. Keratin filaments are fewer in these tumors than in the typical corticotroph adenoma.

Crooke's Cell Adenoma. Rarely, corticotroph tumors may undergo Crooke's hyalinization (222, 227). This morphologic alteration (see chapter 1) is characteristic of nontumorous corticotrophs which are subject to feedback suppression by elevated circulating levels of cortisol and is seen in the adenohypophyses of patients with primary adrenal hypercortisolism or the ectopic ACTH syndrome; in Cushing's disease, it is usually confined to the suppressed nontumorous corticotroph population. Some of the reported Crooke cell adenomas have been associated with clinically typical Cushing's disease, some with intermittent Cushing's syndrome, a few have been reported to be hormonally inactive, and some have had evidence of low hormonal activity (214,217,223). In one case, a Crooke cell adenoma was associated with corticotroph hyperplasia (214).

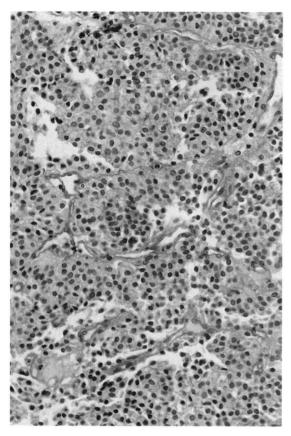

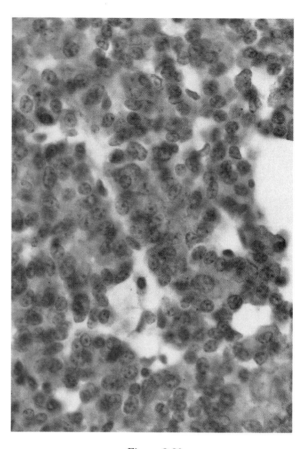

Figure 3-89
HISTOLOGY OF SPARSELY GRANULATED
CORTICOTROPH ADENOMA: PAS STAIN

Sparsely granulated corticotroph adenomas do not exhibit the conspicuous PAS positivity of the more common densely granulated variant; PAS positivity here is focal and hard to identify.

Figure 3-90
IMMUNOHISTOCHEMICAL LOCALIZATION OF
ACTH IN SPARSELY GRANULATED
CORTICOTROPH ADENOMA

The sparsely granulated variant of corticotroph adenoma has less striking immunoreactivity for ACTH in tumor cells, however, cytoplasmic granules are identified on careful examination.

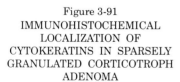

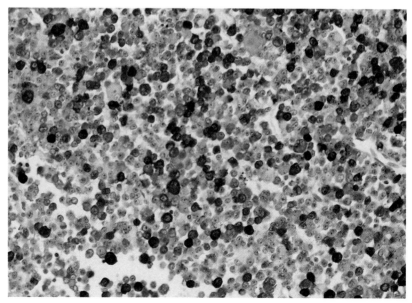

Figure 3-91
IMMUNOHISTOCHEMICAL
LOCALIZATION OF
CYTOKERATINS IN SPARSELY
GRANULATED CORTICOTROPH
ADENOMA

Cytoplasmic immunoreactivity for low molecular weight cytokeratins is identified in many tumor cells of a sparsely granulated corticotroph adenoma.

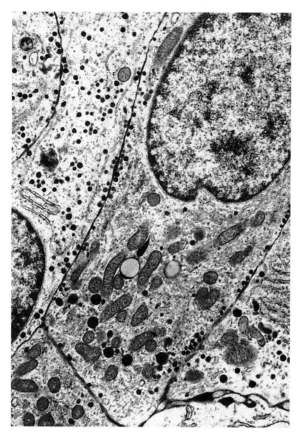

Figure 3-92
ULTRASTRUCTURE OF SPARSELY
GRANULATED CORTICOTROPH ADENOMA

These tumors have unusual ultrastructural features and do not resemble nontumorous corticotrophs. The cells have well-developed rough endoplasmic reticulum and well-formed Golgi complexes, however, the secretory granules are sparser than in normal corticotrophs or in densely granulated corticotroph adenomas. Secretory granules are small but exhibit the marked variability in shape and electron density that is characteristic of corticotrophs. Intermediate filaments are not as conspicuous as in the densely granulated variant and do not accumulate into perinuclear bundles.

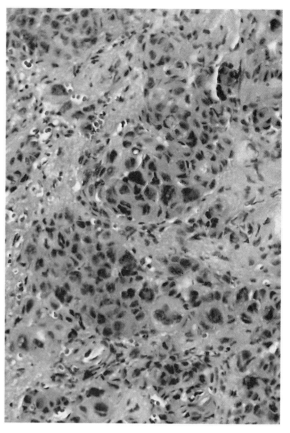

Figure 3-93
HISTOLOGY OF A CROOKE CELL ADENOMA

These tumors are composed of highly atypical, pleomorphic cells with enlarged hyperchromatic nuclei. Because of their highly unusual morphology, the tumor cells can be mistaken for metastatic carcinoma or other rare tumors, such as gangliocytomas, but the pale hyaline material encircling the nucleus indicates the accumulation of keratin filaments.

The tumors are composed of highly atypical cells (fig. 3-93) that can be mistaken for metastatic carcinoma or other unusual neoplasms in the sellar region, such as gangliocytomas. The large tumor cells have cytoplasmic basophilia and PAS positivity limited to the cell periphery while the majority of the cytoplasm is homogeneous, chromophobic, or slightly acidophilic (fig. 3-94). The diagnosis is confirmed by the immunohistochemical detection of weak ACTH reactivity at the cell periphery (fig. 3-95) and abundant low molecular weight cytokeratins throughout the cell cytoplasm (fig. 3-96). Ultrastructural examination confirms that most of the cytoplasm is filled with intermediate filaments; the secretory granules are predominantly pushed to the cell periphery or may be found immediately adjacent to the nucleus (figs. 3-97, 3-98).

Morphologic Effects of Drugs and Hormones. The cells of corticotroph adenomas are known to respond to stimulation and inhibition by several substances: incubation in vitro with cortisol or dexamethasone, cyproheptadine, or reserpine inhibits release of ACTH (224,240,246); CRH, vasopressin, vasoactive intestinal peptide (VIP), and TRH stimulate the release of POMC-derived peptides (224,225,231,240,245,249–251). Hormone synthesis is likewise inhibited by corticosteroids

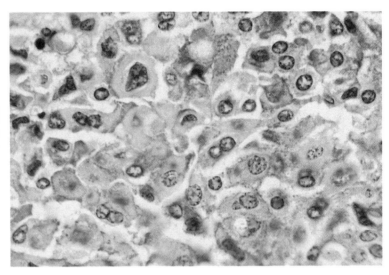

Figure 3-94
HISTOLOGY OF A
CROOKE CELL ADENOMA
Basophilic granules are identified only at the periphery of the cell in a Crooke cell adenoma. The remainder of the cytoplasm is filled with pale acidophilic hyaline material.

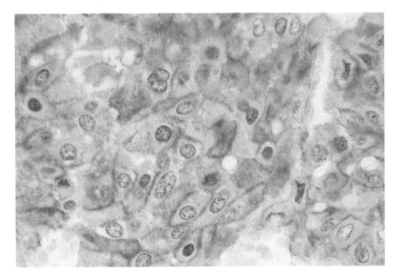

Figure 3-95
IMMUNOHISTOCHEMICAL
LOCALIZATION OF ACTH IN
A CROOKE CELL ADENOMA
These tumor cells stain for ACTH only at the cell periphery, corresponding to the basophilic granularity.

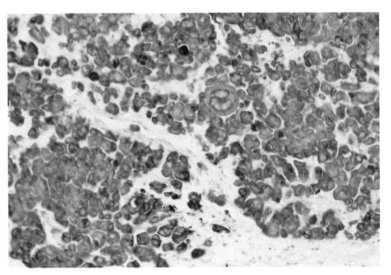

Figure 3-96
IMMUNOHISTOCHEMICAL
LOCALIZATION OF CYTOKERATINS
IN A CROOKE CELL ADENOMA
The bulk of the tumor cell cytoplasm is filled with cytokeratin filaments that correspond to the hyaline area identified on routine histology. Nuclear atypia is striking in this tumor.

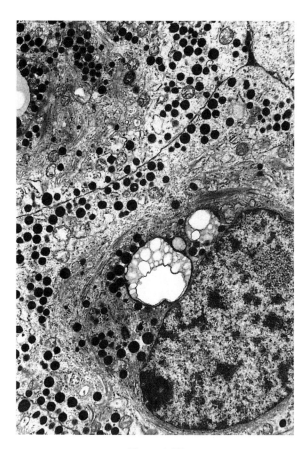

Figure 3-97
ULTRASTRUCTURE OF A CROOKE CELL ADENOMA
Tumor cells in a Crooke cell adenoma have an abundance of perinuclear cytoplasmic intermediate filaments that correspond to keratin. The juxtanuclear complex lysosome is similar to the "enigmatic body" of nontumorous corticotrophs. Secretory granules are either trapped adjacent to the nucleus by the intermediate filaments or are pushed to the cell periphery.

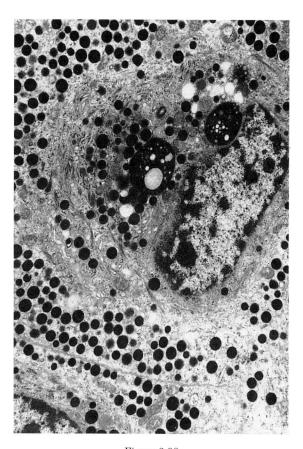

Figure 3-98
ULTRASTRUCTURE OF A CROOKE CELL ADENOMA
A tumor cell in a Crooke cell adenoma harbors abundant perinuclear intermediate filaments which trap lysosomes and secretory granules.

and stimulated by CRH (247). The response to prolonged stimulation is persistent, indicating that there is no down-regulation of the receptors involved (220). The morphologic changes that ensue have been studied in vitro and indicate that there is an increase in synthetic organelles and a reduction in the cytoplasmic volume density of secretory granules during incubation with CRH (224). Accumulation of filaments in adenomatous corticotrophs is the direct effect of cortisol and is associated with reduced ACTH release (224).

Differential Diagnosis. One of the most difficult clinical differential diagnoses involves the determination of the cause of cortisol excess. Even the documentation of ACTH excess does not imply the presence of a causative pituitary adenoma.

The common occurrence of "ectopic ACTH secretion" by endocrine tumors in many sites throughout the body, most commonly lung and usually a small cell carcinoma, has led to the development of a protocol of careful clinical and biochemical investigation (237,241). In patients with no other obvious source of ACTH hypersecretion, inferior petrosal sinus sampling is recommended to confirm and lateralize the pituitary pathology (239).

Ectopic secretion of CRH is rare but clinically significant, since it gives rise to a clinical and biochemical syndrome resembling Cushing's disease (206,210,216,226,244,253). CRH has been reported in endocrine tumors of lung, thyroid, gut and pancreas, and in prostate, and in pheochromocytomas (207,208). A rare case of hypothalamic gangliocytoma containing CRH has also been reported (206). CRH production causes pituitary corticotroph hyperplasia rather than adenoma, but this may be difficult to distinguish from a primary pituitary disorder, since some patients with primary pituitary Cushing's disease have corticotroph hyperplasia with or without adenoma, and pituitary adenomas associated with Cushing's disease may be extremely small and undetectable by radiologic imaging, even MRI. Usually, it is only after surgery, with documentation of corticotroph hyperplasia without adenoma and with persistent disease, that there is an indication to examine the patient for a possible source of CRH overproduction.

Prognosis and Therapy. Left untreated, Cushing's disease can lead to increasing weakness, hypertension, hypokalemia, fasting hyperglycemia, osteopenia, and severe mental disorders which may require psychiatric therapy. The reduced ability to fight infection can also have grave consequences. The major objective of therapy, then, is to reduce ACTH levels to within the normal range and to restore cortisol secretion to normal. As with other tumors, the therapeutic options include radiation, surgery, and selected drugs. Surgery to remove the adrenals may lead to the development of Nelson's syndrome and is no longer used routinely.

Despite the difficulty in localizing pituitary tumors for transsphenoidal adenomectomy, the application of CT scanning, MRI, and inferior petrosal sinus sampling to lateralize the tumor has improved the results of the surgical approach. Selective resection is possible in the majority of patients with small, noninvasive tumors and corrects hypercortisolism with little morbidity in a significant proportion (205,233,241). Nevertheless, those with nodular hyperplasia require complete hypophysectomy for cure, resulting in subsequent hypopituitarism. In patients with larger tumors, the results of surgery are less successful; only a minority of patients with invasive tumors can be cured with surgery alone (209,221).

For surgical failures, radiation therapy, either by external irradiation with either conventional X-ray high voltage photons or heavy particles (212,213,241,248), or by pituitary implantation of radioactive yttrium (^{90}Y) is used (243). Recently, application of the photon knife or gamma knife suggests the possibility of more effective and localized radiation with fewer side effects, but experience is still limited (241).

Some studies have suggested that ACTH secretion can be inhibited by cyproheptadine or reserpine. Cyproheptadine, a serotonin antagonist, has been reported to suppress ACTH release by pituitary tumors in up to 50 percent of patients with Cushing's disease (228), however, this therapy has not gained widespread support. Other neuropharmacologic agents, including reserpine or metergoline, another antiserotoninergic agent, have been used with mild success (228).

In the most severe cases, and while awaiting the effects of radiotherapy, management is directed at blocking cortisol synthesis. Patients can be treated with adrenalectomy, or medically with ketoconazole or aminoglutethimide (241), or rarely with metyrapone or low dose mitotane (o,p'DDD) (205). These drugs have severe side effects and are used as a last resort.

PITUITARY ADENOMAS CAUSING GONADOTROPIN EXCESS

Clinical Features. Gonadotroph adenomas can present with signs or symptoms of gonadal dysfunction but clinical evidence of gonadotropin excess is rare and more often they are detected due to mass effects. Patients generally have large tumors which cause headache and visual field defects or other cranial nerve deficits (275,276). Male patients with suspected clinically nonfunctioning adenomas usually have elevated gonadotropin levels, and the diagnosis of gonadotroph adenoma is suspected on the basis of the biochemical findings. Clinically diagnosed gonadotroph tumors occur mainly in middle-aged men who have a history of normal gonadal function (275). This may reflect the fact that they are more difficult to diagnose in women; perimenopausal or postmenopausal women have physiologically elevated levels of gonadotropins, making the distinction between a gonadotroph adenoma and a nonsecreting adenoma difficult clinically, however, elevated levels of one gonadotropin alone or associated with hypopituitarism may suggest the diagnosis of a gonadotropin-producing adenoma. In premenopausal females, these tumors are rare. Although the tumors generally present in older patients, they have been occasionally reported in younger people; in this situation, they have been frequently associated with underlying hypogonadism (266).

Paradoxically, gonadotroph adenomas are usually associated with gonadal hypofunction; rarely is there evidence of gonadal stimulation (259). Patients who have gonadotroph adenoma unassociated with primary hypogonadism generally have a history of normal pubertal development and sexual function. They generally exhibit normal secondary sexual characteristics and most have a history of normal fertility (275, 276). In contrast, patients with longstanding primary hypogonadism may have a history of normal pubertal development with subsequent gonadal failure or may have a history of primary amenorrhea or eunuchoidism (275). In young women, it has been reported that gonadotropin-secreting tumors can masquerade as primary ovarian failure; persistent supranormal serum gonadotropins may inhibit ovarian function and this is reversible after resection of the tumor (257).

Biochemical Findings. The diagnosis of gonadotroph adenoma requires documentation of elevated serum levels of follicle-stimulating hormone (FSH), luteinizing hormone (LH), or both. In the majority of cases reported, FSH levels alone are elevated; in some cases both hormones are abnormally high. In postmenopausal women, however, elevation of these hormones is physiologic; only if FSH is elevated and LH is suppressed can one establish the existence of tumor hypersecretion and adenohypophysial damage with insufficiency of LH. Only rarely has a tumor produced LH only (263). In some patients, free α- and β-subunits circulate in large quantities; secretion of uncombined subunits by these adenomas has been confirmed in vitro (277). Patients with gonadotroph adenomas generally have subnormal levels of gonadal steroids and a diagnosis of secondary hypogonadism may be entertained in the absence of elevated gonadotropin levels.

In the diagnostic assessment of patients with pituitary gonadotroph adenoma, abnormal hormone responses to stimuli may prove useful. Gonadotropin release by these tumors responds to stimulation by gonadotropin-releasing hormone (GnRH) and also, paradoxically, to TRH. Both FSH and LH are thought to respond to TRH stimulation, however, the FSH response is primarily that of the intact molecule whereas LH usually responds with increased release of a single subunit, usually β-LH (275). This para-

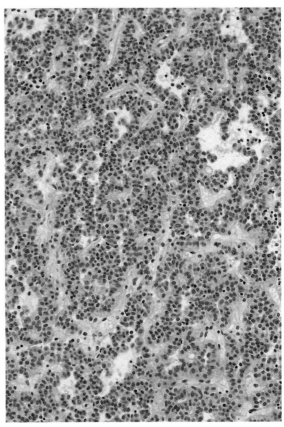

Figure 3-99
HISTOLOGY OF GONADOTROPH ADENOMA
The tumors are characterized by a prominent sinusoidal, trabecular, and papillary architecture. The tumor cells form pseudorosettes around vascular channels.

doxical response has been shown in vitro to be a direct effect of TRH (255,267,270).

Radiologic Findings. These tumors usually present as large macroadenomas with significant suprasellar or parasellar extension. The initial diagnostic evaluation includes CT scanning or MRI to evaluate the degree of invasion.

Gross Findings. The invasive lesions are usually large and well-vascularized soft tumors that may exhibit areas of hemorrhage or necrosis.

Microscopic Findings. Gonadotroph adenomas are usually composed of chromophobic cells with a prominent sinusoidal, trabecular, or papillary architecture and prominent pseudorosette formations around blood vessels (figs. 3-99, 3-100). Oncocytic change is found in this tumor type, usually focally (fig. 3-101). Some tumor cells contain a few PAS-positive cytoplasmic granules

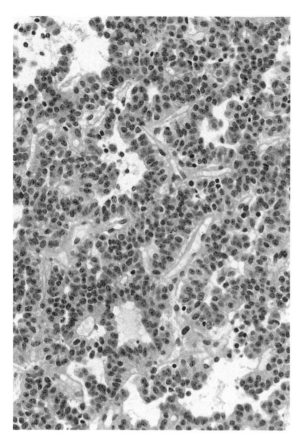

Figure 3-100
HISTOLOGY OF GONADOTROPH ADENOMA
The tumor cells of a gonadotroph adenoma are characteristically elongated; the nucleus tends to be localized preferentially at one pole of the cell and the opposite pole consists of elongated cytoplasm which is usually chromophobic.

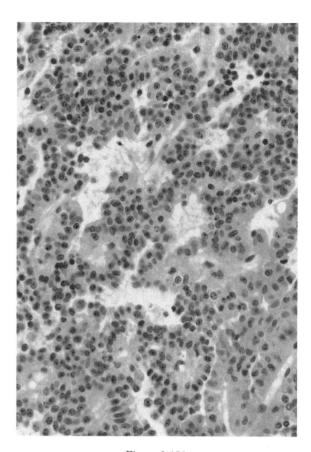

Figure 3-101
HISTOLOGY OF GONADOTROPH ADENOMA
Gonadotroph adenomas frequently contain areas of oncocytic change in which the tumor cells become more round to polygonal, the cytoplasm is granular and eosinophilic, and there may be mild nuclear atypia.

(fig. 3-102). Immunohistochemistry usually localizes α-subunit (fig. 3-103), β-FSH (fig. 3-104), and β-LH (fig. 3-105) within tumor cells; the intensity is extremely variable. Usually, both LH and FSH subunits are found, despite the fact that FSH secretion predominates in vivo. These adenomas also exhibit nuclear staining for SF-1 (254), a steroidogenic transcription factor also found in adrenal cortex and gonadal steroidogenic cells (fig. 3-106).

Most gonadotroph adenomas are heterogeneous ultrastructurally. The tumor cells vary from distinctive polar cells which contain euchromatic nuclei and well-differentiated cytoplasm (figs. 3-107, 3-108) to poorly differentiated round or polygonal cells (fig. 3-109). The rough endoplasmic reticulum can be abundant but is usually found as scattered short profiles; it is usually dilated and contains electron lucent flocculent material. Golgi complexes are often large and globular, usually in a juxtanuclear location. Secretory granules are variable in number; they are small, measuring up to 250 nm in diameter, moderately electron dense, and preferentially localized at the opposite pole from the nucleus. Oncocytic change, often found focally in these lesions, is characterized by accumulation of mitochondria (fig. 3-110).

Gonadotroph adenomas have been reported to occur in patients with longstanding primary hypogonadism. In these patients, the adenoma may be associated with gonadotroph hyperplasia and the formation of "gonadectomy" or "gonadal-deficiency" cells, large gonadotrophs in the nontumorous gland with an abundant vacuolated

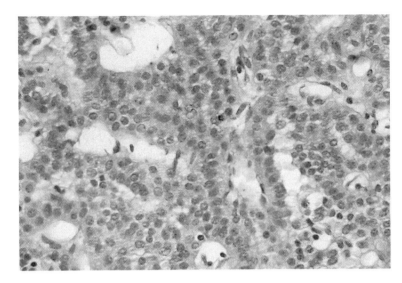

Figure 3-102
HISTOLOGY OF GONADOTROPH
ADENOMA: PAS STAIN
The PAS stain occasionally highlights
PAS-positive cytoplasmic droplets in scat-
tered tumor cells in gonadotropin-producing
adenomas.

Figure 3-103
IMMUNOHISTOCHEMICAL
LOCALIZATION OF α-SUBUNIT
IN GONADOTROPH ADENOMA
Most tumor cells contain some degree of
immunoreactivity for α-subunit but reactiv-
ity tends to be highly variable throughout
the tumor.

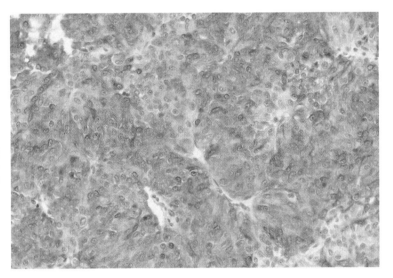

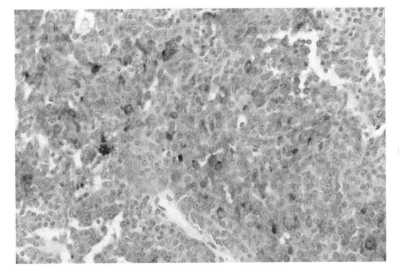

Figure 3-104
IMMUNOHISTOCHEMICAL
LOCALIZATION OF
β-FSH IN GONADOTROPH ADENOMA
β-FSH is found usually in a focal pattern
in the cytoplasm of many tumor cells.

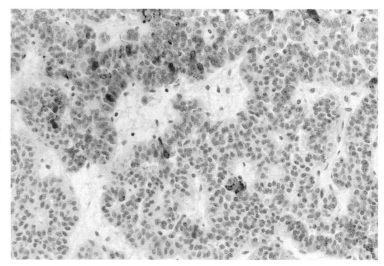

Figure 3-105
IMMUNOHISTOCHEMICAL
LOCALIZATION OF β-LH IN
GONADOTROPH ADENOMA
β-LH is also found in scattered tumor cells but the immunoreactivity for β-LH tends to be less than that for β-FSH.

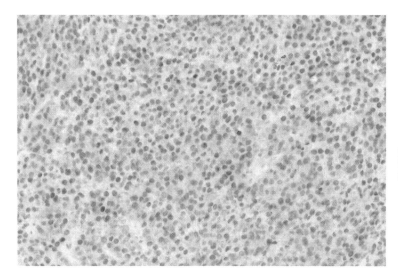

Figure 3-106
IMMUNOHISTOCHEMICAL
LOCALIZATION OF SF-1
IN GONADOTROPH ADENOMA
The nuclei of tumor cells in a gonadotropin-producing pituitary adenoma are usually intensely immunoreactive for steroidogenic factor-1 (SF-1).

Figure 3-107
ULTRASTRUCTURE OF
GONADOTROPH ADENOMA
These tumors are composed of elongated cells with striking polarity. This figure illustrates the cytoplasmic pole of tumor cells preferentially oriented around a vascular channel with accumulation of secretory granules.

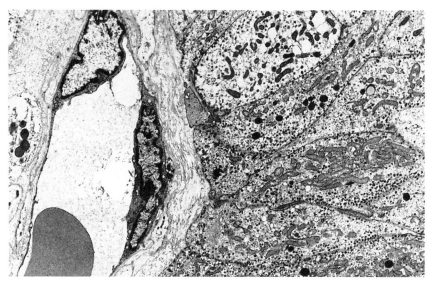

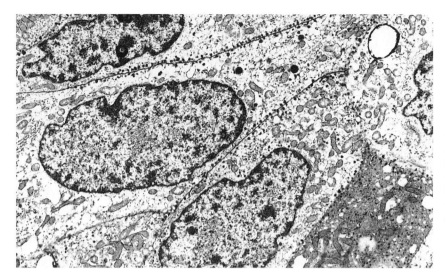

Figure 3-108
ULTRASTRUCTURE OF
GONADOTROPH ADENOMA
The characteristic gonadotroph adenoma is composed of elongated cells with the nucleus preferentially located at one pole. The tumor cells have short profiles of slightly dilated rough endoplasmic reticulum and occasional well-formed Golgi complexes. Secretory granules are few and small and generally accumulate at the cell border.

Figure 3-109
ULTRASTRUCTURE OF
GONADOTROPH ADENOMA
Some gonadotropin-producing adenomas are composed of less well-differentiated cells that are polygonal or round. They contain short profiles of dilated rough endoplasmic reticulum and some have well-formed Golgi complexes. Secretory granules are few and small.

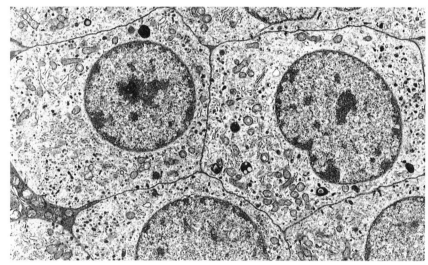

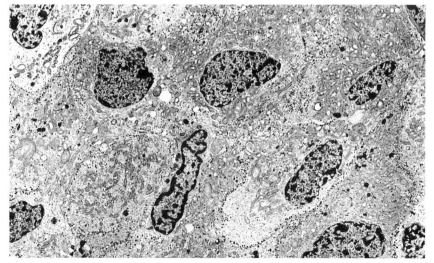

Figure 3-110
ULTRASTRUCTURE OF
GONADOTROPH ADENOMA:
ONCOCYTIC CHANGE
Gonadotroph adenomas often exhibit at least focal oncocytic change. The cytoplasm is filled with numerous dilated mitochondria that displace other cytoplasmic organelles; nevertheless, short profiles of dilated rough endoplasmic reticulum and Golgi complexes are recognized. The small secretory granules accumulate close to the plasmalemma.

cytoplasm that is almost totally filled with dilated endoplasmic reticulum containing flocculent material (see chapter 1).

Differential Diagnosis. The gonadotropins share homology with chorionic gonadotropin (hCG) produced by the placenta. Excess production of hCG is not uncommon in patients with choriocarcinoma and other germ cell tumors, but this is readily distinguished from pituitary gonadotropin secretion by immunoassays. Other situations of ectopic secretion of gonadotropins are not clinically significant.

Gonadotropin excess in children resulting in precocious puberty is almost never due to a pituitary adenoma. True or central precocious puberty, which is gonadotropin dependent, is usually due to germ cell tumors that can produce gonadotropin-like substances (see chapter 7), to hypothalamic hamartomas producing GnRH (see chapter 5), or to other central nervous system tumors or tumor-like lesions that interfere with physiologic suppression of the hypothalamic-pituitary gonadotropic axis in children.

Prognosis and Therapy. Surgery remains the first therapeutic approach to these tumors (262). Given the success of transsphenoidal surgery even for macroadenomas with suprasellar extension, transfrontal surgery is rarely indicated; it is associated with much higher morbidity and mortality and is therefore reserved only for patients with very large tumors in which the bulk of the tumor is suprasellar (260).

In patients with large tumor or with significant extrasellar extension, postoperative radiation is usually offered as an adjuvant to surgery (278).

It has been suggested that treatment with GnRH analogues may be useful, since GnRH is known to down-regulate its receptors when administered continuously. However, down-regulation of GnRH receptors is not seen in these tumors in vitro or in vivo (255,258,267,270,273,274) and therapy with GnRH analogues has been generally abandoned.

These adenomas are known to have dopamine receptors (265,271). Bromocriptine has been reported to reduce elevated serum gonadotropins (256,261,264,268,272,279) and to suppress gonadotropin and α-subunit release in vitro (267,268,270). There is only a single report of reduction in tumor size during bromocriptine treatment (281) and at the present time, there is no morphologic or clinical evidence that the drug is an effective modality for the treatment of these adenomas.

Octreotide may be useful in reducing elevated gonadotropin levels in some patients (269,280). Despite the fact that several patients have reported improvement in visual fields, it has not been conclusively shown to reduce tumor size as determined objectively by radiologic imaging.

CLINICALLY NONFUNCTIONING PITUITARY ADENOMAS

Clinical Features. Approximately 25 percent of pituitary adenomas lack a characteristic clinical syndrome or serum hormone marker. Most patients have macroadenomas with significant suprasellar extension and they present with symptoms of a mass: headache, neuro-ophthalmologic abnormalities such as superior or bitemporal visual field defects, other cranial nerve deficits, or even cavernous sinus syndrome. In some patients, the initial presentation may be due to pituitary apoplexy, hemorrhage within a macroadenoma, or hypopituitarism.

Biochemical Findings. Patients with clinically nonfunctioning adenoma do not usually have evidence of hormone hypersecretion. In most, serum hormone levels are normal or even reduced due to tissue destruction in the sella turcica. The degree of hypopituitarism is variable: GH insufficiency is common and gonadotropin insufficiency is considered to be the second most common endocrine abnormality (293). The reduction of gonadotropin levels has been attributed to tumor mass effect but may also be attributed to the mild hyperprolactinemia that is frequently caused by pituitary stalk compression in patients with large tumors (293). Postmenopausal women generally have elevated gonadotropin levels but in association with a nonfunctioning adenoma there is often evidence of gonadotroph insufficiency. Hypothyroidism or adrenocortical insufficiency are found less frequently but, with dynamic testing, impaired corticotroph or thyrotroph reserve is common (293). Even when serum GH, TSH, FSH, LH, or α-subunit levels are not reduced, they may fail to respond to stimulation with hypothalamic-releasing hormones, indicating a degree of hypopituitarism.

Some patients have evidence of α-subunit hypersecretion, alone or together with intact gonadotropins (294,295).

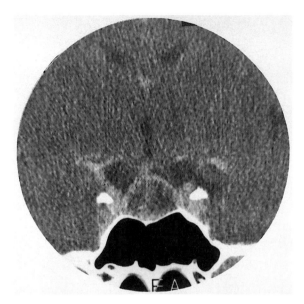

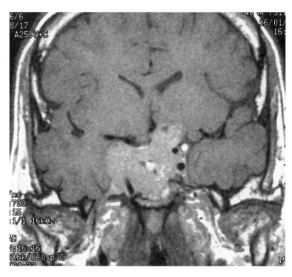

Figure 3-112
RADIOLOGIC FEATURES: CLINICALLY
NONFUNCTIONING ADENOMA

T2-weighted MRI scan with gadolinium of a large invasive grade IV pituitary adenoma that was entirely unassociated with evidence of hormone excess clinically and biochemically. The lesion compresses the 4th and lateral ventricles; there are areas of hypo- and hyperintensity that may reflect liquefaction of the tumor. (Courtesy of Dr. S. Ezzat, Toronto, Canada.)

Figure 3-111
RADIOLOGIC FEATURES OF CLINICALLY
NONFUNCTIONING ADENOMA

CT scan of the sella turcica with contrast enhancement in a patient with a clinically nonfunctioning pituitary adenoma reveals a hypodense grade III lesion with significant suprasellar extension. (Courtesy of Dr. S. Ezzat, Toronto, Canada.)

Radiologic Findings. Because of the lack of a characteristic clinical syndrome, these tumors usually present late, when they have already become large macroadenomas with significant suprasellar or extrasellar extension. The initial diagnostic evaluation must include CT scanning (fig. 3-111) or MRI (fig. 3-112). Digital subtraction angiograms may be useful to exclude the possibility of aneurysm.

Microscopic Findings. Despite the clinical homogeneity, these tumors present as a wide range of morphologic lesions. The diagnosis rests entirely on microscopic features at the light and electron microscopic level.

Silent Somatotroph Adenomas. A few somatotroph adenomas have been unassociated with acromegaly or gigantism. One patient had elevated blood levels of biologically inactive GH (296); others had no detectable alteration of circulating GH (301,308,316,319,325). The silent somatotroph tumors that have been subjected to careful morphologic analysis have been otherwise typical sparsely granulated somatotroph adenomas (figs. 3-113–3-115). Tissue culture has shed some light on the pathophysiology of these

lesions: while some initially release only small quantities of GH, after several days in vitro GH release increases, suggesting that GH secretion may have been suppressed in vivo (301).

Silent Lactotroph Adenomas. Patients with lactotroph adenoma may present with symptoms of a mass lesion that appears to be a nonfunctioning tumor (286,309). In some, there is biochemical evidence of PRL excess, suggesting that the tumors secrete an immunologically recognized hormone that is biologically inactive; in others, hormone secretion appears to be defective. The pattern of immunohistochemical staining and the ultrastructural appearance of silent lactotroph adenomas resemble those of functioning lactotroph adenomas (figs. 3-116–3-118).

Silent Thyrotroph Adenomas. Patients with thyrotroph adenoma may present with symptoms of a mass lesion that appears to be a nonfunctioning tumor (290). The pattern of immunohistochemical staining and the ultrastructural appearance (fig. 3-119) of silent thyrotroph adenomas resemble those of functioning thyrotroph adenomas as described above.

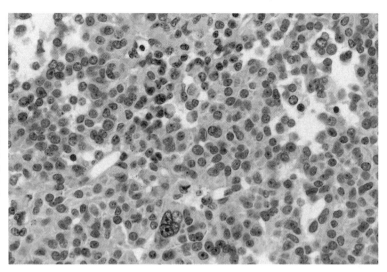

Figure 3-113
HISTOLOGY OF SILENT
SOMATOTROPH ADENOMA

A silent somatotroph adenoma resembles a sparsely granulated somatotroph adenoma but is unassociated with clinical evidence of growth hormone or IGF-1 excess. The tumor is composed of relatively pleomorphic cells with chromophobic cytoplasm and occasional juxtanuclear pale areas corresponding to fibrous bodies.

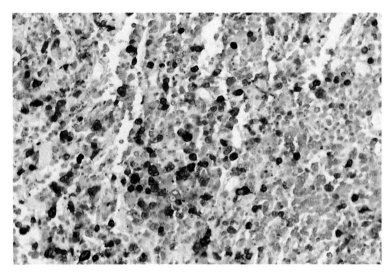

Figure 3-114
IMMUNOHISTOCHEMICAL
LOCALIZATION OF GROWTH
HORMONE IN SILENT
SOMATOTROPH ADENOMA

As in functioning sparsely granulated somatotroph adenomas, the silent variant of this tumor contains focal and variable immunoreactivity for growth hormone in the cytoplasm of tumor cells.

Figure 3-115
IMMUNOHISTOCHEMICAL
LOCALIZATION OF CYTOKERATINS
IN SILENT SOMATOTROPH ADENOMA

The silent somatotroph adenoma, like its functioning counterpart, is composed of cells with conspicuous fibrous bodies which are highlighted by immunostaining for low molecular weight cytokeratins.

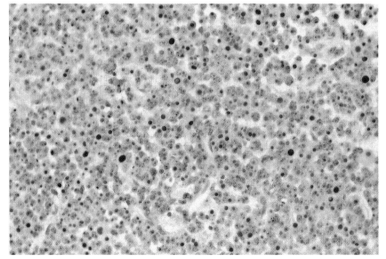

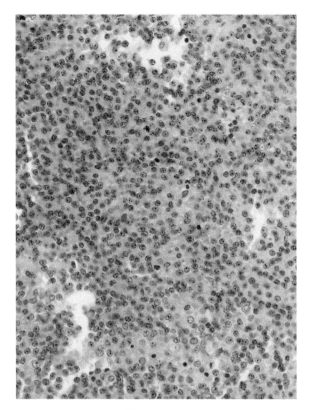

Figure 3-116
HISTOLOGY OF SILENT LACTOTROPH ADENOMA
These rare tumors resemble functioning lactotroph adenomas histologically; they are composed of chromophobic cells which can have either a trabecular or a solid architectural pattern.

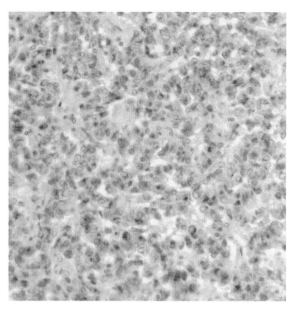

Figure 3-117
IMMUNOHISTOCHEMICAL LOCALIZATION OF PROLACTIN IN SILENT LACTOTROPH ADENOMA
These tumors generally contain immunoreactivity for prolactin in the characteristic juxtanuclear location, despite the lack of clinical evidence of hormone excess.

Silent Corticotroph Adenomas. Not all corticotroph adenomas cause Cushing's disease; some are "silent" (291), tumors unassociated with evidence of ACTH production or release in vivo but which are immunoreactive for ACTH and other POMC derivatives and have characteristic ultrastructural features of corticotrophs. Patients with silent corticotroph adenoma usually have hyperprolactinemia, even without evidence of stalk section effect (300). Several POMC derivatives, in particular β-endorphin, are known to stimulate PRL release and may account for this finding (310). It is important to verify the diagnosis because of the aggressive behavior of these adenomas which recur and have a propensity to undergo hemorrhagic infarction (290,314).

Two morphologic variants of silent corticotroph adenoma have been described (300). Type I adenomas resemble the densely granulated basophilic

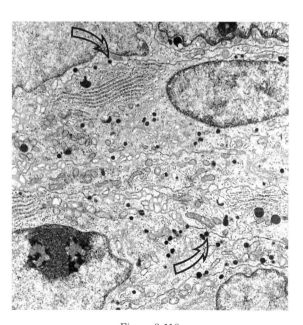

Figure 3-118
ULTRASTRUCTURE OF SILENT
LACTOTROPH ADENOMA
A sparsely granulated lactotroph adenoma is composed of cells with elongated processes, well-developed rough endoplasmic reticulum, and prominent juxtanuclear Golgi complexes that harbor forming secretory granules which may be quite pleomorphic. Extrusion of secretory material at the lateral cell border, "misplaced exocytosis" (arrows), is the hallmark of lactotrophs.

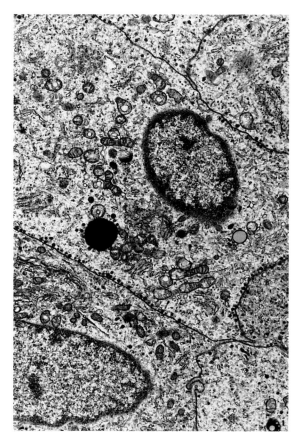

Figure 3-119
ULTRASTRUCTURE OF
SILENT THYROTROPH ADENOMA

This clinically nonfunctioning adenoma is composed of polygonal cells with elongated processes. The cell cytoplasm contains short profiles of slightly dilated rough endoplasmic reticulum, large Golgi complexes, and lysosomal dense bodies. The small and evenly electron dense secretory granules are aligned at the plasma membrane. The tumor was immunoreactive for α-subunit and β-TSH.

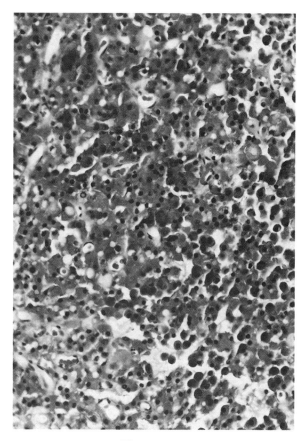

Figure 3-120
HISTOLOGY OF SILENT
CORTICOTROPH ADENOMA, TYPE I

These basophilic adenomas have either a trabecular or solid architecture. The cytoplasm contains basophilic secretory granules. Unlike the functioning tumors which are generally diagnosed early because of hormone excess, these clinically silent tumors generally are diagnosed when they become large and create mass effects. They often have abundant hemorrhage with focal necrosis.

tumors associated with Cushing's disease (fig. 3-120): they have strong ACTH immunoreactivity (fig. 3-121), contain abundant cytokeratin filaments (fig. 3-122), and, by electron microscopy, are composed of typical corticotrophs (fig. 3-123). Type II tumors resemble the uncommon chromophobic tumors (fig. 3-124) but stain for ACTH and other POMC-derived peptides (fig. 3-125) and are usually devoid of cytoplasmic intermediate filaments (fig. 3-126) (291). These adenomas express the POMC gene (307). They are immunoreactive for ACTH and β-endorphin (318) and release ACTH-like substances in vitro (282). Their clinical silence may be due to abnormal cleavage of the POMC molecule. It is thought that they produce either abnormal fragments of POMC (287) or cleave the molecule into smaller derivatives such as α-melanocyte-stimulating hormone (MSH) or corticotropin-like intermediate lobe peptide (CLIP).

Silent Gonadotroph Adenomas. Gonadotroph adenomas are morphologically classified more frequently than they are diagnosed clinically (300, 317), hence the distinction between clinically functioning gonadotroph adenomas that can be diagnosed on the basis of symptoms, clinical setting, and biochemistry, and clinically silent tumors of that category which are detected due to mass effects (311). Gonadotroph adenomas occur mainly in middle-aged patients and are more common in

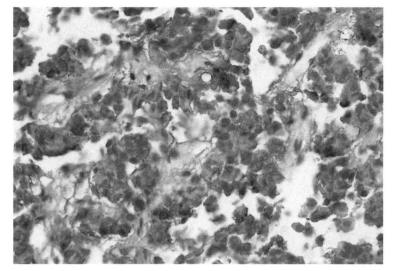

Fig 3-121
IMMUNOHISTOCHEMICAL
LOCALIZATION OF ACTH IN SILENT
CORTICOTROPH ADENOMA, TYPE I
The cytoplasm of the tumor cells is immunoreactive for ACTH.

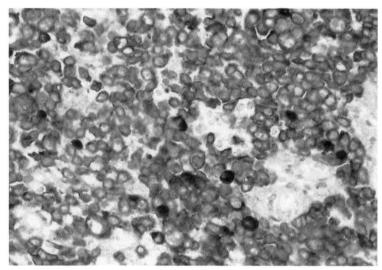

Figure 3-122
IMMUNOHISTOCHEMICAL
LOCALIZATION OF
CYTOKERATINS IN SILENT
CORTICOTROPH ADENOMA, TYPE I
These tumors generally contain abundant cytokeratin filaments which are readily identified immunohistochemically with the Cam 5.2 antibody.

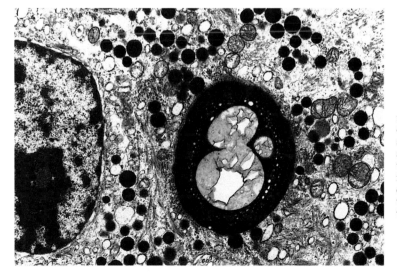

Figure 3-123
ULTRASTRUCTURE OF SILENT
CORTICOTROPH ADENOMA, TYPE I
These tumors are composed of cells that resemble normal corticotrophs. They are characterized by their relatively abundant secretory granules that are highly variable in size, shape, and electron density. In addition, they have conspicuous perinuclear bundles of intermediate filaments that correspond to cytokeratins. Complex lysosomes, resembling the "enigmatic bodies" of normal corticotrophs, are readily identified.

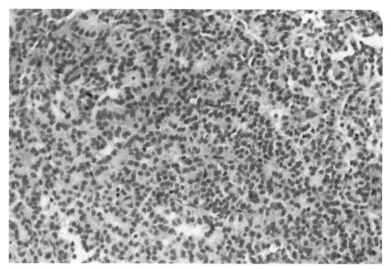

Figure 3-124
HISTOLOGY OF SILENT
CORTICOTROPH ADENOMA, TYPE II
These tumors tend to be chromophobic or
only slightly basophilic. They have a sinusoidal
or solid architecture.

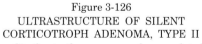

Figure 3-125
IMMUNOHISTOCHEMICAL
LOCALIZATION OF ACTH IN
SILENT CORTICOTROPH
ADENOMA, TYPE II
These tumors have variable immunoreac-
tivity for ACTH and other POMC derivatives,
but generally, hormone products are not dif-
ficult to identify by immunohistochemistry,
allowing recognition of this tumor type.

Figure 3-126
ULTRASTRUCTURE OF SILENT
CORTICOTROPH ADENOMA, TYPE II
Similar to the rare sparsely granulated
corticotroph adenomas associated with
ACTH excess, these tumors have well-developed rough endoplasmic reticulum and secretory granules that tend to be small but
extremely variable in size, shape, and electron density.

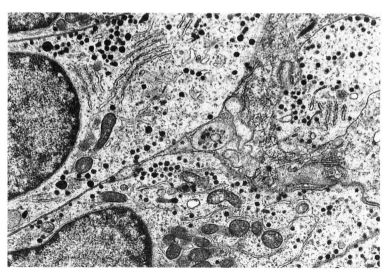

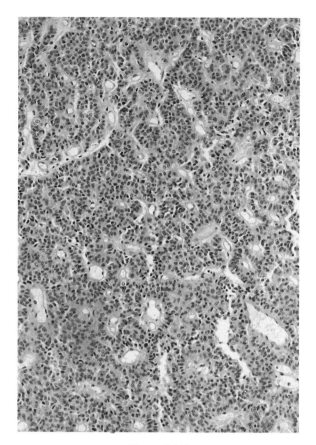

Figure 3-127
HISTOLOGY OF SILENT GONADOTROPH ADENOMA
These tumors are characterized by trabecular architecture and conspicuous pseudorosette formation around vascular channels. Scattered tumor cells contain abundant granular cytoplasm, indicating focal oncocytic change.

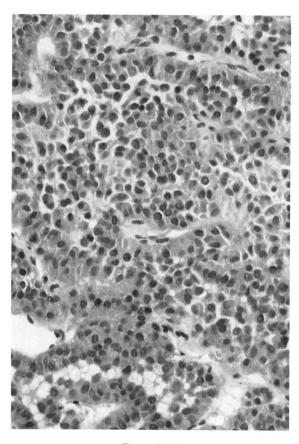

Figure 3-128
HISTOLOGY OF SILENT GONADOTROPH ADENOMA
Around vascular channels the tumor cells are elongated whereas in the center of nests and sheets they are round and polygonal. The cytoplasm varies from chromophobic to eosinophilic and granular, indicating oncocytic change.

men, but failure to diagnose this entity in perimenopausal and postmenopausal females results in most gonadotroph adenomas in women being classified as clinically nonfunctioning tumors (288). This group of tumors represents almost one third of surgically resected adenomas in most series.

Morphologically, the tumors that are diagnosed on the basis of symptoms and biochemistry, and those that are clinically silent are indistinguishable. There is a characteristic histologic appearance of trabecular and papillary architecture forming pseudorosettes around vascular channels (figs. 3-127, 3-128). Oncocytic change can be found in any adenoma type but it is rare in nongonadotrophic tumors, apart from the acidophil stem cell adenoma. Most gonadotroph adenomas have at least focal oncocytic change (fig. 3-129); the

degree of oncocytic change varies and can be extensive. Oncocytic change is characterized histologically by abundant cytoplasm which may be acidophilic and granular.

The tumor cytoplasm is immunoreactive for α-subunit (fig. 3-130) as well as β-subunits of FSH (fig. 3-131) and LH (fig. 3-132). There is strong nuclear positivity for SF-1 (fig. 3-133).

Gonadotroph adenomas show a wide range of differentiation, from highly developed cells with marked polarity and elongated cell processes (figs. 3-134, 3-135) to rounded cells with numerous mitochondria that displace many of the cytoplasmic organelles (figs. 3-136, 3-137). They have characteristic short profiles of dilated rough endoplasmic reticulum, rounded Golgi complexes, and small secretory granules which

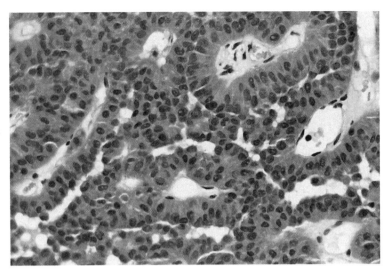

Figure 3-129
HISTOLOGY OF SILENT
GONADOTROPH
ADENOMA: ONCOCYTIC CHANGE
A gonadotroph adenoma is composed of
elongated cells that form pseudorosettes
around vascular channels. These tumor cells
have the characteristic abundant eosinophilic granular cytoplasm of oncocytes.

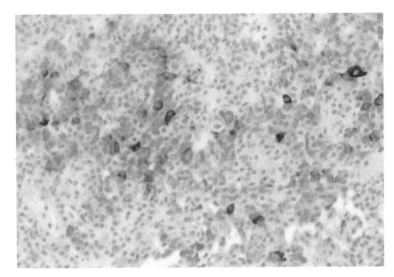

Figure 3-130
IMMUNOHISTOCHEMICAL
LOCALIZATION OF α–SUBUNIT IN
SILENT GONADOTROPH ADENOMA
Scattered tumor cells are strongly immu-
noreactive for α-subunit throughout the cy-
toplasm.

Figure 3-131
IMMUNOHISTOCHEMICAL
LOCALIZATION OF β-FSH IN SILENT
GONADOTROPH ADENOMA
Some tumor cells are immunoreactive for
β-FSH; staining tends to be localized around
vascular channels where the cells also show
histologic evidence of differentiation as
gonadotrophs.

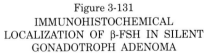
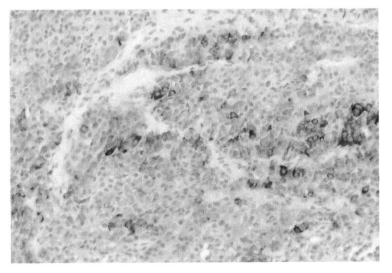

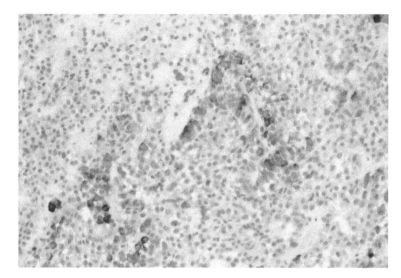

Figure 3-132
IMMUNOHISTOCHEMICAL
LOCALIZATION OF β-LH IN SILENT
GONADOTROPH ADENOMA
Scattered tumor cells throughout the lesion
are immunopositive for β-LH.

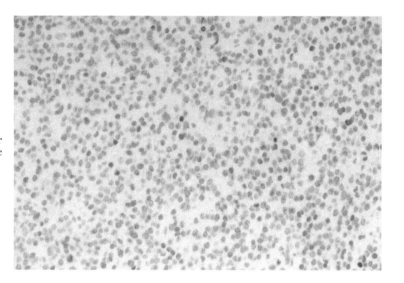

Figure 3-133
IMMUNOHISTOCHEMICAL
LOCALIZATION OF SF-1 IN SILENT
GONADOTROPH ADENOMA
The tumor cells exhibit strong nuclear
positivity for SF-1, indicating gonadotropic
differentiation.

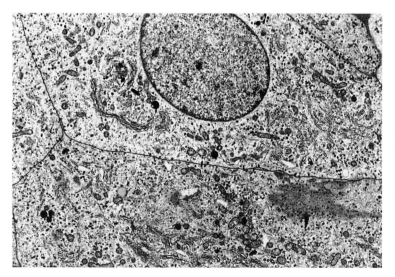

Figure 3-134
ULTRASTRUCTURE OF SILENT
GONADOTROPH ADENOMA
Like their functioning counterparts,
these tumors are composed of elongated cells
that have distinct polarity. They harbor
abundant short profiles of slightly dilated
rough endoplasmic reticulum, prominent
Golgi complexes, and numerous small secretory granules that have flocculent electron
dense contents.

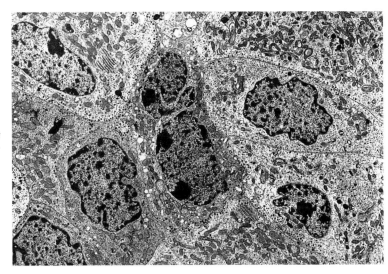

Figure 3-135
ULTRASTRUCTURE OF
SILENT GONADOTROPH
ADENOMA
Silent gonadotroph adenomas generally contain areas of oncocytic change; the accumulation of mitochondria varies from cell to cell.

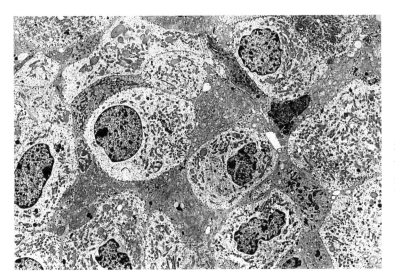

Figure 3-136
ULTRASTRUCTURE OF SILENT
GONADOTROPH ADENOMA:
ONCOCYTIC CHANGE
An oncocytic gonadotroph adenoma is characterized by light and dark cells. The cells harbor numerous mitochondria that occupy the bulk of the cytoplasm. The remainder of the cytoplasm contains other subcellular organelles. The presence of secretory granules indicates the secretory capacity of these cells.

Figure 3-137
ULTRASTRUCTURE OF SILENT
GONADOTROPH
ADENOMA: ONCOCYTIC CHANGE
This gonadotroph adenoma exhibits oncocytic change with accumulation of mitochondria. Nevertheless, other subcellular organelles are readily identified and the small secretory granules are quite numerous.

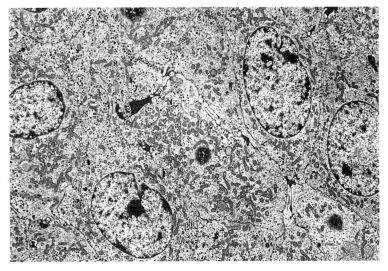

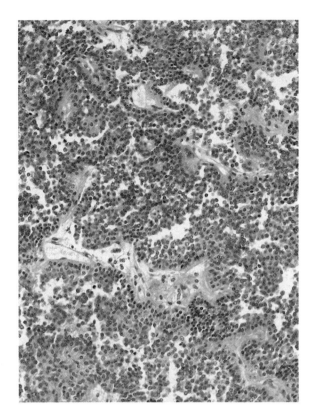

Figure 3-138
HISTOLOGY OF SILENT GONADOTROPH
ADENOMA (NULL CELL TYPE)

A poorly differentiated gonadotroph adenoma is composed of solid sheets of cells that show focal differentiation similar to well-differentiated gonadotroph adenomas, with the formation of pseudorosettes around vascular channels. In more solid areas, the tumor cells are small and have scant cytoplasm.

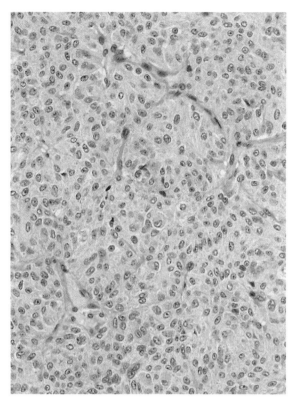

Figure 3-139
HISTOLOGY OF ONCOCYTOMA

This oncocytoma is composed entirely of solid nests and sheets of epithelial cells that have abundant eosinophilic granular cytoplasm.

measure up to 250 nm in diameter and occasionally have peripheral halos surrounding variably electron dense contents.

Null cell adenomas and oncocytomas were considered formerly to be tumors that had no markers allowing characterization of their cytodifferentiation. When first described, almost 25 percent of these pituitary adenomas were devoid of immunoreactivity and the ultrastructural features were considered to be nonspecific. However, it is now known that most release gonadotropins or their subunits (285,323). The quantities of hormone released are low, as they are in cultures of clinically silent gonadotroph adenomas and in cultured nontumorous pituitary tissue where gonadotrophs represent only approximately 5 percent of the cell population (285). The reverse hemolytic plaque assay has shown that hormone release is attribut-

able to only a small percentage of tumor cells and that the quantities of hormones released are exceedingly small (324). Molecular analyses have shown that glycoprotein hormone genes are expressed in these adenomas (292,309) as well as the gonadotroph transcription factor SF-1 (283). Dynamic studies in vitro have shown that these tumors respond to stimulation by GnRH and exhibit paradoxical stimulation by TRH (284,302, 304,305), features consistent with gonadotroph differentiation. These studies suggest that null cell adenomas represent gonadotropin-producing tumors with very low functional activity.

Chromophobic tumors generally have a diffuse or sinusoidal architecture but careful examination usually reveals focal trabecular or papillary architecture and pseudorosette formations around blood vessels (fig. 3-138). In some tumors, oncocytic change is diffuse and the lesions are classified as oncocytomas (fig. 3-139). Modern

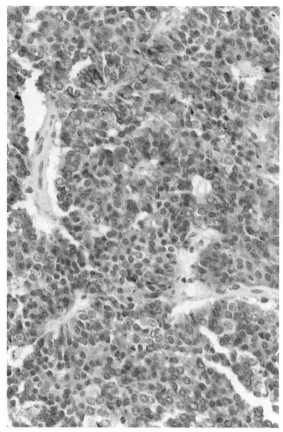

Figure 3-140
IMMUNOHISTOCHEMICAL LOCALIZATION
OF α-SUBUNIT IN SILENT GONADOTROPH
ADENOMA (NULL CELL TYPE)
Despite the lack of clear histologic differentiation, the tumor cells contain focal but very strong cytoplasmic immunopositivity for α-subunit of glycoprotein hormones.

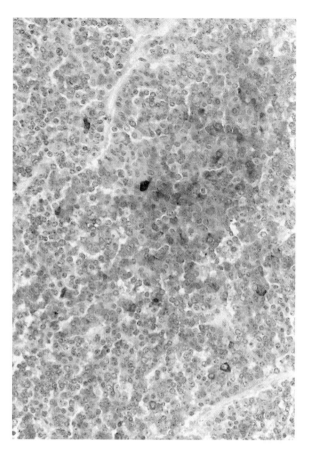

Figure 3-141
IMMUNOHISTOCHEMICAL LOCALIZATION OF
SILENT β-FSH IN GONADOTROPH
ADENOMA (NULL CELL TYPE)
Tumor cells scattered throughout this lesion contain cytoplasmic reactivity for β-FSH; this antigen is found more often than β-LH but either or both can found in the cytoplasm of silent gonadotroph adenomas.

immunohistochemical techniques show these tumors to contain scattered cells with cytoplasmic immunoreactivity for α-subunit (fig. 3-140) and β-subunits of FSH (fig. 3-141), LH, or both as well as nuclear staining for SF-1. There have been attempts to define the distinction between gonadotroph adenomas and null cell adenomas by the percentages of gonadotropin-immunoreactive cells determined by light microscopy (299), but it seems clear from many types of analysis that there is no clinical or biologic difference that correlates with these subclassifications.

By electron microscopy, tumor cells in the less well-differentiated adenomas are small and polygonal; they lack the polarity of well-differentiated gonadotrophs. The scant, poorly developed cytoplasm reflects low hormonal activity (figs. 3-142, 3-143) (286). The cytoplasm contains poorly developed short profiles of rough endoplasmic reticulum, relatively small Golgi complexes, and sparse, small secretory granules. There is a variable accumulation of mitochondria which, in oncocytomas, can occupy up to 50 percent of the cytoplasmic area (figs. 3-144, 3-145) (323). Despite the numerous mitochondria, the cytoplasm in oncocytoma cells contains scant organelles resembling those of the non-oncocytic gonadotroph adenoma. There is a spectrum of oncocytic change in non-oncocytic tumors and increasing oncocytic change may be seen in tumor recurrences in a given patient (299,300).

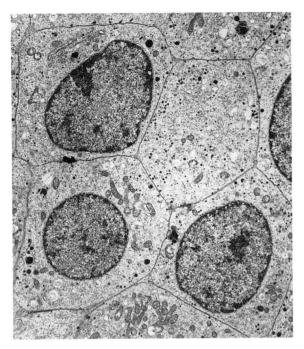

Figure 3-142
ULTRASTRUCTURE OF SILENT GONADOTROPH
ADENOMA (NULL CELL TYPE)
These tumor cells have poorly developed cytoplasmic organelles and scattered small secretory granules.

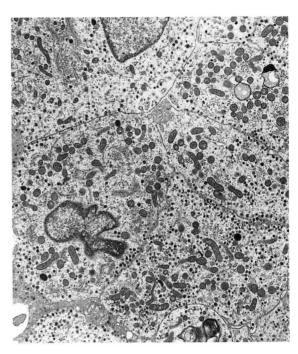

Figure 3-143
ULTRASTRUCTURE OF SILENT GONADOTROPH
ADENOMA (NULL CELL TYPE)
The cells have dilated rough endoplasmic reticulum, conspicuous Golgi complexes, and numerous secretory granules.

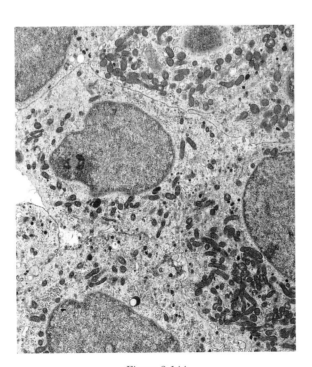

Figure 3-144
ULTRASTRUCTURE OF ONCOCYTOMA
This adenoma is composed of cells with poorly differentiated cytoplasmic organelles but mitochondria are numerous.

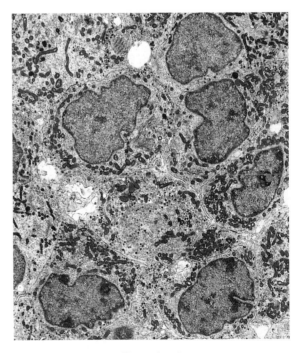

Figure 3-145
ULTRASTRUCTURE OF ONCOCYTOMA
The cytoplasm is almost entirely filled with mitochondria. Other subcellular organelles are identifiable but are sparse.

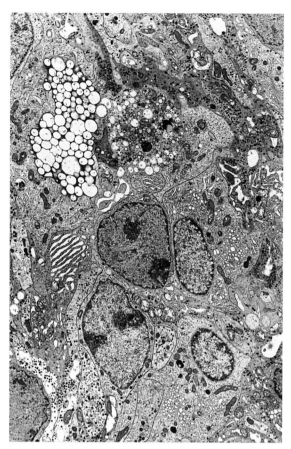

Figure 3-146
ULTRASTRUCTURE OF "FEMALE TYPE"
GONADOTROPH ADENOMA

These tumors are characterized by the presence of dilated profiles of rough endoplasmic reticulum, small secretory granules that are of variable electron density, and a conspicuous Golgi complex which has been described as a "honey-comb Golgi," characterized by vesicular sacculi. These tumors do not generally contain immunoreactive gonadotropins and their true identity remains to be established.

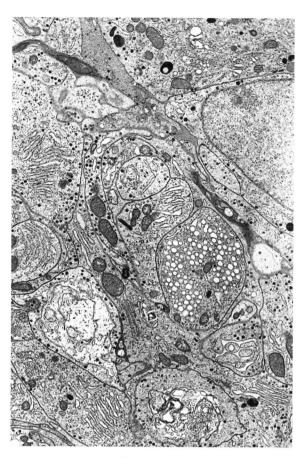

Figure 3-147
ULTRASTRUCTURE OF "FEMALE TYPE"
GONADOTROPH ADENOMA

This tumor type is characterized by an unusual dilated vesicular Golgi complex that has been called a "honey-comb Golgi." The cytoplasm also contains dilated profiles of rough endoplasmic reticulum and numerous small secretory granules that are variable in size and shape. The exact nature of this tumor type remains to be established.

A rare tumor that has been reported to be unique to women is the female type of gonadotroph adenoma (figs. 3-146, 3-147). These tumors have a highly characteristic ultrastructure but rarely contain immunoreactive gonadotropins. In fact, in the author's experience, they most often contain ACTH-like reactivity and release ACTH in vitro rather than gonadotropins. The tumors are composed of moderate-sized cells with distinct polarity. They have euchromatic nuclei and an abundant cytoplasm filled with slightly dilated rough endoplasmic reticulum profiles. The highly distinctive honeycomb Golgi complex has round sacculi containing a homogeneous, moderately electron

dense material. In some tumors, in place of a honeycomb Golgi, there is a tripolar Golgi complex with vesicular sacculi at the center. Secretory granules are generally sparse, small (100 to 200 nm in diameter), and moderately electron dense. These are enigmatic lesions that may represent variants of silent corticotroph adenomas.

Poorly Differentiated Adenomas. Rare adenomas are hormone-negative lesions, composed of poorly differentiated cells (fig. 3-148). They may exhibit focal plurihormonality and plurimorphous differentiation (298). Some null cell adenomas respond in vitro to stimulation by LRH, TRH, CRH, or GRH (284,312,315); the expression of

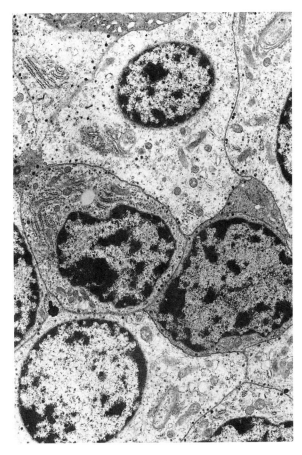

Figure 3-148
PRECURSOR CELL ADENOMA
This tumor is composed of very small, poorly differentiated cells. Some tumor cells contain short profiles of rough endoplasmic reticulum, others contain Golgi complexes, but secretory granules are sparse and small. This tumor contained no hormone immunoreactivity to allow identification of its differentiation, and it released no detectable hormones in vitro.

receptors implicated by these results has been confirmed by measuring cytosolic free calcium and adenyl cyclase activity (313) and by direct measurement of TRH binding sites (305). In contrast to the strong evidence of gonadotroph differentiation in the majority of adenomas that have been classified as null cell adenomas, some of these tumors may be composed of pluripotential progenitor cells that express receptors of various types and are capable of differentiating along different hormone-producing cell lines (299).

Differential Diagnosis. The differential diagnosis for these tumors is wide and includes many tumors and tumor-like lesions in the sellar region. Tumors such as meningiomas, gliomas, germ cell tumors, and metastatic carcinomas can be mistaken for pituitary adenomas; careful examination of the histologic features and appropriate immunohistochemical analyses, detailed in the relevant sections of this text, will provide the correct diagnosis. Other tumors and tumor-like lesions that present clinically as a sellar mass usually have characteristic morphology that allows ready diagnosis; the features of craniopharyngiomas, cysts, and inflammatory lesions are discussed in following chapters. A difficult problem occasionally arises when nontumorous adenohypophysis or neurohypophysis is biopsied; it is important to recognize these tissues and not err by misdiagnosing a tumor.

Prognosis and Therapy. Patients generally present for medical attention at the stage where the tumor has grown to involve surrounding structures and caused compressive symptoms. Surgical decompression and debulking remain the mainstays of treatment (293). The need for surgery is underlined by the necessity for diagnostic assessment of the tumor since it is essential to exclude other tumors which are indistinguishable without morphologic analysis. As for most pituitary adenomas, the success of transsphenoidal surgery, even for extrasellar macroadenomas, has reduced the indication for transfrontal surgery to patients with very large invasive tumors (289). Total or near total removal of the tumor can be achieved in some patients; these tumors, however, have a distinct tendency to recur. Postoperative radiation is usually offered as an adjuvant to surgery to prevent regrowth of large tumors that cannot be completely resected (320).

Despite the fact that these are among the most common pituitary tumors, there is no efficacious substance for medical management. For the group of gonadotroph, null cell, and oncocytic adenomas, treatment with GnRH analogues has been attempted (see Pituitary Adenomas Causing Gonadotropin Excess) but the results have not been promising. These adenomas are also known to have dopamine receptors (297,306), however, with rare exception, bromocriptine has not been efficacious in reducing tumor size (322) which is the main treatment goal for these lesions. Octreotide has been reported to improve visual field defects in some patients (303,321), but it has not been shown to reduce tumor size as determined objectively by imaging analyses.

When surgery is contraindicated due to the general condition of the patient and there are no compressive features, patients may be monitored by serial imaging with CT or MRI, along with formal visual field assessment at 6- to 12-month intervals. Regardless of the management course taken, anterior pituitary reserve must be formally assessed, and complete or selective trophic hormonal deficiencies require appropriate hormonal replacement.

PLURIHORMONAL ADENOMAS

Clinical Features. A number of unusual clinical presentations have been reported in association with plurihormonal tumors. The most common involves production of GH and TSH by tumors that cause acromegaly or gigantism in association with hyperthyroidism (327,340,341,343,345,348, 349). Other tumors have caused hyperthyroidism in association with hyperprolactinemia due to production of both TSH and PRL (328,331,333,336). Rarely, Cushing's disease has been associated with excess GH, PRL, TSH (347), or gonadotropins (346). Gonadotropins have also been reported in association with PRL (330,332) and TSH (337). Most of these tumors are characterized as plurihormonal only on the basis of morphologic studies. In the case of tumors with significant suprasellar extension they may be clinically silent with only mild to moderate hyperprolactinemia but leading to the "stalk section effect" (334).

In many of these tumors, one component is silent and the tumor manifests with only one syndrome or the other. The plurihormonal nature of such lesions is recognized by morphologic studies alone (334).

Biochemical Findings. The biochemistry of these lesions can be very confusing because of the unusual profiles of hormone excess. They may be associated with elevated levels of several hormones and reduced levels of other adenohypophysial substances due to tissue destruction by tumor growth. The details of these biochemical findings cannot be reported in this chapter; each individual case has had a distinct profile and the reader is referred to the individual reports for further elaboration.

Radiologic Findings. This highly variable group of tumors has a wide range of imaging findings, ranging from those of intrasellar macroadenomas to those of widely invasive large tumors.

Microscopic Findings. Plurihormonal pituitary adenomas are recognized with increasing frequency (339). The use of systematic immunohistochemistry has revealed immunoreactivity for multiple adenohypophysial hormones in many tumors. In particular, α-subunit is widely recognized in a number of pituitary adenoma types; it is most commonly associated with GH (326,338, 344) and is expected to be expressed by tumors producing glycoprotein hormones. In addition, pituitary adenomas that produce ACTH and α-subunit have been reported to be more common than detectable by clinical investigation (329).

Plurihormonal tumors that produce GH, PRL and, on occasion, α-subunit have been classified, and represent well-recognized causes of acromegaly or gigantism and hyperprolactinemia; these have been described above. This section is restricted to unusual plurihormonal tumors that produce unexpected combinations of hormones that cannot be accounted for by current concepts of adenohypophysial cytodifferentiation.

Detailed morphologic studies using immunocytochemistry and electron microscopy have shown that plurihormonal tumors can be divided into monomorphous and plurimorphous types. Monomorphous adenomas consist of one cell type that is capable of producing several hormones; multiple hormones can be documented by immunocytochemistry in the cytoplasm of the same cell. Plurimorphous plurihormonal adenomas are composed of two or more cell types, each of which has a characteristic hormonal profile and usually a distinct ultrastructural appearance which resembles that of a nontumorous adenohypophysial cell type. Although this distinction appears relatively simplistic, careful ultrastructural immunocytochemical studies have revealed that even in plurimorphous tumors, unusual plurihormonal profiles within individual cells can be recognized. Extrapolation reveals that tumors associated with acromegaly and hyperthyroidism may be monomorphous, composed of cells resembling somatotrophs or thyrotrophs; the latter appears to be more common, nevertheless, the monomorphous cell type is immunoreactive for GH as well as TSH (327, 340–343,345,348,349). Similarly, tumors producing TSH and PRL have been reported to be bimorphous, composed of thyrotrophs and lactotrophs (333) or monomorphous, composed of cells resembling thyrotrophs (328,331,336). Various other plurihormonal tumors have variable morphologies.

One unusual tumor of note is the silent subtype III adenoma (335): this peculiar tumor type has been associated with hyperprolactinemia or acromegaly or, in some instances, with no clinical evidence of hormone excess. The tumors are macroadenomas, often with parasellar extension. They are histologically diffuse and exhibit focal immunoreactivity for one or more adenohypophysial hormones. The diagnosis relies on electron microscopy (fig. 3-149). These adenomas are composed of large cells whose nuclei are usually found at one pole of the cell and may harbor spheridia. The abundant cytoplasm contains well-developed, widely distributed rough endoplasmic reticulum that may be found in continuity with randomly distributed tubular smooth endoplasmic reticulum. The Golgi complex is usually prominent and tortuous. Mitochondria may be numerous and are found in clusters. The cells have interdigitating attenuated processes in which small secretory granules accumulate. These characteristic ultrastructural features allow their recognition as a distinct entity, although the cell of origin is obscure (335).

Prognosis and Therapy. Plurihormonal tumors are usually managed surgically; the use of medical therapy would be predicated on the hormonal profile of the individual tumor. There is insufficient information to assess whether plurihormonality alters the prognosis compared with usual tumor types. It has been suggested that the silent subtype III adenoma is a more aggressive adenoma that is prone to recurrence but is also relatively radiosensitive (335).

PITUITARY APOPLEXY

Definition. Acute hemorrhagic necrosis of a pituitary adenoma may lead to rapid tumor expansion and cause severe headache, lethargy, coma, or other signs of increased intracranial pressure. The term pituitary apoplexy defines this complex series of clinical events that results from fulminant expansion of a pituitary tumor because of infarction and hemorrhage.

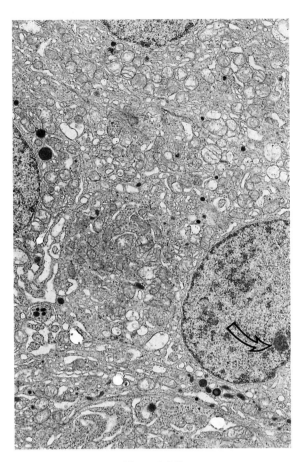

Figure 3-149
ULTRASTRUCTURE OF
SILENT SUBTYPE III ADENOMA

This very unusual and aggressive plurihormonal pituitary tumor is characterized by ultrastructural parameters. The nuclei contain spheridia (arrow), which are unusual in other pituitary adenomas. The cytoplasm is filled with tightly packed endoplasmic reticulum and highly developed, quite tortuous Golgi complexes. Secretory granules tend to be sparse and accumulate in cell processes. Cell membranes show complex interdigitations and are difficult to identify in these tumors. Mitochondria are numerous and sometimes dilated.

Clinical Features. This endocrine emergency is characterized by the sudden onset of headache, visual impairment, and cranial nerve palsies due to acute enlargement and necrosis of a pituitary mass (fig. 3-150). Most patients have no history of a pituitary adenoma prior to the apoplectic episode, however, in some cases the necrosis is precipitated by carotid angiography during the course of investigation of a sellar mass or during radiation therapy of a known pituitary tumor. Other predisposing factors include trauma, coagulopathies, temporal arteritis, diabetes mellitus, and atherosclerosis. The clinical spectrum of presentation ranges from acute headache to sudden death. The patient often complains of diplopia from compression of the oculomotor and abducens cranial nerves due to increased pressure within the cavernous sinus. Other neurologic features include altered consciousness, motor weakness, signs of meningeal irritation, and diabetes insipidus. Acute hypopituitarism often contributes to morbidity and mortality.

Morphologic Findings. Pituitary adenomas can exhibit degenerative features such as infarction and hemorrhage (figs. 3-151, 3-152); some develop cysts and even calcify. The term "apoplexy" is generally reserved for those extreme cases in which clinical signs of compression of perisellar structures or meningeal irritation occur following pituitary infarction or hemorrhage.

Prognosis and Therapy. When pituitary apoplexy is suspected, glucocorticoids should be immediately administered. Fluids and electrolytes should be carefully monitored for either diabetes insipidus or syndrome of inappropriate secretion of antidiuretic hormone (SIADH). The clinical course is often unpredictable and spontaneous recovery may occur (350). Patients with severe visual impairment or altered level of consciousness, however, require urgent surgical decompression. The likelihood of visual recovery depends more on early decompression than the extent of the initial visual deficit. Transsphenoidal decompression is the preferred approach. Postoperative anterior and posterior pituitary function assessment is essential since long-term hormone replacement is often necessary.

ASSOCIATED DISORDERS— MULTIPLE ENDOCRINE NEOPLASIA

The multiple endocrine neoplasia (MEN) syndromes are familial disorders in which neoplasms arise de novo in several endocrine tissues. The syndromes are classified according to their pattern of clinical presentation. Pituitary adenomas are integral components of the type 1 (MEN-1) syndrome; other MEN syndromes are not usually associated with pituitary pathology.

In 1954, Wermer (357) described the syndrome which now bears his name and is characterized by the association of parathyroid hyperplasia, pituitary adenomas, and endocrine

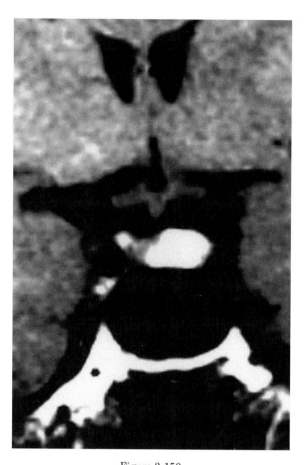

Figure 3-150
RADIOLOGY OF PITUITARY APOPLEXY
A pituitary adenoma has undergone necrosis and recent hemorrhage which is detectable as a hyperintense area on T1-weighted MRI. (Courtesy of Dr. S. Ezzat, Toronto, Canada.)

tumors of the pancreas. This disorder is inherited with an autosomal dominant genetic pattern; the causative gene, localized to chromosome 11 (11q13), was recently cloned (352) and encodes a putative tumor suppressor (see chapter 3). Other neoplasms such as adrenocortical and thyroid adenomas; endocrine tumors of the lung, gut, and other dispersed endocrine cells; lipomas; and pinealomas occur more frequently in patients with the MEN syndromes than in the general population (353,354). The neoplasms may arise synchronously but are more often diagnosed in a metachronous fashion.

Pituitary adenomas occur in approximately two thirds of patients with MEN-1 (353,354). They may be multicentric (355,356), although proof of this can be difficult to obtain. It has been

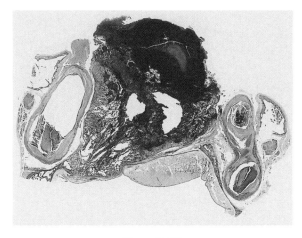

Figure 3-151
PITUITARY APOPLEXY
This autopsy specimen reveals extensive hemorrhage in
a large pituitary adenoma that resulted in clinical features
of apoplexy. (Courtesy of Dr. J.M. Bilbao, Toronto, Canada.)

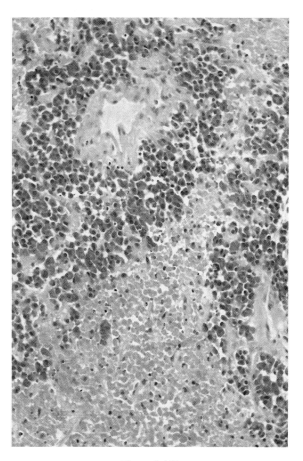

Figure 3-152
PITUITARY APOPLEXY
This surgically resected pituitary adenoma exhibits extensive necrosis, consistent with the clinical presentation of apoplexy in a patient with known acromegaly.

suggested that these patients may have an underlying hyperplastic process similar to that seen in the parathyroids and pancreases of patients with MEN-1 (353,354), however, there is no reported evidence of this change.

Pituitary tumors of all types and producing any of the adenohypophysial hormones occur in patients with MEN-1, however, hormonally active adenomas are more common in this group of patients than in the general population with sporadic pituitary adenomas (353). There is a preponderance of adenomas secreting PRL, GH, or both of those hormones (355). Hypersecretion of ACTH is less frequent than secretion of GH or PRL. Clinically nonfunctioning pituitary adenomas are less common in patients with MEN-1 than in those with sporadic pituitary adenomas. The morphologic features of both adenoma types are indistinguishable.

The pathophysiology of MEN-1–associated adenomas is unknown. It has been suggested that ectopic production of hypophysiotropic hormones by, for example, pancreatic lesions, may play a role in the development of these pituitary adenomas (351). While it is now clear that the tumors have a genetic basis, it may be that hormonal factors are involved in the determination of hormonal activity and account for the more common hypersecretory syndromes of pituitary adenomas associated with MEN-1.

ECTOPIC ADENOMAS

Ectopic pituitary adenomas are rare, but well documented. They have been reported in the sphenoid sinus (fig. 3-153) and parapharyngeal region (359,362,365,367,368). It is not surprising that these tumors can arise in such locations, since remnants of embryonic adenohypophysis may be deposited along the path of the developing Rathke's cleft and these remnants are known to contain all the hormone-producing cell types found in the normal gland. Ectopic adenohypophysial tissue has also been described in a suprasellar location in up to 20 percent of people (361) and suprasellar or parasellar tumors may develop accordingly (360). Curious sites of reported ectopic pituitary adenomata include the middle nasal meatus and the petrous temporal bone

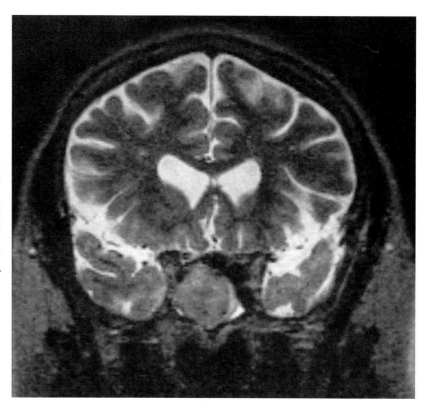

Figure 3-153
MAGNETIC RESONANCE
IMAGING OF AN ECTOPIC
PITUITARY ADENOMA
(T2 WEIGHTED)
This patient had glucocorticoid excess and a biochemical profile that was highly suggestive of Cushing's disease. Scans failed to document an intrasellar mass but a tumor was identified arising in and occupying much of the sphenoid sinus. This was characterized as a corticotroph adenoma by histology, immunohistochemistry, and electron microscopy. (Courtesy of Dr. S. Ezzat, Toronto, Canada.)

(367), the clivus (358), and the hypothalamus (364,366), including the third ventricle (363).

The age and sex of patients with ectopic adenomas are similar to those reported for intrasellar pituitary adenomas. However, the proportion of hormonally active tumors is higher than among sellar lesions and the most common endocrinologic abnormality is Cushing's disease, unlike the situation concerning intrasellar adenomas (359,369).

When clinical syndromes of pituitary hormone excess are not associated with detectable intrasellar pathology, the possibility of ectopic sites of tumor development should be considered (365). CT and MRI examination can be helpful in delineating the lesion and determining its relationship to the sella (369). Occasionally, ectopic pituitary adenomas are associated with intrasellar pituitary tumors (367). Clinically nonfunctioning ectopic pituitary adenomas may present with local mass effects (365). The diagnosis of pituitary adenoma in these unusual sites requires rigorous confirmation by immunohistochemistry and electron microscopy.

PATHOGENESIS OF PITUITARY ADENOMAS

For many years there has been controversy regarding the basis of pituitary tumorigenesis. The two prevailing theories have pitted hormonal stimulation against an intrinsic pituitary defect (378,441,450).

The evidence supporting a hormonal etiology includes: 1) paradoxical pituitary hormone responses to exogenous hormonal stimulation that are characteristic of pituitary adenomas; 2) the development of pituitary adenomas in situations of excessive hypothalamic hormone stimulation or reduced feedback suppression by target gland hormones; and 3) hypothalamic hormone production within the anterior pituitary that suggests a role for local excess stimulation.

Persuasive arguments against a hormonal etiology are: 1) the rarity of hyperplastic changes associated with adenomas; 2) the lack of true adenomatous changes in the pituitary even after long and sustained exposure to hypothalamic hormone stimulation in some instances; and 3) the low

128

frequency of recurrence following successful tumor resection. Additionally, some pituitary adenomas have been shown to lack hypothalamic hormone receptor synthesis (375). Most compelling, however, is the growing body of evidence in favor of intrinsic pituitary cell defects accounting for the development of these lesions.

An integrated approach reconciling the two proposed theories of tumorigenesis applies the multistep theory of carcinogenesis. It is likely that the majority of pituitary adenomas develop from transformed cells that are, nevertheless, dependent on hormonal stimulation for tumor promotion (378).

Hormonal Basis of Pituitary Tumorigenesis

This theory has received support from a substantial body of evidence that GRH can cause somatotroph proliferation (387) and from the well-documented development of somatotroph hyperplasia in patients with extrahypothalamic tumors secreting GRH (454,467). In addition, hypothalamic tumors containing GRH have been associated with sparsely granulated somatotroph adenomas (384). In vitro, human somatotroph adenoma cells are known to respond to GRH stimulation (371,372,423,435, 464,474), indicating the presence of GRH receptors on these tumors, but they lack the down-regulation characteristic of normal somatotrophs (423,464). Thus it would appear that GRH stimulation may play a role in the development of these tumors. Moreover, an animal model of GRH excess, transgenic mice overexpressing GRH, has proven that chronic overstimulation alone can result in tumor formation (381,433). However, in situations of GRH excess, the pituitary GH-producing adenomas were associated with hyperplasia of GH-producing cells, a phenomenon that is distinctly rare in patients with sporadic pituitary GH-producing adenomas (452). Moreover, in humans, continuous overstimulation by ectopic GRH does not alone result in adenoma formation (396).

The pathogenesis of lactotroph adenomas may involve defective inhibition by hypothalamic dopamine or excessive stimulation by a putative PRL-releasing factor such as TRH or vasoactive intestinal peptide (VIP) (441). The presence of lactotroph hyperplasia in the tissue surrounding lactotroph adenomas in some cases (383,452) supports this theory. Lactotrophs are known to proliferate during pregnancy (383,458) and estrogen has also been implicated as a PRL-stimulating factor. In the late 1970s administration of oral contraceptives was implicated in rapid increases in size and secretion of some lactotroph adenomas (412) and was thought to be responsible for a possible increase in the incidence of lactotroph adenomas; it is more likely that the latter reflects increased awareness of the entity soon after the discovery of PRL. Although high doses of estrogen undoubtedly stimulate lactotrophs, and a few lactotroph adenomas may grow during pregnancy (388), these tumors are not more numerous or larger during gestation (458) and there is little evidence that low dose oral contraceptives play a significant role in tumor pathogenesis.

The role of decreased hypothalamic inhibition was supported by some authors who found vascular changes, including arteriogenesis, in lactotroph adenomas. They speculated that the neovascularization from the systemic circulation, which has negligible levels of dopamine, allowed lactotrophs to escape dopaminergic tonic inhibition (456); it was also shown that estrogens stimulate vascular reorganization and arteriogenesis (455). However, systemic blood is known to contribute to the adenohypophysial blood supply in normals (409) and the implication of neovascularization as a causative factor in the pathogenesis of lactotroph adenomas remains unproven. Moreover, knockout mice lacking pituitary dopaminergic D_2 receptors develop lactotroph hyperplasia but not adenoma (424).

The hormonal regulation of thyrotroph adenomas has been shown to be abnormal as well as highly variable (386,402,463,469). While some tumors can be suppressed by dopamine (402, 463), the dopaminergic resistance may implicate altered or absent dopamine receptors as an etiologic factor (386). Patients with longstanding primary hypothyroidism develop pituitary thyrotroph hyperplasia and associated lactotroph hyperplasia; this proliferation has been attributed to TRH stimulation. These patients exhibit a spectrum of hyperplasias and neoplasias (406,457), suggesting that continuous stimulation leads to thyrotroph adenoma (417).

The postulated etiology of Cushing's disease has shown tremendous flux since Cushing's description in the 1930s of a primary pituitary disorder (428). In the 1940s, the documentation of adrenal hyperresponsiveness to ACTH and the presence of Crooke's hyalinization in the pituitary brought a primary adrenal etiology to the fore. In contrast, the autopsy documentation of lesions in the paraventricular nucleus of patients with Cushing's disease suggested that the hypothalamus may be the site of primary pathology; this was supported by reports of Cushing's disease associated with increased intracranial pressure due to intracranial tumors and regression of Cushingoid symptomatology following tumor removal. In the 1950s, the trend implicating the pituitary as the site of primary pathology returned, with the recognition of the therapeutic efficacy of pituitary irradiation or microsurgical removal of an adenoma. Nevertheless, it has been recognized in the last two decades that patients with Cushing's disease may have other associated neuroendocrine and electroencephalogram abnormalities. Reports of a therapeutic response to antiserotoninergic or antidopaminergic agents reverted attention to the hypothalamus (427). Long-term follow-up of patients who have undergone transsphenoidal resection of microadenomas has indicated recurrence of disease in some. A few patients with pituitary Cushing's disease have corticotroph hyperplasia as the cause of the disorder in the absence of a discrete adenoma (425). These findings have implicated CRH excess in the pathogenesis of Cushing's disease (428).

Lack of suppressibility of corticotroph adenomas by glucocorticoids was suggested by one study (436) as a mechanism involved in the pathologic ACTH secretion in Cushing's disease and Nelson's syndrome. This report has not been confirmed by other investigators. The characterization of CRH in 1981 permitted its identification in a number of extra-pituitary tumors associated with a clinical picture resembling Cushing's disease; in some of those tumors there was corticotroph hyperplasia (393,404). In one instance, a hypothalamic gangliocytoma producing CRH was associated with corticotroph hyperplasia and Cushing's disease (382). These experiments suggested that CRH may play a role in the proliferation of corticotrophs, and animal studies using continuous infusion of CRH have confirmed that prolonged exposure to CRH leads to increased numbers of corticotrophs (379,405,440). However, it is yet to be proved that CRH alone causes pituitary corticotroph adenoma. As is the case with GH-producing tumors, the pathogenesis is probably multifactorial and CRH may play a role in the promotion of tumor cell proliferation (378).

The occurrence of gonadotroph adenomas in patients with hypogonadism has suggested that the chronic stimulation resulting from primary gonadal failure may play a role in the formation and growth of these adenomas (461). Animal models have supported this theory (444); nevertheless, the majority of gonadotroph adenomas are not associated with underlying hypogonadism or evidence of chronic hypothalamic stimulation in the adjacent nontumorous adenohypophysis (452) and appear to arise spontaneously.

Molecular Basis of Pituitary Tumorigenesis

Clonality Studies in Pituitary Adenomas. The technique of clonality assessment using X chromosome inactivation patterns evolved from the Lyon hypothesis, which states that only one X chromosome is active in any female somatic cell; the inactivation occurs early in embryogenesis and persists throughout the lifespan of the cell and its progeny. Several studies have shown that pituitary adenomas exhibit a pattern of monoclonality based on X chromosome inactivation (373,416). Most lesions that displayed a polyclonal pattern were contaminated with normal pituitary tissue; the small size of adenomas associated with Cushing's syndrome in particular has confounded the interpretation of the clonal status of these tumors (407,416,459).

Oncogenes and Tumor Suppressor Genes in Pituitary Adenomas. Although pituitary adenomas are monoclonal proliferations, somatic mutations that have been identified in other malignancies are usually absent in these tumors and the events leading to pituitary tumorigenesis remain unknown. A few candidate oncogenes and tumor suppressor genes have been implicated.

G-proteins are heterotrimeric membrane-anchored peptides which are involved in transducing signals from cell surface ligand-receptor complexes to downstream effectors. The α-subunit dissociates from the β- and γ-subunits of Gs when guanosine triphosphate (GTP) displaces bound guanosine diphosphate (GDP), stimulating adenylyl cyclase to produce adenosine monophosphate (AMP) from adenosine triphosphate (ATP). Cyclic AMP (cAMP) in turn activates cAMP-dependent protein kinases, increases intracellular calcium transport, and may potentiate the effect of activated inositol phospholipid-dependent protein kinases. The weak intrinsic GTPase activity of Gsα and the action of GTPase activating peptides (GAP) dissociates GTP from Gsα and terminates the response. Single point mutations in two critical domains of the Gsα subunit resulted in constitutive activation and were identified in several endocrine tumors; a codon 201 change from arginine to cysteine or a codon 227 mutation resulting in an arginine substitution for glycine inhibited hydrolysis of GTP. These G-protein or *Gsp* mutations were first described in a subset of somatotroph adenomas (437,470). Subsequent studies, however, have identified this highly conserved mutation in a small number of nonfunctional pituitary adenomas as well (468). In patients with acromegaly, *Gsp* mutations were found to be associated with higher GH levels by some investigators (429) but not others (414). Furthermore, the presence of this mutation appears to correlate with a densely granulated ultrastructural appearance (462) and possibly greater responsiveness to inhibition by the somatostatin analog, octreotide (397).

Supportive evidence for the pivotal role of cAMP in mediating somatotroph differentiation and tumorigenesis is provided by an animal model. Targeted overexpression of the cholera toxin in the somatotroph results in pituitary tumors and gigantism in transgenic mice (390).

Mutations of the *ras* genes are uncommon in pituitary adenomas (392,415,447), however there is one report of a highly aggressive prolactinoma with a mutation of codon 12 of *H-ras* (421). In contrast, *ras* mutations have been detected in pituitary carcinomas, suggesting that this mutation may be a requisite event for malignant transformation. Conserved mutations in the V3 region of the α-isoform of the signaling kinase, protein kinase-C (PKC), have been described in a selected series of invasive pituitary adenomas (377).

Inactivation of both alleles of the putative MEN-1 tumor suppressor site at 11q13 was initially regarded as a potential "hot spot" for sporadic pituitary adenomas. Indeed, deletions of significant portions of this locus were described in some early reports (391). Subsequent studies, however, have shown allelic deletions in only a minority of sporadic functional and nonfunctional adenomas (389,415). In some instances, this genetic material loss was associated with Gsα mutations (415,466) or *ras* heterozygosity. Only a relatively small number of pituitary adenomas from patients with MEN-1 have been examined for loss of chromosome 11q13 genetic material. While most pituitary adenomas are composed of a monoclonal cell population, there is evidence that loss of heterozygosity (LOH) at the 11q13 site is a rare event in sporadic adenomas (476). Since the recent cloning and characterization of the gene responsible for MEN-1 (394) it has been possible to determine that germline mutations of the menin gene are associated with LOH of the normal allele in pituitary adenomas of patients with MEN-1, but that mutations and LOH of this gene are rare in sporadic pituitary adenomas, occurring in only approximately 5 percent of such lesions (478).

The retinoblastoma (*Rb*) gene is another member of the family of tumor suppressor genes that has been implicated in several neoplasms including retinoblastoma and osteosarcoma. Mice heterozygous for an *Rb* mutation develop pituitary tumors of intermediate lobe corticotroph differentiation (418,419). Paradoxically, however, no such mutations have been identified in human pituitary adenomas (395,477). Instead, preliminary data shows LOH at sites telomeric and centromeric to the *Rb* locus in some aggressive pituitary adenomas (446). These data argue for an independent tumor suppressor gene on 13q which is closely linked with but is not *Rb*.

Another interesting finding is the absence of mutations or deletions in the p53 tumor suppressor gene (415,465) and lack of mutations or overexpression of the c-*erb*B-2/*neu* proto-oncogene (401) in pituitary adenomas.

Growth Factors and Pituitary Tumorigenesis

Growth factors are polypeptides which activate growth-promoting pathways to induce cells to enter and proceed through the cell cycle. They are considered to play an important role in the multistep pathway of tumorigenesis. A number of oncogene products are homologous to growth factors, their receptors, or enzymes that participate in the mitogenic process. In several systems, growth factors have been shown to interact with specific membrane receptors in regulating cell growth and gene expression in an autocrine or paracrine manner.

A number of peptide growth factors, classified into several major families, regulate cell replication and functional differentiation by directly altering the expression of specific genes (451). Some are known to affect hormone production and some are, in turn, modulated by hormones (398). A few have been identified in the hypothalamus and play a physiologic role in pituitary regulation (380).

The pituitary is also a site of both synthesis and action of growth factors (398,471). A number of growth factors have been identified in adenohypophysial cells, including insulin-like growth factors-I and -II (IGF-I, IGF-II), epidermal growth factor (EGF), nerve growth factor (NGF) (445), transforming growth factor-alpha (TGF-α), transforming growth factor-beta (TGF-β), and basic fibroblast growth factor (bFGF). Several partially characterized pituitary-derived growth factors have also been described (398,471), including thyroid hormone-inducible growth factor, vascular endothelial growth factor (410), mammary cell growth factor (443), adrenal growth factor (453), chondrocyte growth factor (420,422), and adipocyte growth factor. Some of these are released by pituitary cells in vitro. These substances may modulate hormone production as well as cell growth in human pituitary adenomas. The regulation of circulating or pituitary-derived growth factors and their respective receptors may, therefore, be important determinants of pituitary cell function and trophic hormone secretion. Limited preliminary evidence suggests that human pituitary tumor cells produce multiple peptides which stimulate rat adenohypophysial cell replication in vitro (472). The relative significance of these different growth factors in human pituitary adenomas remains to be established, however, several have been implicated in the pathogenesis of these tumors.

TGF-α is expressed as a membrane-anchored protein by human adenohypophysial cells and tumors (400). TGF-α may alter pituitary production of GH, PRL, and TSH as well as cell proliferation (403). Estrogen stimulation has been implicated in pituitary tumorigenesis (426) and

TGF-α appears to mediate some estrogenic effects (442). Targeted overexpression of TGF-α under the control of the PRL promoter results in lactotroph adenomas (439), providing compelling evidence for the significance of this growth factor in pituitary tumorigenesis.

EGF is expressed by human pituitary tumors (431). It is detectable by immunohistochemistry in most adenohypophysial cells and its mRNA is expressed with marked variation in all types of functional and nonfunctional adenomas. Like TGF-α with which it shares a receptor, it may have a paracrine or autocrine mechanism for regulation of pituitary cell growth and hormone production (431).

The common receptor of EGF and TGF-α, EGF-R, is a 170-kD plasma membrane protein product of the proto-oncogene v-*erb*β. Its cytoplasmic domain requires intrinsic tyrosine kinase activation. This activating signal may arrive from ligand-induced conformational change in the extracellular domain. Alternatively, the kinase site is regulated by interoceptor association-dissociation in a homodimeric or heterodimeric fashion. EGF-R is overexpressed in several types of human cancers and in most instances this overexpression is accompanied by TGF-α expression; expression of this receptor appears to correlate with tumor aggressiveness. EGF-R is expressed by pituitary adenomas, with the highest levels detected in recurrent somatotroph adenomas and aggressive silent subtype III adenomas, suggesting a selective mechanism for the EGF/EGF-R family in the growth of aggressive pituitary tumors (431).

The TGF-β family is represented in at least three different forms in the pituitary. Inhibins and activins consist of 2 homodimeric or heterodimeric polypeptide subunits derived from a common precursor (475); inhibin A (α-βA) and inhibin B (α-βB) selectively inhibit the release of FSH from pituitary gonadotroph cells whereas activin (βA-βB), activin A (βA-βA), and activin B (βB-βB) stimulate its release. Inhibin subunits are expressed by pituitary gonadotroph adenomas (376,413) and activin is known to stimulate hormone secretion by these tumors (374). Activin effects are mediated by two kinds of binding proteins, activin receptors and follistatin (475); the former are required for activin binding, but follistatin binds the protein resulting in decreased activity. Activin receptors are expressed in gonadotroph adenomas and interestingly, follistatin expression is reduced or absent in some, suggesting the possibility of enhanced activin stimulation as a pathogenetic mechanism in the development of these common pituitary tumors (448).

Basic fibroblast growth factor (bFGF, also known as FGF-2) is 1 of 9 members of the FGF family that has potent mitogenic, angiogenic, and hormone regulatory functions (438). bFGF immunoreactivity was described originally in the nonhormone-producing bovine pituitary folliculo-stellate cells that have been implicated in paracrine regulation within the adenohypophysis (411). bFGF has been shown to regulate GH, PRL, and TSH secretion by the hormone-producing adenohypophysial cells of the rodent pituitary (385,430). bFGF is produced by human pituitary adenomas (399,432,434). Pituitary-derived bFGF stimulates replication of PRL-secreting cells but also may inhibit DNA synthesis in pituitary adenoma cells (449), suggesting that some forms of the growth factor or its receptor may act as a growth inhibitor. Elevated blood concentrations of bFGF-like immunoreactivity have been noted in patients with multiple endocrine neoplasia (MEN)-1 (479) and in patients with sporadic pituitary adenomas (399). The FGF-related *hst* gene has been found in transforming DNA of human PRL-secreting tumors (408) and transfection studies have shown that *hst* facilitates lactotroph proliferation in vivo and in vitro (460). Transgenic mice expressing bFGF under the control of the GH and α-subunit promoters developed hyperplasia of several adenohypophysial cell types but not frank adenomatous changes (473). Recently, altered FGF receptors were identified in pituitary adenomas, including a novel truncated kinase isoform of FGFR4 (370). These data suggest that a member of the FGF family or the FGF receptor family may play an important role in pituitary tumorigenesis.

REFERENCES

Epidemiology of Pituitary Adenomas

1. Apel RL, Wilson RJ, Asa SL. A composite somatotroph-corticotroph pituitary adenoma. Endocr Pathol 1994;5:240–6.
2. Burrow GN, Wortzman G, Rewcastle NB, Holgate RC, Kovacs K. Microadenomas of the pituitary and abnormal sellar tomograms in an unselected autopsy series. N Engl J Med 1981;304:156–8.
3. Costello RT. Subclinical adenoma of the pituitary gland. Am J Pathol 1936;12:205–15.
4. Elster AD. Modern imaging of the pituitary. Radiology 1993;187:1–14.
5. Gold EB. Epidemiology of pituitary adenomas. Epid Rev 1981;3:163–83.
6. Hardy J. Transsphenoidal microsurgery of the normal and pathological pituitary. In: Clinical neurosurgery. Proceedings of the Congress of Neurological Surgeons, 1968. Baltimore: Williams & Wilkins, 1969:185–217.
7. Kane LA, Leinung MC, Scheithauer BW, et al. Pituitary adenomas in childhood and adolescence. J Clin Endocrinol Metab 1994;79:1135–40.
8. Klibanski A, Zervas NT. Diagnosis and management of hormone-secreting pituitary adenomas. N Engl J Med 1991;324:822–31.
9. Kontogeorgos G, Kovacs K, Horvath E, Scheithauer BW. Multiple adenomas of the human pituitary. A retrospective autopsy study with clinical implications. J Neurosurg 1991;74:243–7.
10. Kontogeorgos G, Scheithauer BW, Horvath E, et al. Double adenomas of the pituitary: a clinicopathological study of 11 tumors. Neurosurgery 1992;31:840–9.
11. Kovacs K, Horvath E. Tumors of the pituitary gland. Atlas of Tumor Pathology, 2nd Series, Fascicle 21. Washington, D.C.: Armed Forces Institute of Pathology, 1986.
12. Kovacs K, Ryan N, Horvath E, Singer W, Ezrin C. Pituitary adenomas in old age. J Gerontol 1980;35:16–22.
13. McComb DJ, Ryan N, Horvath E, Kovacs K. Subclinical adenomas of the human pituitary. New light on old problems. Arch Pathol Lab Med 1983;107:488–91.
14. Mindermann T, Wilson CB. Age-related and gender-related occurrence of pituitary adenomas. Clin Endocrinol 1994;41:359–64.
15. Mukai K, Seljeskog EL, Dehner LP. Pituitary adenomas in patients under 20 years old. A clinicopathological study of 12 cases. J Neurooncol 1986;4:79–89.
16. Parent AD, Brown B, Smith EE. Incidental pituitary adenomas: a retrospective study. Surgery 1982;92:880–3.
17. Scheithauer BW. Surgical pathology of the pituitary: the adenomas. Part I. Pathol Ann 1984;19:317–74.
18. Terada T, Kovacs K, Stefaneanu L, Horvath E. Incidence, pathology, and recurrence of pituitary adenomas: study of 647 unselected surgical cases. Endocr Pathol 1995;6:301–10.
19. Thodou E, Kontogeorgos G, Horvath E, Kovacs K, Smyth HS, Ezzat S. Asynchronous pituitary adenomas with differing morphology. Arch Pathol Lab Med 1995;119:748–50.
20. Wilson CB, Dempsey LC. Transsphenoidal microsurgical removal of 250 pituitary adenomas. J Neurosurg 1978;48:13–22.

Classifications of Pituitary Adenomas

21. Anniko M, Tribukait B, Wersäll J. DNA ploidy and cell phase in human pituitary tumors. Cancer 1984;53:1708–13.
22. Fitzgibbons PL, Appley AJ, Turner RR, et al. Flow cytometric analysis of pituitary tumors. Correlation of nuclear antigen p105 and DNA content with clinical behavior. Cancer 1988;62:1556–60.
23. Gandour-Edwards R, Kapadia SB, Janecka IP, Martinez AJ, Barnes L. Biologic markers of invasive pituitary adenomas involving the sphenoid sinus. Mod Pathol 1995;8:160–4.
24. Hardy J. Transsphenoidal surgery of hypersecreting pituitary tumors. In: Kohler PO, Ross GT, eds. Diagnosis and treatment of pituitary tumors. Int Congress Series No. 303. Amsterdam: Exerpta Medica, 1973:179–98.
25. Horvath E, Kovacs K, Smyth HS, et al. A novel type of pituitary adenoma: morphological features and clinical correlations. J Clin Endocrinol Metab 1988;66:1111–8.
26. Hsu DW, Hakim F, Biller BM, et al. Significance of proliferating cell nuclear antigen index in predicting pituitary adenoma recurrence. J Neurosurg 1993;78:753–61.
27. Knosp E, Kitz K, Perneczky A. Proliferation activity in pituitary adenomas: measurement by monoclonal antibody Ki-67. Neurosurgery 1989;25:927–30.
28. Kovacs K, Horvath E. Tumors of the pituitary gland. Atlas of Tumor Pathology, 2nd Series, Fascicle 21. Washington, D.C.: Armed Forces Institute of Pathology, 1986.
29. Kovacs K, Horvath E, Ryan N, Ezrin C. Null cell adenoma of the human pituitary. Virchows Arch [Pathol Anat] 1980;387:165–74.
30. Landolt AM, Shibata T, Kleihues P. Growth rate of human pituitary adenomas. J Neurosurg 1987;67:803–6.
31. Thapar K, Kovacs K, Scheithauer BW, et al. Proliferative activity and invasiveness among pituitary adenomas and carcinomas: an analysis using the MIB-1 antibody. Neurosurgery 1996;38:99–107.
32. Sautner D, Saeger W. Invasiveness of pituitary adenomas. Pathol Res Pract 1991;187:632–6.
33. Scheithauer BW, Kovacs KT, Laws ER Jr, Randall RV. Pathology of invasive pituitary tumors with special reference to functional classification. J Neurosurg 1986;65:733–44.
34. Selman WR, Laws ER Jr, Scheithauer BW, Carpenter SM. The occurrence of dural invasion in pituitary adenomas. J Neurosurg 1986;64:402–7.
35. Takino H, Herman V, Weiss M, Melmed S. Purine-binding factor (nm23) gene expression in pituitary tumors: marker of adenoma invasiveness. J Clin Endocrinol Metab 1995;80:1733–8.
36. van der Mey AG, van Krieken JH, Van Dulken H, van Seters AP, Vielvoye J, Hulshof JH. Large pituitary adenomas with extension into the nasopharynx. Report of three cases with a review of the literature. Ann Otol Rhinol Laryngol 1989;98:618–24.
37. Wong K, Raisanen J, Taylor SL, McDermott MW, Wilson CB, Gutin PH. Pituitary adenoma as an unsuspected clival tumor. Am J Surg Pathol 1995;19:900–3.

Pituitary Adenomas Causing Growth Hormone Excess

38. Arafah BM, Brodkey JS, Kaufman B, Velasco M, Manni A, Pearson OH. Transsphenoidal microsurgery in the treatment of acromegaly and gigantism. J Clin Endocrinol Metab 1980;50:578–85.
39. Arafah BM, Rosenzweig JL, Fenstermaker R, Salazar R, McBride CE, Selman W. Value of growth hormone dynamics and somatomedin C (insulin-like growth factor 1) levels in predicting the long-term benefit after transsphenoidal surgery for acromegaly. J Lab Clin Med 1987;109:346–54.
40. Asa SL, Felix I, Kovacs K, Ramyar L. Effects of somatostatin on somatotroph adenomas of the human pituitary: an in vitro functional and morphological study. Endocr Pathol 1990;1:228–35.
41. Asa SL, Kovacs K, Horvath E, Singer W, Smyth HS. Hormone secretion in vitro by plurihormonal pituitary adenomas of the acidophil cell line. J Clin Endocrinol Metab 1992;75:68–75.
42. Asa SL, Puy LA, Lew AM, Sundmark VC, Elsholtz HP. Cell type-specific expression of the pituitary transcription activator Pit-1 in the human pituitary and pituitary adenomas. J Clin Endocrinol Metab 1993;77:1275–80.
43. Asa SL, Scheithauer BW, Bilbao JM, et al. A case for hypothalamic acromegaly: a clinicopathological study of six patients with hypothalamic gangliocytomas producing growth hormone-releasing factor. J Clin Endocrinol Metab 1984;58:796–803.
44. Barakat S, Melmed S. Reversible shrinkage of a growth hormone-secreting pituitary adenoma by a long-acting somatostatin analogue, octreotide. Arch Intern Med 1989;149:1443–5.
45. Barkan AL, Kelch RP, Hopwood NJ, Beitins IZ. Treatment of acromegaly with the long-acting somatostatin analog SMS 201-995. J Clin Endocrinol Metab 1988;66:16–23.
46. Barkan AL, Lloyd RV, Chandler WF, et al. Preoperative treatment of acromegaly with long-acting somatostatin analog SMS 201-995: shrinkage of invasive pituitary macroadenomas and improved surgical remission rate. J Clin Endocrinol Metab 1988;67:1040–8.
47. Barnard LB, Grantham WG, Lamberton P, O'Dorisio TM, Jackson IM. Treatment of resistant acromegaly with a long-acting somatostatin analogue (SMS 201-995). Ann Intern Med 1986;105:856–61.
48. Baumann G. Acromegaly. Endocrinol Metab Clin North Am 1987;16:685–703.
49. Beck-Peccoz P, Bassetti M, Spada A, et al. Glycoprotein hormone α-subunit response to growth hormone (GH)-releasing hormone in patients with active acromegaly. Evidence for α-subunit and GH coexistence in the same tumoral cell. J Clin Endocrinol Metab 1985;61:541–6.
50. Berelowitz M, Szabo M, Frohman LA, Firestone S, Chu L, Hintz RL. Somatomedin-C mediates growth hormone negative feedback by effects on both the hypothalamus and the pituitary. Science 1981;212:1279–81.
51. Bevan JS, Asa SL, Rossi ML, Esiri MM, Adams CB, Burke CW. Intrasellar gangliocytoma containing gastrin and growth hormone-releasing hormone associated with a growth hormone-secreting pituitary adenoma. Clin Endocrinol (Oxf) 1989;30:213–24.
52. Chanson P, Timsit J, Masquet C, et al. Cardiovascular effects of the somatostatin analog octreotide in acromegaly. Ann Intern Med 1990;113:921–5.

53. Chiodini PG, Cozzi R, Dallabonzana D, et al. Medical treatment of acromegaly with SMS 201-995, a somatostatin analog: a comparison with bromocriptine. J Clin Endocrinol Metab 1987;64:447–53.

54. Christensen SE, Weeke J, Orskov H, et al. Continuous subcutaneous pump infusion of somatostatin analogue SMS201-995 versus subcutaneous injection schedule in acromegalic patients. Clin Endocrinol (Oxf) 1987;27:297–306.

55. Corenblum B, Sirek AM, Horvath E, Kovacs K, Ezrin C. Human mixed somatotrophic and lactotrophic pituitary adenomas. J Clin Endocrinol Metab 1976;42:857–63.

56. Dons RF, Rieth KG, Gordon P, Roth J. Size and erosive features of the sella turcica in acromegaly as predictors of therapeutic response to supervoltage irradiation. Am J Med 1983;74:69–72.

57. Eastman RC, Gorden P, Glatstein E, Roth J. Radiation therapy of acromegaly. Endocrinol Metab Clin North Am 1992;21:693–712.

58. Eastman RC, Gorden P, Roth J. Conventional supervoltage irradiation is an effective treatment for acromegaly. J Clin Endocrinol Metab 1979;48:931–40.

59. Evans HM, Long JA. The effect of the anterior lobe administered intraperitoneally upon growth, maturity, and oestrous cycles of the rat. Anat Rec 1921;21:62–3.

60. Ezzat S, Asa SL, Stefaneanu L, et al. Somatotroph hyperplasia without pituitary adenoma associated with a long standing growth hormone-releasing hormone-producing bronchial carcinoid. J Clin Endocrinol Metab 1994;78:555–60.

61. Ezzat S, Ezrin C, Yamashita S, Melmed S. Recurrent acromegaly resulting from ectopic growth hormone gene expression by a metastatic pancreatic tumor. Cancer 1993;71:66–70.

62. Ezzat S, Horvath E, Harris AG, Kovacs K. Morphological effects of octreotide on growth hormone-producing pituitary adenomas. J Clin Endocrinol Metab 1994;79:113–8.

63. Ezzat S, Kontogeorgos G, Redelmeier DA, Horvath E, Harris AG, Kovacs K. In vivo responsiveness of morphological variants of growth hormone-producing pituitary adenomas to octreotide. Eur J Endocr 1995;133:686–90.

64. Ezzat S, Redelmeier DA, Gnehm M, Harris AG. A prospective multicenter octreotide dose response study in the treatment of acromegaly. J Endocrinol Invest 1995;18:364–9.

65. Ezzat S, Snyder PJ, Young WF, et al. Octreotide treatment of acromegaly. A randomized, multicenter study. Ann Intern Med 1992;117:711–8.

66. Faglia G, Arosio M, Bazzoni N. Ectopic acromegaly. Endocrinol Metab Clin North Am 1992;21:575–95.

67. Felix IA, Horvath E, Kovacs K, Smyth HS, Killinger DW, Vale J. Mammosomatotroph adenoma of the pituitary associated with gigantism and hyperprolactinemia. A morphological study including immunoelectron microscopy. Acta Neuropathol (Berl) 1986;71:76–82.

68. Frawley LS, Boockfor FR. Mammosomatotropes: presence and functions in normal and neoplastic pituitary tissue. Endocr Rev 1991;12:337–55.

69. Frohman LA. Therapeutic options in acromegaly. J Clin Endocrinol Metab 1991;72:1175–81.

70. García-Uría J, Del Pozo JM, Bravo G. Functional treatment of acromegaly by transsphenoidal microsurgery. J Neurosurg 1978;49:36–40.

71. George SR, Kovacs K, Asa SL, Horvath E, Cross EG, Burrow GN. Effect of SMS 201-995, a long-acting somatostatin analogue, on the secretion and morphology of a pituitary growth hormone cell adenoma. Clin Endocrinol (Oxf) 1987;26:395–405.

72. Giovanelli MA, Motti ED, Paracchi A, Beck-Peccoz P, Ambrosi B, Faglia G. Treatment of acromegaly by transsphenoidal microsurgery. J Neurosurg 1976;44:677–86.

73. Glikson M, Gil-Ad I, Galun E, et al. Acromegaly due to ectopic growth hormone-releasing hormone secretion by a bronchial carcinoid tumour. Dynamic hormonal responses to various stimuli. Acta Endocrinol (Copenh) 1991;125:366–71.

74. Gorden P, Comi RJ, Maton PN, Go VL. NIH conference. Somatostatin and somatostatin analogue (SMS 201-995) in treatment of hormone-secreting tumors of the pituitary and gastrointestinal tract and non-neoplastic diseases of the gut. Ann Intern Med 1989;110:35–50.

75. Grunstein RR, Ho KK, Sullivan CE. Effect of octreotide, a somatostatin analog, on sleep apnea in patients with acromegaly. Ann Intern Med 1994;121:478–83.

76. Halse J, Harris AG, Kvistborg A, et al. A randomized study of SMS 201-995 versus bromocriptine treatment in acromegaly: clinical and biochemical effects. J Clin Endocrinol Metab 1990;70:1254–61.

77. Harris AG, Kokoris SP, Ezzat S. Continuous versus intermittent subcutaneous infusion of octreotide in the treatment of acromegaly. Endocrinology 1995;35:59–71.

78. Herman V, Weiss M, Becker D, Melmed S. Hypothalamic hormonal regulation of human growth hormone gene expression in somatotroph adenoma cell cultures. Endocr Pathol 1990;1:236–44.

79. Ho KY, Evans WS, Thorner MO. Disorders of prolactin and growth hormone secretion. Clin Endocrinol Metab 1985;14:1–32.

80. Ho KY, Weissberger AJ, Marbach P, Lazarus L. Therapeutic efficacy of the somatostatin analog SMS 201-995 (octreotide) in acromegaly. Effects of dose and frequency and long-term safety. Ann Intern Med 1990;112:173–81.

81. Horvath E, Kovacs K. The adenohypophysis. In: Kovacs K, Asa SL, eds. Functional endocrine pathology. Boston: Blackwell Scientific Publications, 1991:245–81.

82. Horvath E, Kovacs K, Killinger DW, Smyth HS, Weiss MH, Ezrin C. Mammosomatotroph cell adenoma of the human pituitary: a morphologic entity. Virchows Arch [A] 1983;398:277–89.

83. Jaffe CA, Barkan AL. Treatment of acromegaly with dopamine agonists. Endocrinol Metab Clin North Am 1992;21:713–35.

84. Kawakita S, Asa SL, Kovacs K. Effects of growth hormone-releasing hormone (GHRH) on densely granulated somatotroph adenomas and sparsely granulated somatotroph adenomas in vitro: a morphological and functional investigation. J Endocrinol Invest 1989;12:443–8.

85. Klijn JG, Lamberts SW, de Jong FH, van Dongen KJ, Birkenhäger JC. Interrelationships between tumour size, age, plasma growth hormone and incidence of extrasellar extension in acromegalic patients. Acta Endocrinol (Copenh) 1980;95:289–97.

86. Kontogeorgos G, Asa SL, Kovacs K, Smyth HS, Singer W. Production of alpha-subunit of glycoprotein hormones by pituitary somatotroph adenomas in vitro. Acta Endocrinol (Copenh) 1993;129:565–72.

87. Kontogeorgos G, Kovacs K, Scheithauer BW, Rologis D, Orphanidis G. Alpha-subunit immunoreactivity in plurihormonal pituitary adenomas of patients with acromegaly. Mod Pathol 1991;4:191–5.

88. Kovacs K, Horvath E. Tumors of the pituitary gland. Atlas of Tumor Pathology, 2nd Series, Fascicle 21. Washington, DC: Armed Forces Institute of Pathology, 1986.

89. Kvistborg-Flogstad A, Halse J, Graass P, et al. A comparison of octreotide, bromocriptine, or a combination of both drugs in acromegaly. J Clin Endocrinol Metab 1994;79:461–5.

90. Lamberts SW. The role of somatostatin in the regulation of anterior pituitary hormone secretion and the use of its analogs in the treatment of human pituitary tumors. Endocr Rev 1988;9:417–36.

91. Lamberts SW, Krenning EP, Reubi JC. The role of somatostatin and its analogs in the diagnosis and treatment of tumors. Endocr Rev 1991;12:450–82.

92. Lamberts SW, Zweens M, Klijn JG, van Vroonhoven CC, Stefanko SZ, Del Pozo E. The sensitivity of growth hormone and prolactin secretion to the somatostatin analogue SMS 201-995 in patients with prolactinomas and acromegaly. Clin Endocrinol (Oxf) 1986;25:201–12.

93. Landolt AM, Osterwalder V, Stuckmann G. Preoperative treatment of acromegaly with SMS 201-995: surgical and pathological observations. In: Lüdecke DK, Tolis G, eds. Growth hormone, growth factors, and acromegaly. New York: Raven Press, 1987:229–44.

94. Laws ER Jr, Piepgras DG, Randall RV, Abboud CF. Neurosurgical management of acromegaly. Results in 82 patients treated between 1972 and 1977. J Neurosurg 1979;50:454–61.

95. Li J, Stefaneanu L, Kovacs K, Horvath E, Smyth HS. Growth hormone (GH) and prolactin (PRL) gene expression and immunoreactivity in GH- and PRL-producing human pituitary adenomas. Virchows Arch [A] 1993;422:193–201.

96. Li JY, Racadot O, Kujas M, Kouadri M, Peillon F, Racadot J. Immunocytochemistry of four mixed pituitary adenomas and intrasellar gangliocytomas associated with different clinical syndromes: acromegaly, amenorrheagalactorrhea, Cushing's disease and isolated tumoral syndrome. Acta Neuropathol (Berl) 1989;77:320–8.

97. Lim MJ, Barkan AL, Buda AJ. Rapid reduction of left ventricular hypertrophy in acromegaly after suppression of growth hormone hypersecretion. Ann Intern Med 1992;117:719–26.

98. Lloyd RV, Anagnostou D, Cano M, Barkan AL, Chandler WF. Analysis of mammosomatotropic cells in normal and neoplastic human pituitary tissues by the reverse hemolytic plaque assay and immunocytochemistry. J Clin Endocrinol Metab 1988;66:1103–10.

99. Loras B, Li JY, Durand A, Trouillas J, Sassolas G, Girod C. GRF et adénomes somatotropes humains. Corrélations in vivo et in vitro entre la libération de GH et les aspects morphologiques et immunocytochimiques. Ann Endocrinol (Paris) 1985;46:373–82.

100. Loras B, Trouillas J, Li Y, Durand A, Girod C, Bertrand J. Inversely related evolution of growth hormone and prolactin secretions in long-term tissue cultures of human pituitary adenomas from acromegalic patients. In Vitro Cell Dev Biol 1988;24:1064–70.

101. Losinski NE, Horvath E, Kovacs K, Asa SL. Immunoelectron microscopic evidence of mammosomatotrophs in human adult and fetal adenohypoph-yses, rat adenohypophyses and human and rat pituitary adenomas. Anat Anz 1991;172:11–6.

102. Lüdecke D, Kautzky R, Saeger W, Schrader D. Selective removal of hypersecreting pituitary adenomas? An analysis of endocrine function, operative and microscopical findings in 101 cases. Acta Neurochir 1976;35:27–42.

103. Marie P. Sur deux cas d'acromégalie. Hypertrophie singulière non congénitale des extremités supérieures, inférieures et céphaliques. Rev Méd 1986;6:297–333.

104. McKnight JA, McCance DR, Sheridan B, et al. A long term dose-response study of somatostatin analogue (SMS 201-995, octreotide) in resistant acromegaly. Clin Endocrinol (Oxf) 1991;34:119–25.

105. Melmed S, Braunstein GD, Chang RJ, Becker DP. Pituitary tumors secreting growth hormone and prolactin. Ann Intern Med 1986;105:238–53.

106. Minkowski O. Ueber einen Fall von Akromegalie. Berl Klin Wochenschr 1987;24:371–4.

107. Nabarro JD. Acromegaly. Clin Endocrinol (Oxf) 1987;26:481–512.

108. Neumann PE, Goldman JE, Horoupian DS, Hess MA. Fibrous bodies in growth hormone-secreting adenomas contain cytokeratin filaments. Arch Pathol Lab Med 1985;109:505–8.

109. Oppenheim DS, Kana AR, Sangha JS, Klibanski A. Prevalence of α-subunit hypersecretion in patients with pituitary tumors: clinically nonfunctioning and somatotroph adenomas. J Clin Endocrinol Metab 1990;70:859–64.

110. Oppizzi G, Liuzzi A, Chiodini P, et al. Dopaminergic treatment of acromegaly: different effects on hormone secretion and tumor size. J Clin Endocrinol Metab 1984;58:988–92.

111. Osamura RY. Immunoelectron microscopic studies of GH and α-subunit in GH secreting pituitary adenomas. Pathol Res Pract 1988;183:569–71.

112. Osamura RY, Watanabe K. Immunohistochemical colocalization of growth hormone (GH) and alpha subunit in human GH secreting pituitary adenomas. Virchows Arch [A] 1987;411:323–30.

113. Phillips LS, Vassilopoulou-Sellin R. Somatomedins. N Engl J Med 1980;302:371–80.

114. Quabbe HJ. Treatment of acromegaly by trans-sphenoidal operation, 90-yttrium implantation and bromocriptine: results in 230 patients. Clin Endocrinol (Oxf) 1982;16:107–19.

115. Rhodes RH, Dusseau JJ, Boyd AS Jr, Knigge KM. Intrasellar neural-adenohypophyseal choristoma. A morphological and immunocytochemical study. J Neuropathol Exp Neurol 1982;41:267–80.

116. Richmond W, Seviour PW, Teal TK, Elkeles RS. Analgesic effect of somatostatin analogue (octreotide) in headache associated with pituitary tumours. Br Med J 1987;295:248–9.

117. Roelfsema F, Van Dulken H, Frölich M. Long-term results of transsphenoidal pituitary microsurgery in 60 acromegalic patients. Clin Endocrinol (Oxf) 1985;23:555–65.

118. Ross DA, Wilson CB. Results of transphenoidal microsurgery for growth hormone-secreting pituitary adenoma in a series of 214 patients. J Neurosurg 1988;68:854–67.

119. Sano T, Asa SL, Kovacs K. Growth hormone-releasing hormone-producing tumors: clinical, biochemical, and morphological manifestations. Endocr Rev 1988;9:357–73.

120. Sano T, Ohshima T, Yamada S. Expression of glycoprotein hormones and intracytoplasmic distribution of cytokeratin in growth hormone-producing pituitary adenomas. Pathol Res Pract 1991;187:530–3.

121. Schulte HM, Benker G, Windeck R, Olbricht T, Reinwein D. Failure to respond to growth hormone releasing hormone (GHRH) in acromegaly due to a GHRH secreting pancreatic tumor: dynamics of multiple endocrine testing. J Clin Endocrinol Metab 1985;61:585–7.

122. Serri O, Somma M, Comtois R, et al. Acromegaly: biochemical assessment of cure after long term follow-up of transsphenoidal selective adenomectomy. J Clin Endocrinol Metab 1985;61:1185–9.

123. Singer W. Does pituitary stalk compression cause hyperprolactinemia? Endocr Pathol 1990;1:65–7.

124. Spada A, Arosio M, Bochicchio D, et al. Clinical, biochemical and morphological correlates in patients bearing growth hormone-secreting pituitary tumors with or without constitutively active adenylyl cyclase. J Clin Endocrinol Metab 1990;71:1421–6.

125. Spada A, Bassetti M, Reza-Elahi F, Arosio M, Gil-del-Alamo P, Vallar L. Differential transduction of dopamine signal in different subtypes of human growth hormone-secreting adenomas. J Clin Endocrinol Metab 1994;78:411–7.

126. Spada A, Elahi FR, Arosio M, et al. Lack of desensitization of adenomatous somatotrophs to growth hormone-releasing hormone in acromegaly. J Clin Endocrinol Metab 1987;64:585–91.

127. Stolar MW, Amburn K, Baumann G. Plasma "big" and "big-big" growth hormone (GH) in man: an oligomeric series composed of structurally diverse GH monomers. J Clin Endocrinol Metab 1984;59:212–8.

128. Teitelman G, Alpert S, Polak JM, Martinez A, Hanahan D. Precursor cells of mouse endocrine pancreas coexpress insulin, glucagon and the neuronal proteins tyrosine hydroxylase and neuropeptide Y, but not pancreatic polypeptide. Development 1993;118:1031–9.

129. Thorner MO, Frohman LA, Leong DA, et al. Extrahypothalamic growth hormone-releasing factor (GRF) secretion is a rare cause of acromegaly: plasma GRF levels in 177 acromegalic patients. J Clin Endocrinol Metab 1984;59:846–9.

130. Thorner MO, Perryman RL, Cronin MJ, et al. Somatotroph hyperplasia. Successful treatment of acromegaly by removal of a pancreatic islet tumor secreting a growth hormone-releasing factor. J Clin Invest 1982;70:965–77.

131. Trouillas J, Girod C, Lhéritier M, Claustrat B, Dubois MP. Morphological and biochemical relationships in 31 human pituitary adenomas with acromegaly. Virchows Arch [Pathol Anat] 1980;389:127–42.

132. Trouillas J, Loras B, Guigard MP, Girod C. Alpha-subunit secretion by normal and tumoral growth hormone cells in humans [Abstract]. Endocr Pathol 1992;3:S53.

133. Ur E, Mather SJ, Bomanji J, et al. Pituitary imaging using a labelled somatostatin analogue in acromegaly. Clin Endocrinol (Oxf) 1992;36:147–50.

134. Vance ML, Harris AG. Long-term treatment of 189 acromegalic patients with the somatostatin analog octreotide. Results of the International Multicenter Acromegaly Study Group. Arch Intern Med 1991;151:1573–8.

135. Wass JA, Laws ER Jr, Randall RV, Sheline GE. The treatment of acromegaly. Clin Endocrinol Metab 1986;15:683–707.

136. Zafar M, Ezzat S, Ramyar L, Pan N, Smyth HS, Asa SL. Cell-specific expression of estrogen receptor in the human pituitary and its adenomas. J Clin Endocrinol Metab 1995;80:3621–7.

Pituitary Adenomas Causing Prolactin Excess

137. Ahumada JC, del Castillo EB. Amenorrea y galactorrhea. Bol Soc Gin Y Obstet. 1932;11:64.

137a. Argonz J, Del Castillo EB. A syndrome characterized by estrogenic insufficiency, galactorrhea and decreased urinary gonadotropin. J Clin Endocrinol Metab 1953;13:79–87.

138. Asa SL, Kovacs K, Horvath E, Singer W, Smyth HS. Hormone secretion in vitro by plurihormonal pituitary adenomas of the acidophil cell line. J Clin Endocrinol Metab 1992;75:68–75.

139. Asa SL, Puy LA, Lew AM, Sundmark VC, Elsholtz HP. Cell type-specific expression of the pituitary transcription activator Pit-1 in the human pituitary and pituitary adenomas. J Clin Endocrinol Metab 1993;77:1275–80.

140. Blackwell RE. Diagnosis and management of prolactinomas. Fertil Steril 1985;43:5–16.

141. Burrow GN, Wortzman G, Rewcastle NB, Holgate RC, Kovacs K. Microadenomas of the pituitary and abnormal sellar tomograms in an unselected autopsy series. N Engl J Med 1981;304:156–8.

142. Ciric I, Mikhael M, Stafford T, Lawson L, Garces R. Transsphenoidal microsurgery of pituitary macroadenomas with long-term follow-up results. J Neurosurg 1983;59:395–1.

143. Domingue JN, Richmond IL, Wilson CB. Results of surgery in 114 patients with prolactin-secreting pituitary adenomas. Am J Obstet Gynecol 1980;137:102–8.

144. Fahlbusch R, Buchfelder M, Schrell U. Short-term preoperative treatment of macroprolactinomas by dopamine agonists. J Neurosurg 1987;67:807–15.

145. Fields K, Kulig E, Lloyd RV. Detection of prolactin messenger RNA in mammary and other normal and neoplastic tissues by polymerase chain reaction. Lab Invest 1993;68:354–60.

146. Forbes AP, Henneman PH, Griswold GC, Albright F. Syndrome characterized by galactorrhea, amenorrhea and low urinary FSH: comparison with acromegaly and normal lactation. J Clin Endocrinol Metab 1954;14:265–71.

147. Frommel R. Ueber puerperale Atrophie des Uterus. Z Geburtshilfe Gynakol 1882;7:305–13.

148. Gellersen B, Kempf R, Telgmann R, DiMattia GE. Nonpituitary human prolactin gene transcription is independent of Pit-1 and differentially controlled in lymphocytes and in endometrial stroma. Mol Endocrinol 1994;8:356–73.

149. Grisoli F, Vincentelli F, Jaquet P, Guibout M, Hassoun J, Farnarier P. Prolactin secreting adenoma in 22 men. Surg Neurol 1980;13:241–7.

150. Grossman A, Besser GM. Prolactinomas. Br Med J 1985;290:182–4.

151. Guyda H, Hwang P, Friesen H. Immunologic evidence for monkey and human prolactin (MPr and HPr). J Clin Endocrinol Metab 1971;32:120–3.

152. Heitz PU, Landolt AM, Zenklusen HR, et al. Immunocytochemistry of pituitary tumors. J Histochem Cytochem 1987;35:1005–11.

153. Ho KY, Evans WS, Thorner MO. Disorders of prolactin and growth hormone secretion. Clin Endocrinol Metab 1985;14:1–32.

154. Hoffman WH, Gala RR, Kovacs K, Subramanian MG. Ectopic prolactin secretion from a gonadoblastoma. Cancer 1987;60:2690–5.

155. Homburg R, West C, Brownell J, Jacobs HS. A double-blind study comparing a new non-ergot, long-acting dopamine agonist, CV 205-502, with bromocriptine in women with hyperprolactinemia. Clin Endocrinol (Oxf) 1990;32:565–71.

156. Horvath E, Kovacs K. The adenohypophysis. In: Kovacs K, Asa SL, eds. Functional endocrine pathology. Boston: Blackwell Scientific Publications, 1991:245–81.

157. Horvath E, Kovacs K, Singer W, Ezrin C, Kerenyi NA. Acidophil stem cell adenoma of the human pituitary. Arch Pathol Lab Med 1977;101:594–9.

158. Horvath E, Kovacs K, Singer W, et al. Acidophil stem cell adenoma of the human pituitary: clinicopathologic analysis of 15 cases. Cancer 1981;47:761–71.

159. Hubbard JL, Scheithauer BW, Abboud CF, Laws ER Jr. Prolactin-secreting adenomas: the preoperative response to bromocriptine treatment and surgical outcome. J Neurosurg 1987;67:816–21.

160. Jay V, Kovacs K, Horvath E, Lloyd RV, Smyth HS. Idiopathic prolactin cell hyperplasia of the pituitary mimicking prolactin cell adenoma: a morphological study including immunocytochemistry, electron microscopy, and in situ hybridization. Acta Neuropathol (Berl) 1991;82:147–51.

161. Klibanski A. Osteoporosis and hyperprolactinemia. Semin Reprod Endocrinol 1984;2:93–8.

162. Koppelman MC, Kurtz DW, Morrish KA, et al. Vertebral body bone mineral content in hyperprolactinemic women. J Clin Endocrinol Metab 1984;59:1050–3.

163. Kovacs K, Horvath E. Tumors of the pituitary gland. Atlas of Tumor Pathology, 2nd Series, Fascicle 21. Washington, D.C.: Armed Forces Institute of Pathology, 1986.

164. Kovacs K, Ryan N, Horvath E, Singer W, Ezrin C. Pituitary adenomas in old age. J Gerontol 1980;35:16–22.

165. Kovacs K, Stefaneanu L, Horvath E, et al. Effect of dopamine agonist medication on prolactin producing pituitary adenomas. A morphological study including immunocytochemistry, electron microscopy and in situ hybridization. Virchows Arch [A] 1991;418:439–46.

166. Laws ER Jr, Fode NC, Redmond MJ. Transsphenoidal surgery following unsuccessful prior therapy. An assessment of benefits and risks in 158 patients. J Neurosurg 1985;63:823–9.

167. Lewis UJ, Singh RN, Sinha YN, VanderLaan WP. Electrophoretic evidence for human prolactin. J Clin Endocrinol Metab 1971;23:153–6.

168. Lipper S, Isenberg HD, Kahn LB. Calcospherites in pituitary prolactinomas. A hypothesis for their formation. Arch Pathol Lab Med 1984;108:31–4.

169. McComb DJ, Ryan N, Horvath E, Kovacs K. Subclinical adenomas of the human pituitary. New light on old problems. Arch Pathol Lab Med 1983;107:488–91.

170. Mehta AE, Reyes FI, Faiman C. Primary radiotherapy of prolactinomas. Eight- to 15-year follow-up. Am J Med 1987;83:49–58.

171. Melmed S, Braunstein GD, Chang RJ, Becker DP. Pituitary tumors secreting growth hormone and prolactin. Ann Intern Med 1986;105:238–53.

172. Molitch ME, Elton RL, Blackwell RE, et al. Bromocriptine as primary therapy for prolactin-secreting macroadenomas: results of a prospective multicenter study. J Clin Endocrinol Metab 1985;60:698–705.

173. Nabarro JD. Pituitary prolactinomas. Clin Endocrinol (Oxf) 1982;17:129–55.

174. Parent AD, Brown B, Smith EE. Incidental pituitary adenomas: a retrospective study. Surgery 1982;92:880–3.

175. Peillon F, Dupuy M, Li JY, et al. Pituitary enlargement with suprasellar extension in functional hyperprolactinemia due to lactotroph hyperplasia: a pseudotumoral disease. J Clin Endocrinol Metab 1991;73:1008–15.

176. Randall RV, Laws ER Jr, Abboud CF, Ebersold MJ, Kao PC, Scheithauer BW. Transsphenoidal microsurgical treatment of prolactin-producing pituitary adenomas. Results in 100 patients. Mayo Clin Proc 1983;58:108–21.

177. Serri O, Rasio E, Beauregard H, Hardy J, Somma M. Recurrence of hyperprolactinemia after selective transsphenoidal adenomectomy in women with prolactinoma. N Engl J Med 1983;309:280–3.

178. Soares MJ, Faria TN, Roby KF, Deb S. Pregnancy and the prolactin family of hormones: coordination of anterior pituitary, uterine, and placental expression. Endocr Rev 1991;12:402–23.

179. Thorner MO, Martin WH, Rogol AD, et al. Rapid regression of pituitary prolactinomas during bromocriptine treatment. J Clin Endocrinol Metab 1980;51:438–45.

180. Tindall GT, Kovacs K, Horvath E, Thorner MO. Human prolactin-producing adenomas and bromocriptine: a histological, immunocytochemical, ultrastructural and morphometric study. J Clin Endocrinol Metab 1982;55:1178–83.

181. Tindall GT, McLanahan CS, Christy JH. Transsphenoidal microsurgery for pituitary tumors associated with hyperprolactinemia. J Neurosurg 1978;48:849–60.

182. Vance ML, Thorner MO. Prolactinomas. Endocrinol Metab Clin North Am 1987;16:731–53.

183. Weiss MH, Wycoff RR, Yadley R, Gott P, Feldon S. Bromocriptine treatment of prolactin-secreting tumors: surgical implications. Neurosurgery 1983;12:640–2.

184. Zafar M, Ezzat S, Ramyar L, Pan N, Smyth HS, Asa SL. Cell-specific expression of estrogen receptor in the human pituitary and its adenomas. J Clin Endocrinol Metab 1995;80:3621–7.

Pituitary Adenomas Causing Thyrotropin Excess

185. Asa SL. Tissue culture in the diagnosis and study of pituitary adenomas. In: Lloyd RV, ed. Surgical pathology of the pituitary gland. Philadelphia: WB Saunders, 1993:94–115.

186. Bevan JS, Burke CW, Esiri MM, et al. Studies of two thyrotrophin-secreting pituitary adenomas: evidence for dopamine receptor deficiency. Clin Endocrinol (Oxf) 1989;31:59–70.

187. Comi RJ, Gesundheit N, Murray L, Gorden P, Weintraub BD. Response of thyrotropin-secreting pituitary adenomas to a long-acting somatostatin analogue. N Engl J Med 1987;317:12–7.

188. Filetti S, Rapoport B, Aron DC, Greenspan FC, Wilson CB, Fraser W. TSH and TSH-subunit production by human thyrotrophic tumour cells in monolayer culture. Acta Endocrinol (Copenh) 1982;99:224–31.

189. Gershengorn MC, Weintraub BD. Thyrotropin-induced hyperthyroidism caused by selective pituitary resistance to thyroid hormone. A new syndrome of "inappropriate secretion of TSH." J Clin Invest 1975;56:633–42.

190. Hershman JM, Higgins HP. Hydatidiform mole—a cause of clinical hyperthyroidism. Report of two cases with evidence that the molar tissue secreted a thyroid stimulator. N Engl J Med 1971;284:573–7.

191. Hill SA, Falko JM, Wilson CB, Hunt WE. Thyrotrophin-producing pituitary adenomas. J Neurosurg 1982;57:515–9.

192. Horvath E, Kovacs K. The adenohypophysis. In: Kovacs K, Asa SL, eds. Functional endocrine pathology. Boston: Blackwell Scientific Publications, 1991:245–81.

193. Khalil A, Kovacs K, Sima AA, Burrow GN, Horvath E. Pituitary thyrotroph hyperplasia mimicking prolactin-secreting adenoma. J Endocrinol Invest 1984;7:399–404.

194. Kourides IA, Ridgway EC, Weintraub BD, Bigos ST, Gershengorn MC, Maloof F. Thyrotropin-induced hyperthyroidism: use of alpha and beta subunit levels to identify patients with pituitary tumors. J Clin Endocrinol Metab 1977;45:534–43.

195. Kovacs K, Horvath E. Tumors of the pituitary gland. Atlas of Tumor Pathology, 2nd Series, Fascicle 21. Washington, D.C.: Armed Forces Institute of Pathology, 1986.

196. Lamberts SW. The role of somatostatin in the regulation of anterior pituitary hormone secretion and the use of its analogs in the treatment of human pituitary tumors. Endocr Rev 1988;9:417–36.

197. Mashiter K, van Noorden S, Fahlbusch R, Fill H, Skrabal K. Hyperthyroidism due to a TSH secreting pituitary adenoma: case report, treatment and evidence for adenoma TSH by morphological and cell culture studies. Clin Endocrinol (Oxf) 1983;18:473–83.

198. Orme SM, Lamb JT, Nelson M, Belchetz PE. Shrinkage of thyrotrophin secreting pituitary adenoma treated with octreotide. Postgrad Med J 1991;67:466–8.

199. Scheithauer BW, Kovacs K, Randall RV, Ryan N. Pituitary gland in hypothyroidism. Histologic and immunocytologic study. Arch Pathol Lab Med 1985;109:499–504.

200. Smallridge RC. Thyrotropin-secreting pituitary tumors. Endocrinol Metab Clin North Am 1987;16:765–92.

201. Smallridge RC, Smith CE. Hyperthyroidism due to thyrotropin-secreting pituitary tumors. Diagnostic and therapeutic considerations. Arch Intern Med 1983;143:503–7.

202. Takamatsu J, Mozai T, Kuma K. Bromocriptine therapy for hyperthyroidism due to increased thyrotropin secretion. J Clin Endocrinol Metab 1984;58:934–6.

203. Trouillas J, Girod C, Loras B, et al. The TSH secretion in the human pituitary adenomas. Pathol Res Pract 1988;183:596–600.

204. Yovos JG, Falko JM, O'Dorisio TM, Malarkey WB, Cataland S, Capen CC. Thyrotoxicosis and a thyrotropin-secreting pituitary tumor causing unilateral exophthalmos. J Clin Endocrinol Metab 1981;53:338–43.

Pituitary Adenomas Causing ACTH Excess

205. Aron DC, Findling JW, Tyrrell JB. Cushing's disease. Endocrinol Metab Clin North Am 1987;16:705–30.

206. Asa SL, Kovacs K, Tindall GT, Barrow DL, Horvath E, Vecsei P. Cushing's disease associated with an intrasellar gangliocytoma producing corticotrophin-releasing factor. Ann Intern Med 1984;101:789–93.

207. Asa SL, Kovacs K, Vale W, Petrusz P, Vecsei P. Immunohistologic localization of corticotrophin-releasing hormone in human tumors. Am J Clin Pathol 1987;87:327–33.

208. Birkenhäger JC, Upton GV, Seldenrath HJ, Krieger DT, Tashjian AH Jr. Medullary thyroid carcinoma: ectopic production of peptides with ACTH-like, corticotrophin releasing factor-like and prolactin production-stimulating activities. Acta Endocrinol (Copenh) 1976;83:280–92.

209. Boggan JE, Tyrrell JB, Wilson CB. Transsphenoidal microsurgical management of Cushing's disease. Report of 100 cases. J Neurosurg 1983;59:195–200.

210. Carey RM, Varma SK, Drake CR Jr, et al. Ectopic secretion of corticotropin-releasing factor as a cause of Cushing's syndrome. A clinical, morphologic, and biochemical study. N Engl J Med 1984;311:13–20.

211. Cushing H. The basophil adenomas of the pituitary body and their clinical manifestations (pituitary basophilism). Bull Johns Hopkins Hosp 1932;50:137–95.

212. Dons RF, Rieth KG, Gordon P, Roth J. Size and erosive features of the sella turcica in acromegaly as predictors of therapeutic response to supervoltage irradiation. Am J Med 1983;74:69–72.

213. Eastman RC, Gorden P, Roth J. Conventional supervoltage irradiation is an effective treatment for acromegaly. J Clin Endocrinol Metab 1979;48:931–40.

214. Felix IA, Horvath E, Kovacs K. Massive Crooke's hyalinization in corticotroph cell adenomas of the human pituitary. A histological, immunocytological and electron microscopic study of three cases. Acta Neurochir 1981;58:235–43.

215. Findling JW, Aron DC, Tyrrell JB, et al. Selective venous sampling for ACTH in Cushing's syndrome: differentiation between Cushing's disease and the ectopic ACTH syndrome. Ann Intern Med 1981;94:647–52.

216. Fjellestad-Paulsen A, Abrahamsson PA, Bjartell A, et al. Carcinoma of the prostate with Cushing's syndrome. A case report with immunohistochemical and chemical demonstration of immunoreactive corticotropin-releasing hormone in plasma and tumor tissue. Acta Endocrinol (Copenh) 1988;119:506–16.

217. Franscella S, Favod-Coune CA, Pizzolato G, et al. Pituitary corticotroph adenoma with Crooke's hyalinization. Endocr Pathol 1991;2:111–6.

218. Gold EM. The Cushing syndromes: changing views of diagnosis and treatment. Ann Intern Med 1979;90:829–44.

219. Gold PW, Loriaux DL, Roy A, et al. Responses to corticotropin-releasing hormone in the hypercortisolism of depression and Cushing's disease. Pathophysiologic and diagnostic implications. N Engl J Med 1986;314:1329–35.

220. Grino M, Boudouresque F, Conte-Devolx B, et al. In vitro corticotropin-releasing hormone (CRH) stimulation of adrenocorticotropin release from corticotroph adenoma cells: effect of prolonged exposure to CRH and its interaction with cortisol. J Clin Endocrinol Metab 1988;66:770–5.

221. Hardy J. Cushing's disease: 50 years later. Can J Neurol Sci 1982;9:375–80.

222. Horvath E, Kovacs K. The adenohypophysis. In: Kovacs K, Asa SL, eds. Functional endocrine pathology. Boston: Blackwell Scientific Publications, 1991:245–81.

223. Horvath E, Kovacs K, Josse R. Pituitary corticotroph cell adenoma with marked abundance of microfilaments. Ultrastruct Pathol 1983;5:249–55.

224. Horvath SE, Asa SL, Kovacs K, Adams LA, Singer W, Smyth HS. Human pituitary corticotroph adenomas in vitro: morphologic and functional responses to corticotropin-releasing hormone and cortisol. Neuroendocrinology 1990;51:241–8.

225. Ishibashi M, Yamaji T. Direct effects of thyrotropin-releasing hormone, cyproheptadine, and dopamine on adrenocorticotropin secretion from human corticotroph adenoma cells in vitro. J Clin Invest 1981;68:1018–27.

226. Jessop DS, Cunnah D, Millar JG, et al. A phaeochromocytoma presenting with Cushing's syndrome associated with increased concentrations of circulating corticotrophin-releasing factor. J Endocrinol 1987;113:133–8.

227. Kovacs K, Horvath E. Tumors of the pituitary gland. Atlas of Tumor Pathology, 2nd Series, Fascicle 21. Washington, D.C.: Armed Forces Institute of Pathology, 1986.

228. Krieger DT. Medical treatment of Cushing disease. In: Tolis G, Labrie F, Martin JB, Naftolin F, eds. Clinical neuroendocrinology: a pathophysiological approach. New York: Raven Press, 1979:423–7.

229. Krieger DT, Luria M. Plasma ACTH and cortisol responses to TRF, vasopressin or hypoglycemia in Cushing's disease and Nelson's syndrome. J Clin Endocrinol Metab 1977;44:361–8.

230. Lamberts SW, de Quijada M, Visser TJ. Regulation of prolactin secretion in patients with Cushing's disease. A comparative study on the effects of dexamethasone, lysine vasopressin and ACTH on prolactin secretion by the rat pituitary gland in vitro. Neuroendocrinology 1981;32:150–4.

231. Lamberts SW, Verleun T, Oosterom R, De Jong F, Hackeng WH. Corticotropin-releasing factor (ovine) and vasopressin exert a synergistic effect on adrenocorticotropin release in man. J Clin Endocrinol Metab 1984;58:298–303.

232. Landolt AM, Valvanis A, Girard J, Eberle AN. Corticotrophin-releasing factor-test used with bilateral, simultaneous inferior petrosal sinus blood-sampling for the diagnosis of pituitary-dependent Cushing's disease. Clin Endocrinol (Oxf) 1986;25:687–96.

233. Mampalam TJ, Tyrrell JB, Wilson CB. Transsphenoidal microsurgery for Cushing disease. A report of 216 cases. Ann Intern Med 1988;109:487–93.

234. Nelson DH, Meakin JW, Thorn GW. ACTH-producing pituitary tumors following adrenalectomy for Cushing's syndrome. Ann Intern Med 1960;52:560–9.

235. Neumann PE, Horoupian DS, Goldman JE, Hess MA. Cytoplasmic filaments of Crooke's hyaline change belong to the cytokeratin class. An immunocytochemical and ultrastructural study. Am J Pathol 1984;116:214–22.

236. Nieman LK, Chrousos GP, Oldfield EH, Avgerinos P, Cutler GB Jr, Loriaux DL. The ovine corticotropin-releasing hormone stimulation test and the dexamethasone suppression test in the differential diagnosis of Cushing's syndrome. Ann Intern Med 1986;105:862–7.

237. Nieman LK, Oldfield EH, Wesley R, Chrousos GP, Loriaux DL, Cutler GB Jr. A simplified morning ovine corticotropin-releasing hormone stimulation test for the differential diagnosis of adrenocorticotropin-dependent Cushing's syndrome. J Clin Endocrinol Metab 1993;77:1308–12.

238. Oldfield EH, Chrousos GP, Schulte HM, et al. Preoperative lateralization of ACTH-secreting pituitary microadenomas by bilateral and simultaneous inferior petrosal venous sinus sampling. N Engl J Med 1985;312:100–3.

239. Oldfield EH, Doppman JL, Nieman LK, et al. Petrosal sinus sampling with and without corticotropin-releasing hormone for the differential diagnosis of Cushing's syndrome. N Engl J Med 1991;325:897–905.

240. Oosterom R, Verleun T, Uitterlinden P, et al. ACTH and β-endorphin secretion by three corticotrophic adenomas in culture. Effects of culture time, dexamethasone, vasopressin and synthetic corticotrophin releasing factor. Acta Endocrinol (Copenh) 1984;106:21–9.

241. Orth DN. Cushing's syndrome. N Engl J Med 1995;332:791–803.

242. Orth DN, DeBold CR, DeCherney GS, et al. Pituitary microadenomas causing Cushing's disease respond to corticotropin-releasing factor. J Clin Endocrinol Metab 1982;55:1017–9.

243. Quabbe HJ. Treatment of acromegaly by trans-sphenoidal operation, 90-yttrium implantation and bromocriptine: results in 230 patients. Clin Endocrinol (Oxf) 1982;16:107–19

244. Schteingart DE, Lloyd RV, Akil H, et al. Cushing's syndrome secondary to ectopic corticotropin-releasing hormone-adrenocorticotropin secretion. J Clin Endocrinol Metab 1986;63:770–5.

245. Suda T, Tomori N, Tozawa F, Demura H, Shizume K. Effects of corticotropin-releasing factor and other materials on adrenocorticotropin secretion from pituitary glands of patients with Cushing's disease in vitro. J Clin Endocrinol Metab 1984;59:840–5.

246. Suda T, Tozawa F, Mouri T, et al. Effects of cyproheptadine, reserpine, and synthetic corticotropin-releasing factor on pituitary glands from patients with Cushing's disease. J Clin Endocrinol Metab 1983;56:1094–9.

247. Suda T, Tozawa F, Yamada M, et al. Effects of corticotropin-releasing hormone and dexamethasone on proopiomelanocortin messenger RNA level in human corticotroph adenoma cells in vitro. J Clin Invest 1988;82:110–4.

248. Wass JA, Laws ER Jr, Randall RV, Sheline GE. The treatment of acromegaly. Clin Endocrinol Metab 1986;15:683–707.

249. White MC, Adams EF, Loizou M, Mashiter K. Vasoactive intestinal peptide stimulates adrenocorticotropin release from human corticotropinoma cells in culture: interaction with arginine vasopressin and hydrocortisone. J Clin Endocrinol Metab 1982;55:967–72.

250. White MC, Adams EF, Loizou M, Mashiter K, Fahlbusch R. Corticotropin releasing factor stimulates ACTH release from human pituitary corticotropic tumour cell in culture. Lancet 1982;1:1251–2.

251. White MC, Adams EF, Loizou M, Mashiter K, Fahlbusch R. Ovine corticotrophin releasing factor stimulates ACTH release from human corticotrophinoma cells in culture; interaction with hydrocortisone and arginine vasopressin. Clin Endocrinol (Oxf) 1985;23:295–302.

252. Yamaji T, Ishibashi M, Teramoto A, Fukushima T. Hyperprolactinemia in Cushing's disease and Nelson's syndrome. J Clin Endocrinol Metab 1984;58:790–5.

253. Zárate A, Kovacs K, Flores M, Morán C, Félix I. ACTH and CRF-producing bronchial carcinoid associated with Cushing's syndrome. Clin Endocrinol (Oxf) 1986;24:523–9.

Pituitary Adenomas Causing Gonadotropin Excess

254. Asa SL, Bamberger AM, Cao B, Wong M, Parker KL, Ezzat S. The transcription factor steroidogenic factor-1 is preferentially expressed in the human pituitary gonadotroph. J Clin Endocrinol Metab 1996;81:2165–70.

255. Asa SL, Gerrie BM, Kovacs K, et al. Structure-function correlations of human pituitary gonadotroph adenomas in vitro. Lab Invest 1988;58:403–10.

256. Berezin M, Olchovsky D, Pines A, Tadmor R, Lunenfeld B. Reduction of follicle-stimulating hormone (FSH) secretion in FSH-producing pituitary adenoma by bromocriptine. J Clin Endocrinol Metab 1984;59:1220–3.

257. Cook DM, Watkins S, Snyder PJ. Gonadotrophin-secreting pituitary adenomas masquerading as primary ovarian failure. Clin Endocrinol (Oxf) 1986;25:729–38.

258. Daniels M, Newland P, Dunn J, Kendall-Taylor P, White MC. Long-term effects of a gonadotrophin-releasing hormone agonist ([D-Ser([But)6]GnRH(1-9)nonapeptide-ethylamide) on gonadotrophin secretion from human pituitary gonadotroph cell adenomas in vitro. J Endocrinol 1988;118:491–6.

259. Djerassi A, Coutifaris C, West VA, et al. Gonadotroph adenoma in a premenopausal woman secreting follicle-stimulating hormone and causing ovarian hyperstimulation. J Clin Endocrinol Metab 1995;80:591–4.

260. Ebersold MJ, Quast LM, Laws ER Jr, Scheithauer B, Randall RV. Long-term results in transsphenoidal removal of nonfunctioning pituitary adenomas. J Neurosurg 1986;64:713–9.

261. Gasser RW, Mueller-Holzner E, Skrabal F, et al. Macroprolactinomas and functionless pituitary tumours. Immunostaining and effect of dopamine agonist therapy. Acta Endocrinol (Copenh) 1987;116:253–9.

262. Klibanski A. Nonsecreting pituitary tumors. Endocrinol Metab Clin North Am 1987;16:793–804.

263. Klibanski A, Deutsch PJ, Jameson JL, et al. Luteinizing hormone-secreting pituitary tumor: biosynthetic characterization and clinical studies. J Clin Endocrinol Metab 1987;64:536–42.

264. Klibanski A, Shupnik MA, Bikkal HA, Black PM, Kliman B, Zervas NT. Dopaminergic regulation of α-subunit secretion and messenger ribonucleic acid levels in α-secreting pituitary tumors. J Clin Endocrinol Metab 1988;66:96–102.

265. Koga M, Nakao H, Arao M, et al. Demonstration of specific dopamine receptors on human pituitary adenomas. Acta Endocrinol (Copenh) 1987;114:595–602.

266. Kovacs K, Horvath E, Rewcastle NB, Ezrin C. Gonadotroph cell adenoma of the pituitary in a woman with long-standing hypogonadism. Arch Gynecol 1980;229:57–65.

267. Kwekkeboom DJ, de Jong FH, Lamberts SW. Gonadotropin release by clinically nonfunctioning and gonadotroph pituitary adenomas in vivo and in vitro: relation to sex and effects of thyrotropin-releasing hormone, gonadotropin-releasing hormone, and bromocriptine. J Clin Endocrinol Metab 1989;68:1128–35.

268. Kwekkeboom DJ, Hofland LJ, van Koetsveld PM, Singh R, van den Berge JH, Lamberts SW. Bromocriptine increasingly suppresses the in vitro gonadotropin and α-subunit release from pituitary adenomas during long term culture. J Clin Endocrinol Metab 1990;71:718–24.

269. Lamberts SW. The role of somatostatin in the regulation of anterior pituitary hormone secretion and the use of its analogs in the treatment of human pituitary tumors. Endocr Rev 1988;9:417–36.

270. Lamberts SW, Verleun T, Oosterom R, et al. The effects of bromocriptine, thyrotropin-releasing hormone, and gonadotropin-releasing hormone on hormone secretion by gonadotropin-secreting pituitary adenomas in vivo and in vitro. J Clin Endocrinol Metab 1987;64:524–30.

271. Lloyd RV, Anagnostou D, Chandler WF. Dopamine receptors in immunohistochemically characterized null cell adenomas and normal human pituitaries. Mod Pathol 1988;1:51–6.

272. Oppenheim DS, Klibanski A. Medical therapy of glycoprotein hormone-secreting pituitary tumors. Endocrinol Metab Clin North Am 1989;18:339–58.

273. Roman SH, Goldstein M, Kourides IA, Comite F, Bardin CW, Krieger DT. The luteinizing hormone-releasing hormone (LHRH) agonist [D-Trp6-Pro9-NEt]LHRH increased rather than lowered LH and α-subunit levels in a patient with an LH-secreting pituitary tumor. J Clin Endocrinol Metab 1984;58:313–9.

274. Sassolas G, LeJeune H, Trouillas J, et al. Gonadotropin-releasing hormone agonists are unsuccessful in reducing tumoral gonadotropin secretion in two patients with gonadotropin-secreting pituitary adenomas. J Clin Endocrinol Metab 1988;67:180–5.

275. Snyder PJ. Gonadotroph cell adenomas of the pituitary. Endocr Rev 1985;6:552–63.

276. Snyder PJ. Gonadotroph cell pituitary adenomas. Endocrinol Metab Clin North Am 1987;16:755–64.

277. Snyder PJ, Bashey HM, Kim SU, Chappel SC. Secretion of uncombined subunits of luteinizing hormone by gonadotroph cell adenomas. J Clin Endocrinol Metab 1984;59:1169–75.

278. Tsang RW, Brierley JD, Panzarella T, Gospodarowicz MK, Sutcliffe SB, Simpson WJ. Radiation therapy for pituitary adenoma: treatment outcome and prognostic factors. Int J Radiat Oncol Biol Phys 1994;30:557–65.

279. Vance ML, Ridgway EC, Thorner MO. Follicle-stimulating hormone- and α-subunit-secreting pituitary tumor treated with bromocriptine. J Clin Endocrinol Metab 1985;61:580–4.

280. Vos P, Croughs RJ, Thijssen JH, van't Verlaat JW, van Ginkel LA. Response of luteinizing hormone secreting pituitary adenoma to a long-acting somatostatin analogue. Acta Endocrinol (Copenh) 1988;118:587–90.

281. Wollesen F, Andersen T, Karle A. Size reduction of extrasellar pituitary tumors during bromocriptine treatment. Ann Intern Med 1982;96:281–6.

Clinically Nonfunctioning Pituitary Adenomas

282. Asa SL. Tissue culture in the diagnosis and study of pituitary adenomas. In: Lloyd RV, ed. Surgical pathology of the pituitary gland. Philadelphia: WB Saunders, 1993:94–115.

283. Asa SL, Bamberger AM, Cao B, Wong M, Parker KL, Ezzat S. The transcription factor steroidogenic factor-1 is preferentially expressed in the human pituitary gonadotroph. J Clin Endocrinol Metab 1996;81:2165–70.

284. Asa SL, Cheng Z, Ramyar L, et al. Human pituitary null cell adenomas and oncocytomas in vitro: effects of adenohypophysiotropic hormones and gonadal steroids on hormone secretion and tumor cell morphology. J Clin Endocrinol Metab 1992;74:1128–34.
285. Asa SL, Gerrie BM, Singer W, Horvath E, Kovacs K, Smyth HS. Gonadotropin secretion in vitro by human pituitary null cell adenomas and oncocytomas. J Clin Endocrinol Metab 1986;62:1011–9.
286. Black PM, Hsu DW, Klibanski A, et al. Hormone production in clinically nonfunctioning pituitary adenomas. J Neurosurg 1987;66:244–50.
287. Chabre O, Martinie M, Vivier J, Eimin-Richard E, Bertagna X, Bachelot I. A clinically silent corticotrophic pituitary adenoma (CSCPA) secreting a biologically inactive but immunoreactive assayable ACTH [Abstract]. J Endocrinol Invest 1991;14(suppl 1):87.
288. Daneshdoost L, Gennarelli TA, Bashey HM, et al. Recognition of gonadotroph adenomas in women. N Engl J Med 1991;324:589–94.
289. Ebersold MJ, Quast LM, Laws ER Jr, Scheithauer B, Randall RV. Long-term results in transsphenoidal removal of nonfunctioning pituitary adenomas. J Neurosurg 1986;64:713–9.
290. Horvath E, Kovacs K. The adenohypophysis. In: Kovacs K, Asa SL, eds. Functional endocrine pathology. Boston: Blackwell Scientific Publications, 1991:245–81.
291. Horvath E, Kovacs K, Killinger DW, Smyth HS, Platts ME, Singer W. Silent corticotropic adenomas of the human pituitary gland: a histologic, immunocytologic, and ultrastructural study. Am J Pathol 1980;98:617–38.
292. Jameson JL, Klibanski A, Black PM, et al. Glycoprotein hormone genes are expressed in clinically nonfunctioning pituitary adenomas. J Clin Invest 1987;80:1472–8.
293. Klibanski A. Nonsecreting pituitary tumors. Endocrinol Metab Clin North Am 1987;16:793–804.
294. Klibanski A, Deutsch PJ, Jameson JL, et al. Luteinizing hormone-secreting pituitary tumor: biosynthetic characterization and clinical studies. J Clin Endocrinol Metab 1987;64:536–42.
295. Klibanski A, Ridgway EC, Zervas NT. Pure alpha subunit-secreting pituitary tumors. J Neurosurg 1983;59:585–9.
296. Klibanski A, Zervas NT, Kovacs K, Ridgway EC. Clinically silent hypersecretion of growth hormone in patients with pituitary tumors. J Neurosurg 1987;66:806–11.
297. Koga M, Nakao H, Arao M, et al. Demonstration of specific dopamine receptors on human pituitary adenomas. Acta Endocrinol (Copenh) 1987;114:595–602.
298. Kontogeorgos G, Horvath E, Kovacs K, Killinger DW, Smyth HS. Null cell adenoma of the pituitary with features of plurihormonality and plurimorphous differentiation. Arch Pathol Lab Med 1991;115:61–4.
299. Kovacs K, Asa SL, Horvath E, et al. Null cell adenomas of the pituitary: attempts to resolve their cytogenesis. In: Lechago J, Kameya T, eds. Endocrine pathology update. New York: Field and Wood, 1990:17–31.
300. Kovacs K, Horvath E. Tumors of the pituitary gland. Atlas of Tumor Pathology, 2nd Series, Fascicle 21. Washington, D.C.: Armed Forces Institute of Pathology, 1986.
301. Kovacs K, Lloyd R, Horvath E, et al. Silent somatotroph adenomas of the human pituitary. A morphologic study of three cases including immunocytochemistry, electron microscopy, in vitro examination, and in situ hybridization. Am J Pathol 1989;134:345–53.
302. Kwekkeboom DJ, de Jong FH, Lamberts SW. Gonadotropin release by clinically nonfunctioning and gonado-troph pituitary adenomas in vivo and in vitro: relation to sex and effects of thyrotropin-releasing hormone, gonadotropin-releasing hormone, and bromocriptine. J Clin Endocrinol Metab 1989;68:1128–35.
303. Lamberts SW. The role of somatostatin in the regulation of anterior pituitary hormone secretion and the use of its analogs in the treatment of human pituitary tumors. Endocr Rev 1988;9:417–36.
304. Lamberts SW, Verleun T, Oosterom R, et al. The effects of bromocriptine, thyrotropin-releasing hormone, and gonadotropin-releasing hormone on hormone secretion by gonadotropin-secreting pituitary adenomas in vivo and in vitro. J Clin Endocrinol Metab 1987;64:524–30.
305. Le Dafniet M, Grouselle D, Li JY, et al. Evidence of thyrotropin-releasing hormone (TRH) and TRH-binding sites in human nonsecreting pituitary adenomas. J Clin Endocrinol Metab 1987;65:1014–9.
306. Lloyd RV, Anagnostou D, Chandler WF. Dopamine receptors in immunohistochemically characterized null cell adenomas and normal human pituitaries. Mod Pathol 1988;1:51–6.
307. Lloyd RV, Fields K, Jin L, Horvath E, Kovacs K. Analysis of endocrine active and clinically silent corticotropic adenomas by in situ hybridization. Am J Pathol 1990;137:479–88.
308. Pagesy P, Li JY, Kujas M, et al. Apparently silent somatotroph adenomas. Pathol Res Pract 1991;187:950–6.
309. Sakurai T, Seo H, Yamamoto N, et al. Detection of mRNA of prolactin and ACTH in clinically nonfunctioning pituitary adenomas. J Neurosurg 1988;69:653–9.
310. Singer W. Does pituitary stalk compression cause hyperprolactinemia? Endocr Pathol 1990;1:65–7.
311. Snyder PJ. Gonadotroph cell adenomas of the pituitary. Endocr Rev 1985;6:552–63.
312. Song JY, Jin L, Chandler WF, et al. Gonadotropin-releasing hormone regulates gonadotropin β-subunit and chromogranin-B messenger ribonucleic acids in cultured chromogranin-A-positive pituitary adenomas. J Clin Endocrinol Metab 1990;71:622–30.
313. Spada A, Reza-Elahi F, Lania A, Gil-del-Alamo P, Bassetti M, Faglia G. Hypothalamic peptides modulate cytosolic free Ca2+ levels and adenylyl cyclase activity in human nonfunctioning pituitary adenomas. J Clin Endocrinol Metab 1991;73:913–8.
314. Stefaneanu L, Kovacs K. Light microscopic special stains and immunohistochemistry in the diagnosis of pituitary adenomas. In: Lloyd RV, ed. Surgical pathology of the pituitary gland. Philadelphia: WB Saunders, 1993:34–51.
315. Surmont DW, Winslow CL, Loizou M, White MC, Adams EF, Mashiter K. Gonadotrophin and alpha subunit secretion by human functionless pituitary adenomas in cell culture: long term effects of luteinizing hormone releasing hormone and thyrotrophin releasing hormone. Clin Endocrinol (Oxf) 1983;19:325–36.
316. Tourniaire J, Trouillas J, Chalendar D, Bonneton-Emptoz A, Goutelle A, Girod C. Somatotropic adenoma manifested by galactorrhea without acromegaly. J Clin Endocrinol Metab 1985;61:451–3.
317. Trouillas J, Girod C, Sassolas G, Claustrat B. The human gonadotropic adenoma: pathologic diagnosis and hormonal correlations in 26 tumors. Semin Diagn Pathol 1986;3:42–57.
318. Trouillas J, Girod C, Sassolas G, et al. A human β-endorphin pituitary adenoma. J Clin Endocrinol Metab 1984;58:242–9.

319. Trouillas J, Sassolas G, Loras B, et al. Somatotropic adenomas without acromegaly. Pathol Res Pract 1991;187:943–9.

320. Tsang RW, Brierley JD, Panzarella T, Gospodarowicz MK, Sutcliffe SB, Simpson WJ. Radiation therapy for pituitary adenoma: treatment outcome and prognostic factors. Int J Radiat Oncol Biol Phys 1994;30:557–65.

321. Vos P, Croughs RJ, Thijssen JH, van't Verlaat JW, van Ginkel LA. Response of luteinizing hormone secreting pituitary adenoma to a long-acting somatostatin analogue. Acta Endocrinol (Copenh) 1988;118:587–90.

322. Wollesen F, Andersen T, Karle A. Size reduction of extrasellar pituitary tumors during bromocriptine treatment. Ann Intern Med 1982;96:281–6.

323. Yamada S, Asa SL, Kovacs K. Oncocytomas and null cell adenomas of the human pituitary: morphometric and in vitro functional comparison. Virchows Arch [A] 1988;413:333–9.

324. Yamada S, Asa SL, Kovacs K, Muller P, Smyth HS. Analysis of hormone secretion by clinically nonfunctioning human pituitary adenomas using the reverse hemolytic plaque assay. J Clin Endocrinol Metab 1989;68:73–80.

325. Yamada S, Sano T, Stefaneanu L, et al. Endocrine and morphological study of a clinically silent somatotroph adenoma of the human pituitary. J Clin Endocrinol Metab 1993;76:352–6.

Plurihormonal Adenomas

326. Beck-Peccoz P, Bassetti M, Spada A, et al. Glycoprotein hormone α-subunit response to growth hormone (GH)-releasing hormone in patients with active acromegaly. Evidence for α-subunit and GH coexistence in the same tumoral cell. J Clin Endocrinol Metab 1985;61:541–6.

327. Beck-Peccoz P, Piscitelli G, Amr S, et al. Endocrine, biochemical, and morphological studies of a pituitary adenoma secreting growth hormone, thyrotropin (TSH), and α-subunit: evidence for secretion of TSH with increased bioactivity. J Clin Endocrinol Metab 1986;62:704–11.

328. Benoit R, Pearson-Murphy BE, Robert F, et al. Hyperthyroidism due to a pituitary TSH secreting tumour with amenorrhoea-galactorrhoea. Clin Endocrinol (Oxf) 1980;12:11–9.

329. Berg KK, Scheithauer BW, Felix I, et al. Pituitary adenomas that produce adrenocorticotropic hormone and alpha-subunit: clinicopathological, immunohistochemical, ultrastructural, and immunoelectron microscopic studies in nine cases. Neurosurgery 1990;26:397–403.

330. Cunningham GR, Huckins C. An FSH and prolactin-secreting pituitary tumor: pituitary dynamics and testicular histology. J Clin Endocrinol Metab 1977;44:248–53.

331. Duello TM, Halmi NS. Pituitary adenoma producing thyrotropin and prolactin. An immunocytochemical and electron microscopic study. Virchows Arch [Pathol Anat] 1977;376:255–65.

332. Faggiano M, Criscuolo T, Perrone L, Quarto C, Sinisi AA. Sexual precocity in a boy due to hypersecretion of LH and prolactin by a pituitary adenoma. Acta Endocrinol (Copenh) 1983;102:167–72.

333. Horn K, Erhardt F, Fahlbusch R, Pickardt CR, von Werder K, Scriba PC. Recurrent goiter, hyperthyroidism, galactorrhea and amenorrhea due to a thyrotropin and prolactin-producing pituitary tumor. J Clin Endocrinol Metab 1976;43:137–43.

334. Horvath E, Kovacs K. The adenohypophysis. In: Kovacs K, Asa SL, eds. Functional endocrine pathology. Boston: Blackwell Scientific Publications, 1991:245–81.

335. Horvath E, Kovacs K, Smyth HS, et al. A novel type of pituitary adenoma: morphological feature and clinical correlations. J Clin Endocrinol Metab 1988;66:1111–8.

336. Jaquet P, Hassoun J, Delori P, Gunz G, Grisoli F, Weintraub BD. A human pituitary adenoma secreting thyrotropin and prolactin: immunohistochemical, biochemical, and cell culture studies. J Clin Endocrinol Metab 1984;59:817–24.

337. Koide Y, Kugai N, Kimura S, et al. A case of pituitary adenoma with possible simultaneous secretion of thyrotropin and follicle-stimulating hormone. J Clin Endocrinol Metab 1982;54:397–403.

338. Kontogeorgos G, Kovacs K, Scheithauer BW, Rologis D, Orphanidis G. Alpha-subunit immunoreactivity in plurihormonal pituitary adenomas of patients with acromegaly. Mod Pathol 1991;4:191–5.

339. Kovacs K, Horvath E, Asa SL, Stefaneanu L, Sano T. Pituitary cells producing more than one hormone. Human pituitary adenomas. Trends Endocrinol Metab 1989;1:104–7.

340. Kovacs K, Horvath E, Ezrin C, Weiss MH. Adenoma of the human pituitary producing growth hormone and thyrotropin. A histologic, immunocytologic and fine-structural study. Virchows Arch [Pathol Anat] 1982;395:59–68.

341. Kuzuya N, Inoue K, Ishibashi M, et al. Endocrine and immunohistochemical studies on thyrotropin (TSH)-secreting pituitary adenomas: responses of TSH, α-subunit, and growth hormone to hypothalamic releasing hormones and their distribution in adenoma cells. J Clin Endocrinol Metab 1990;71:1103–11.

342. Lamberts SW, Oosterom R, Verleun T, Krenning EP, Assies H. Regulation of hormone release by cultured cells from a thyrotropin-growth hormone-secreting pituitary tumor. Direct inhibiting effects of 3,5,3'-triiodothyronine and dexamethasone on thyrotropin secretion. J Endocrinol Invest 1984;7:313–7.

343. Malarkey WB, Kovacs K, O'Dorisio TM. Response of a GH- and TSH-secreting pituitary adenoma to a somatostatin analogue (SMS 201-995): evidence that GH and TSH coexist in the same cell and secretory granules. Neuroendocrinology 1989;49:267–74.

344. Osamura RY, Watanabe K. Immunohistochemical colocalization of growth hormone (GH) and alpha subunit in human GH secreting pituitary adenomas. Virchows Arch [A] 1987;411:323–30.

345. Saeger W, Lüdecke DK. Pituitary adenomas with hyperfunction of TSH. Frequency, histologic classification, immunocytochemistry and ultrastructure. Virchows Arch [Pathol Anat] 1982;394:255–67.

346. Sano T, Kovacs K, Asa SL, Smyth HS. Immunoreactive luteinizing hormone in functioning corticotroph adenomas of the pituitary. Immunohistochemical and tissue culture studies of two cases. Virchows Arch [A] 1990;417:361–7.

347. Sherry SH, Guay AT, Lee AK, et al. Concurrent production of adrenocorticotropin and prolactin from two distinct cell lines in a single pituitary adenoma: a detailed immunohistochemical analysis. J Clin Endocrinol Metab 1982;55:947–55.

348. Simard M, Mirell CJ, Pekary AE, Drexler J, Kovacs K, Hershman JM. Hormonal control of thyrotropin and growth hormone secretion in a human thyrotrope pituitary adenoma studied in vitro. Acta Endocrinol (Copenh) 1988;119:283–90.

349. Trouillas J, Girod C, Loras B, et al. The TSH secretion in the human pituitary adenomas. Pathol Res Pract 1988;183:596–600.

Pituitary Apoplexy

350. Cardoso ER, Peterson EW. Pituitary apoplexy: a review. Neurosurgery 1984;14:363–73.

Associated Disorders - Multiple Endocrine Neoplasia

351. Asa SL, Singer W, Kovacs K, et al. Pancreatic endocrine tumour producing growth hormone-releasing hormone associated with multiple endocrine neoplasia type I syndrome. Acta Endocrinol (Copenh) 1987;115:331–7.

352. Chandrasekharappa SC, Guru SC, Manickam P, et al. Positional cloning of the gene for multiple endocrine neoplasia-type 1. Science 1997;276:404–7.

353. DeLellis RA. Multiple endocrine neoplasia syndromes revisited. Clinical, morphologic and molecular features. Lab Invest 1995;72:494–505.

354. Ezzat S, Asa SL. Syndromes of multiple endocrine neoplasia and hyperplasia. In: Kovacs K, Asa SL, eds.

Functional endocrine pathology. 2nd ed. Boston: Blackwell Science, 1998: in press.

355. Scheithauer BW, Laws ER Jr, Kovacs K, Horvath E, Randall RV, Carney JA. Pituitary adenomas of the multiple endocrine neoplasia type I syndrome. Semin Diagn Pathol 1987;4:205–11.

356. Shintani Y, Yoshimoto K, Horie H, et al. Two different pituitary adenomas in a patient with multiple endocrine neoplasia type 1 associated with growth hormone-releasing hormone-producing pancreatic tumor: clinical and genetic features. Endocr J 1995;42:331–40.

357. Wermer P. Genetic aspects of adenomatosis of endocrine glands. Am J Med 1954;16:363–71.

Ectopic Adenomas

358. Anand NK, Osborne CM, Harkey HL III. Infiltrative clival pituitary adenoma of ectopic origin. Head Neck Surg 1993;108:178–83.

359. Coire CI, Horvath E, Kovacs K, Smyth HS, Ezzat S. Cushing's syndrome from an ectopic pituitary adenoma with peliosis. A histological, immunohistochemical and ultrastructural study and review of the literature. Endocr Pathol 1997;8:65–74.

360. Dyer EH, Civit T, Abecassis JP, Derome PJ. Functioning ectopic supradiaphragmatic pituitary adenomas. Neurosurgery 1994;43:529–32.

361. Hori A. Suprasellar peri-infundibular ectopic adenohypophysis in fetal and adult brains. J Neurosurg 1985;62:113–5.

362. Kikuchi K, Kowada M, Sasaki J, Sageshima M. Large pituitary adenoma of the sphenoid sinus and the nasopharynx: report of a case with ultrastructural evaluations. Surg Neurol 1994;42:330–4.

363. Kleinschmidt-De Masters BK, Winston KR, Rubinstein D, Samuels MH. Ectopic pituitary adenomas of the third ventricle. Case report. J Neurosurg 1990;72:139–42.

364. Lindboe CF, Unsgard G, Myhr G, Scott H. ACTH and TSH producing ectopic suprasellar pituitary adenoma of the hypothalamic region: case report. Clin Neuropathol 1993;12:138–41.

365. Lloyd RV, Chandler WF, Kovacs K, Ryan N. Ectopic pituitary adenomas with normal anterior pituitary glands. Am J Surg Pathol 1986;108:546–52.

366. Matsumura A, Meguro K, Doi M, Tsurushima H, Tomono Y. Suprasellar ectopic pituitary adenoma: case report and review of the literature. Neurosurgery 1990;26:681–5.

367. Rasmussen P, Lindholm J. Ectopic pituitary adenomas. Clin Endocrinol (Oxf) 1979;11:69–74.

358. Shenker Y, Lloyd RV, Weatherbee L, Port FK, Grekin RJ, Barkan AL. Ectopic prolactinoma in a patient with hyperparathyroidism and abnormal sellar radiography. J Clin Endocrinol Metab 1986;62:1065–9.

369. Slonim SM, Haykal HA, Cushing GW, Freidberg SR, Lee AK. MRI appearances of an ectopic pituitary adenoma: case report and review of the literature. Neuroradiology 1993;35:546–8.

Pathogenesis of Pituitary Adenomas

370. Abbass SA, Asa SL, Ezzat S. Altered expression of fibroblast growth factor receptors in human pituitary adenomas. J Clin Endocrinol Metab 1997;82:1160–6.

371. Adams EF, Bhuttacharji SC, Halliwell CL, Loizou M, Birch G, Mashiter K. Effect of pancreatic growth hormone releasing factors on GH secretion by human somatotrophic pituitary tumours in cell culture. Clin Endocrinol (Oxf) 1984;21:709–18.

372. Adams EF, Winslow CL, Mashiter K. Pancreatic growth hormone releasing factor stimulates growth hormone secretion by pituitary cells. Lancet 1983;1:1100–1.

373. Alexander JM, Biller BM, Bikkal H, Zervas NT, Arnold A, Klibanski A. Clinically nonfunctioning pituitary tumors are monoclonal in origin. J Clin Invest 1990;86:336–40.

374. Alexander JM, Jameson JL, Bikkal HA, Schwall RH, Klibanski A. The effects of activin on follicle-stimulating hormone secretion and biosynthesis in human glycoprotein hormone-producing pituitary adenomas. J Clin Endocrinol Metab 1991;72:1261–7.

375. Alexander JM, Klibanski A. Gonadotropin-releasing hormone receptor mRNA expression by human pituitary tumors in vitro. J Clin Invest 1994;93:2332–9.

376. Alexander JM, Swearingen B, Tindall GT, Klibanski A. Human pituitary adenomas express endogenous inhibin subunit and follistatin messenger ribonucleic acids. J Clin Endocrinol Metab 1995;80:147–52.

377. Alvaro V, Lévy L, Dubray C, et al. Invasive human pituitary tumors express a point-mutated α-protein kinase-C. J Clin Endocrinol Metab 1993;77:1125–9.

378. Asa SL, Kovacs K. Pathogenesis of endocrine tumors. In: Kovacs K, Asa SL, eds. Functional endocrine pathology. Boston: Blackwell Scientific Publications, 1991:1005–13.

379. Asa SL, Kovacs K, Hammer GD, Liu B, Roos BA, Low MJ. Pituitary corticotroph hyperplasia in rats implanted with a medullary thyroid carcinoma cell line transfected with a corticotropin-releasing hormone complementary deoxyribonucleic acid expression vector. Endocrinology 1992;131:715–20.

380. Asa SL, Kovacs K, Melmed S. The hypothalamic-pituitary axis. In: Melmed S, ed. The pituitary. Boston: Blackwell Scientific, 1995:3–44.

381. Asa SL, Kovacs K, Stefaneanu L, et al. Pituitary adenomas in mice transgenic for growth hormone-releasing hormone. Endocrinology 1992;131:2083–9.

382. Asa SL, Kovacs K, Tindall GT, Barrow DL, Horvath E, Vecsei P. Cushing's disease associated with an intrasellar gangliocytoma producing corticotrophin-releasing factor. Ann Intern Med 1984;101:789–93.

383. Asa SL, Penz G, Kovacs K, Ezrin C. Prolactin cells in the human pituitary. A quantitative immunocytochemical analysis. Arch Pathol Lab Med 1982;106:360–3.

384. Asa SL, Scheithauer BW, Bilbao JM, et al. A case for hypothalamic acromegaly: a clinicopathological study of six patients with hypothalamic gangliocytomas producing growth hormone-releasing factor. J Clin Endocrinol Metab 1984;58:796–803.

385. Baird A, Mormède P, Ying S-Y, et al. A nonmitogenic pituitary function of fibroblast growth factor: regulation of thyrotropin and prolactin secretion. Proc Natl Acad Sci USA 1985;82:5545–9.

386. Bevan JS, Burke CW, Esiri MM, et al. Studies of two thyrotrophin-secreting pituitary adenomas: evidence for dopamine receptor deficiency. Clin Endocrinol (Oxf) 1989;31:59–70.

387. Billestrup N, Swanson LW, Vale W. Growth hormone-releasing factor stimulates proliferation of somatotrophs in vitro. Proc Natl Acad Sci USA 1986;83:6854–7.

388. Blackwell RE. Diagnosis and management of prolactinomas. Fertil Steril 1985;43:5–16.

389. Boggild MD, Jenkinson S, Pistorello M, et al. Molecular genetic studies of sporadic pituitary tumors. J Clin Endocrinol Metab 1994;78:387–92.

390. Burton FH, Hasel KW, Bloom FE, Sutcliffe JG. Pituitary hyperplasia and gigantism in mice caused by a cholera toxin transgene. Nature 1991;350:74–7.

391. Bystrom C, Larsson C, Blomberg C, et al. Localization of the MEN-1 gene to a small region within chromosome 11q13 by deletion mapping in tumors. Proc Natl Acad Sci USA 1990;87:1968–72.

392. Cai WY, Alexander JM, Hedley-Whyte ET, et al. *Ras* mutations in human prolactinomas and pituitary carcinomas. J Clin Endocrinol Metab 1994;78:89–93.

393. Carey RM, Varma SK, Drake CR Jr, et al. Ectopic secretion of corticotropin-releasing factor as a cause of Cushing's syndrome. A clinical, morphologic, and biochemical study. N Engl J Med 1984;311:13–20.

394. Chandrasekharappa SC, Guru SC, Manickam P, et al. Positional cloning of the gene for multiple endocrine neoplasia-type 1. Science 1997;276:404–7.

395. Cryns VL, Alexander JM, Klibanski A, Arnold A. The retinoblastoma gene in human pituitary tumors. J Clin Endocrinol Metab 1993;77:644–6.

396. Ezzat S, Asa SL, Stefaneanu L, et al. Somatotroph hyperplasia without pituitary adenoma associated with a long standing growth hormone-releasing hormone-producing bronchial carcinoid. J Clin Endocrinol Metab 1994;78:555–60.

397. Ezzat S, Kontogeorgos G, Redelmeier DA, Horvath E, Harris AG, Kovacs K. In vivo responsiveness of morphological variants of growth hormone-producing pituitary adenomas to octreotide. Eur J Endocr 1995;133:686–90.

398. Ezzat S, Melmed S. The role of growth factors in the pituitary. J Endocrinol Invest 1990;13:691–8.

399. Ezzat S, Smyth HS, Ramyar L, Asa SL. Heterogenous in vivo and in vitro expression of basic fibroblast growth factor by human pituitary adenomas. J Clin Endocrinol Metab 1995;80:878–84.

400. Ezzat S, Walpola IA, Ramyar L, Smyth HS, Asa SL. Membrane-anchored expression of transforming growth factor-α in human pituitary adenoma cells. J Clin Endocrinol Metab 1995;80:534–9.

401. Ezzat S, Zheng L, Smyth HS, Asa SL. The c-*erb*B-2/*neu* proto-oncogene in human pituitary tumors. Clin Endocrinol 1997;46:599–606.

402. Filetti S, Rapoport B, Aron DC, Greenspan FC, Wilson CB, Fraser W. TSH and TSH-subunit production by human thyrotrophic tumour cells in monolayer culture. Acta Endocrinol (Copenh) 1982;99:224–31.

403. Fisher DA, Lakshmanan J. Metabolism and effects of epidermal growth factor and related growth factors in mammals. Endocr Rev 1990;11:418–42.

404. Fjellestad-Paulsen A, Abrahamsson PA, Bjartell A, et al. Carcinoma of the prostate with Cushing's syndrome. A case report with immunohistochemical and chemical demonstration of immunoreactive corticotropin-releasing hormone in plasma and tumor tissue. Acta Endocrinol (Copenh) 1988;119:506–16.

405. Gertz BJ, Contreras LN, McComb DJ, Kovacs K, Tyrrell JB, Dallman MF. Chronic administration of corticotropin-releasing factor increases pituitary corticotroph number. Endocrinology 1987;120:381–8.

406. Gesundheit N, Petrick PA, Nissim M, et al. Thyrotropin-secreting pituitary adenomas: clinical and biochemical heterogeneity. Case reports and follow-up of nine patients [see comments]. Ann Intern Med 1989;111:827–35.

407. Gicquel C, LeBouc Y, Luton JP, Girad F, Bertagna X. Monoclonality of corticotroph macroadenomas in Cushing's disease. J Clin Endocrinol Metab 1992;75:472–5.

408. Gonsky R, Herman V, Melmed S, Fagin J. Transforming DNA sequences present in human prolactin-secreting pituitary tumors. Mol Endocrinol 1991;5:1687–95.

409. Gorczyca W, Hardy J. Arterial supply of the human anterior pituitary gland. Neurosurgery 1987;20:369–78.

410. Gospodarowicz D, Abraham JA, Schilling J. Isolation and characterization of a vascular endothelial cell mitogen produced by pituitary-derived folliculostellate cells. Proc Natl Acad Sci USA 1989;86:7311–5.

411. Gospodarowicz D, Ferrara N, Schweigerer L, Neufeld G. Structural characterization and biological functions of fibroblast growth factor. Endocr Rev 1987;8:95–114.

412. Grossman A, Besser GM. Prolactinomas. Br Med J 1985;290:182–4.
413. Haddad G, Penabad JL, Bashey HM, et al. Expression of activin/inhibin subunit messenger ribonucleic acids by gonadotroph adenomas. J Clin Endocrinol Metab 1994;79:1399–403.
414. Harris PE, Alexander JM, Bikkal HA, et al. Glycoprotein hormone α-subunit production in somatotroph adenomas with and without Gsα mutations. J Clin Endocrinol Metab 1992;75:918–23.
415. Herman V, Drazin NZ, Gonsky R, Melmed S. Molecular screening of pituitary adenomas for gene mutations and rearrangements. J Clin Endocrinol Metab 1993;77:50–5.
416. Herman V, Fagin J, Gonsky R, Kovacs K, Melmed S. Clonal origin of pituitary adenomas. J Clin Endocrinol Metab 1990;71:1427–33.
417. Horvath E, Kovacs K. The adenohypophysis. In: Kovacs K, Asa SL, eds. Functional endocrine pathology. Boston: Blackwell Scientific Publications, 1991:245–81.
418. Hu N, Gutsmann A, Herbert DC, Bradley A, Lee WH, Lee EY. Heterozygous Rb^{120}/+ mice are predisposed to tumors of the pituitary gland with a nearly complete penetrance. Oncogene 1994;9:1021–7.
419. Jacks T, Fazeli A, Schmitt EM, Bronson RT, Goodell MA, Weinberg RA. Effects of an *Rb* mutation in the mouse. Nature 1992;359:295–300.
420. Jones KL, Villela JF, Lewis UJ. The growth of cultured rabbit articular chondrocytes is stimulated by pituitary growth factors but not by purified human growth hormone or ovine prolactin. Endocrinology 1986;118:2588–93.
421. Karga HJ, Alexander JM, Hedley-Whyte ET, Klibanski A, Jameson JL. *Ras* mutations in human pituitary tumors. J Clin Endocrinol Metab 1992;74:914–9.
422. Kasper S, Friesen HG. Human pituitary tissue secretes a potent growth factor for chondrocyte proliferation. J Clin Endocrinol Metab 1986;62:70–6.
423. Kawakita S, Asa SL, Kovacs K. Effects of growth hormone-releasing hormone (GHRH) on densely granulated somatotroph adenomas and sparsely granulated somatotroph adenomas in vitro: a morphological and functional investigation. J Endocrinol Invest 1989;12:443–8.
424. Kelly MA, Rubinstein M, Asa SL, et al. Pituitary lactotroph hyperplasia and chronic hyperprolactinemia in dopamine D2 receptor-deficient mice. Neuron 1997;19:103–13.
425. Kovacs K, Horvath E. Tumors of the pituitary gland. Atlas of Tumor Pathology, 2nd Series, Fascicle 21. Washington, D.C.: Armed Forces Institute of Pathology, 1986.
426. Kovacs K, Stefaneanu L, Ezzat S, Smyth HS. Prolactin-producing pituitary adenoma in a male-to-female transsexual patient with protracted estrogen administration. A morphologic study. Arch Pathol Lab Med 1994;118:562–5.
427. Krieger DT. Medical treatment of Cushing disease. In: Tolis G, Labrie F, Martin JB, Naftolin F, eds. Clinical neuroendocrinology: a pathophysiological approach. New York: Raven Press, 1979:423–7.
428. Krieger DT. Physiopathology of Cushing's disease. Endocr Rev 1983;4:22–43.
429. Landis CA, Harsh G, Lyons J, Davis RL, McCormick F, Bourne HR. Clinical characteristics of acromegalic patients whose pituitary tumors contain mutant Gs protein. J Clin Endocrinol Metab 1990;71:1416–20.
430. Larson GH, Koos RD, Sortino MA, Wise PM. Acute effect of basic fibroblast growth factor on secretion of prolactin as assessed by the reverse hemolytic plaque assay. Endocrinology 1990;126:927–32.
431. LeRiche VK, Asa SL, Ezzat S. Epidermal growth factor and its receptor (EGF-R) in human pituitary adenomas: EGF-R correlates with tumor aggressiveness. J Clin Endocrinol Metab 1995;81:656–62.
432. Li Y, Koga M, Kasayama S, et al. Identification and characterization of high molecular weight forms of basic fibroblast growth factor in human pituitary adenomas. J Clin Endocrinol Metab 1992;75:1436–41.
433. Lloyd RV, Jin L, Chang A, et al. Morphologic effects of hGRH gene expression on the pituitary, liver, and pancreas of MT-hGRH transgenic mice. An in situ hybridization analysis. Am J Pathol 1992;141:895–906.
434. Jin L, Chandler WF, Lloyd RV. Localization of basic fibroblast growth factor (bFGF) protein and mRNA in human pituitaries: regulation of bFGF mRNA by gonadotropin-releasing hormone. Endocr Pathol 1994;5:27–34.
435. Loras B, Li JY, Durand A, Trouillas J, Sassolas G, Girod C. GRF et adénomes somatotropes humains. Corrélations in vivo et in vitro entre la libération de GH et les aspects morphologiques et immunocytochimiques. Ann Endocrinol (Paris) 1985;46:373–82.
436. Lüdecke DK, Westphal M, Schabet M, Höllt V. In vitro secretion of ACTH, β-endorphin and β-lipotropin in Cushing's disease and Nelson's syndrome. Horm Res 1980;13:259–79.
437. Lyons J, Landis CA, Harsh G, et al. Two G protein oncogenes in human endocrine tumors. Science 1990;249:655–9.
438. Mason IJ. The ins and outs of fibroblast growth factors. Cell 1994;78:547–52.
439. McAndrew J, Paterson AJ, Asa SL, McCarthy KJ, Kudlow JE. Targeting of transforming growth factor-expression to pituitary lactotrophs in transgenic mice results in selective lactotroph proliferation and adenomas. Endocrinology 1995;136:4479–88.
440. McNicol AM, Kubba MA, McTeague E. The mitogenic effects of corticotrophin-releasing factor on the anterior pituitary gland of the rat. J Endocrinol 1988;118:237–41.
441. Molitch ME. Pathogenesis of pituitary tumors. Endocrinol Metab Clin North Am 1987;16:503–27.
442. Nelson KG, Takahashi T, Lee DC, et al. Transforming growth factor-α is a potential mediator of estrogen action in the mouse uterus. Endocrinology 1992;131:1657–64.
443. Newman CB, Cosby H, Friesen HG, et al. Evidence for a nonprolactin, non-growth-hormone mammary mitogen in the human pituitary gland. Proc Natl Acad Sci USA 1987;84:8110–4.
444. Nicolis G, Shimshi M, Allen C, Halmi NS, Kourides IA. Gonadotropin-producing pituitary adenoma in a man with long-standing primary hypogonadism. J Clin Endocrinol Metab 1988;66:237–41.
445. Patterson J, Childs GV. Interleukin-1 beta stimulates secretion of nerve growth factor from anterior pituitary cells [Abstract]. Endocrinology 1993;[suppl]:88.
446. Pei L, Melmed S, Scheithauer B, Kovacs K, Benedict WF, Prager D. Frequent loss of heterozygosity at the retinoblastoma susceptibility gene (*RB*) locus in aggressive pituitary tumors: evidence for a chromosome 13 tumor suppressor gene other than *RB*. Cancer Res 1995;55:1613–6.
447. Pei L, Melmed S, Scheithauer B, Kovacs K, Prager D. H-*ras* mutations in human pituitary carcinoma metastases. J Clin Endocrinol Metab 1994;78:842–6.

448. Penabad JL, Bashey HM, Asa SL, et al. Decreased follistatin gene expression in gonadotroph adenomas. J Clin Endocrinol Metab 1996;81;3397–403.

449. Prysor-Jones RA, Silverlight JJ, Jenkins JS. Oestradiol, vasoactive intestinal peptide and fibroblast growth factor in the growth of human pituitary tumour cells in vitro. J Endocrinol 1989;120:171–7.

450. Reichlin S. Pathogenesis of pituitary tumors. In: Faglia G, Beck-Peccoz P, Ambrosi B, Travaglini P, Spada A, eds. Pituitary adenomas: new trends in basic and clinical research. Amsterdam: Elsevier, 1991:113–21.

451. Rizzino A. Growth factors. In: Kovacs K, Asa SL, eds. Functional endocrine pathology. Boston: Blackwell Scientific Publications, 1991:979–89.

452. Saeger W. Die Morphologie der paraadenomatösen Adenohypophyse. Ein Beitrag zur Pathogenese der Hypophysenadenome. Virchows Arch [Pathol Anat] 1977;372:299–314.

453. Samsoondar J, Kudlow JE. Partial purification of an adrenal growth factor produced by normal bovine anterior pituitary cells in culture. Endocrinology 1987;120:929–35.

454. Sano T, Asa SL, Kovacs K. Growth hormone-releasing hormone-producing tumors: clinical, biochemical, and morphological manifestations. Endocr Rev 1988;9:357–73.

455. Schechter J, Ahmad N, Elias K, Weiner R. Estrogen-induced tumors: changes in the vasculature in two strains of rat. Am J Anat 1987;179:315–23.

456. Schechter J, Goldsmith P, Wilson C, Weiner R. Morphological evidence for the presence of arteries in human prolactinomas. J Clin Endocrinol Metab 1988;67:713–9.

457. Scheithauer BW, Kovacs K, Randall RV, Ryan N. Pituitary gland in hypothyroidism. Histologic and immunocytologic study. Arch Pathol Lab Med 1985;109:499–50.

458. Scheithauer BW, Sano T, Kovacs KT, Young WF Jr, Ryan N, Randall RV. The pituitary gland in pregnancy: a clinicopathologic and immunohistochemical study of 69 cases. Mayo Clin Proc 1990;65:461–74.

459. Schulte HM, Oldfield EH, Allolio B, Katz DA, Berkman RA, Ali IU. Clonal composition of pituitary adenomas in patients with Cushing's disease: determination by X-chromosome inactivation analysis. J Clin Endocrinol Metab 1991;73:1302–8.

460. Shimon I, Hüttner A, Said J, Spirna OM, Melmed S. Heparin-binding secretory transforming gene (*hst*) facilitates rat lactotrope cell tumorigenesis and induces prolactin gene transcription. J Clin Invest 1996;97:187–95.

461. Snyder PJ. Gonadotroph cell adenomas of the pituitary. Endocr Rev 1985;6:552–63.

462. Spada A, Arosio M, Bochicchio D, et al. Clinical, biochemical and morphological correlates in patients bearing growth hormone-secreting pituitary tumors with or without constitutively active adenylyl cyclase. J Clin Endocrinol Metab 1990;71:1421–6.

463. Spada A, Bassetti M, Martino E, et al. In vitro studies on TSH secretion and adenylate cyclase activity in a human TSH-secreting pituitary adenoma. Effects of somatostatin and dopamine. J Endocrinol Invest 1985;8:193–8.

464. Spada A, Elahi FR, Arosio M, et al. Lack of desensitization of adenomatous somatotrophs to growth hormone-releasing hormone in acromegaly. J Clin Endocrinol Metab 1987;64:585–91.

465. Sumi T, Stefaneanu L, Kovacs K, Asa SL, Rindi G. Immunohistochemical study of p53 protein in human and animal pituitary tumors. Endocr Pathol 1993;4:95–9.

466. Thakker RV, Pook MA, Wooding C, Boscaro M, Scanarini M, Clayton RN. Association of somatotrophinoma with loss of alleles on chromosome 11 and with *gsp* mutations. J Clin Invest 1993;91:2815–21.

467. Thorner MO, Perryman RL, Cronin MJ, et al. Somatotroph hyperplasia. Successful treatment of acromegaly by removal of a pancreatic islet tumor secreting a growth hormone-releasing factor. J Clin Invest 1982;70:965–77.

468. Tordjman K, Stern N, Ouaknine G, et al. Activating mutations of the Gs-gene in nonfunctioning pituitary tumors. J Clin Endocrinol Metab 1993;77:765–9.

469. Trouillas J, Girod C, Loras B, et al. The TSH secretion in the human pituitary adenomas. Pathol Res Pract 1988;183:596–600.

470. Vallar L, Spada A, Giannattasio G. Altered Gs and adenylate cyclase activity in human GH-secreting pituitary adenomas. Nature 1987;330:566–8.

471. Webster J, Ham J, Bevan JS, Scanlon MF. Growth factors and pituitary tumors. Trends Endocrinol Metab 1989;1:95–8.

472. Webster J, Ham J, Bevan JS, ten Horn CD, Scanlon MF. Preliminary characterization of growth factors secreted by human pituitary tumors. J Clin Endocrinol Metab 1991;72:687–92.

473. Weiner RI, Windle J, Mellon P, Schechter J. Role of FGF in tumorigenesis of the anterior pituitary [Abstract]. J Endocrinol Invest 1991;14(suppl):S13.

474. White MC, Daniels M, Kendall-Taylor P, Turner SJ, Mathias D, Teasdale G. Effects of growth hormone-releasing factor (1-44) on growth hormone release from human somatotrophinomas in vitro: interaction with somatostatin, dopamine, vasoactive intestinal peptide and cycloheximide. J Endocrinol 1985;105:269–76.

475. Ying SY. Inhibins, activins, and follistatins: gonadal proteins modulating the secretion of follicle-stimulating hormone. Endocr Rev 1988;9:267–93.

476. Yoshimoto K, Iwahana H, Kubo K, et al. Allele loss on chromosome 11 in a pituitary tumor from a patient with multiple endocrine neoplasia type 1. Jpn J Cancer Res 1991;82:886–9.

477. Zhu J, Leon SP, Beggs AH, Busque L, Gilliland DG, Black PM. Human pituitary adenomas show no loss of heterozygosity at the retinoblastoma gene locus. J Clin Endocrinol Metab 1994;78:922–7.

478. Zhuang Z, Ezzat SZ, Vortmeyer AO, et al. Mutations of the MEN1 tumor suppressor gene in pituitary tumors. Cancer Research 1997;57:5446–51.

479. Zimmering MB, Katsumata N, Sato Y, et al. Increased basic fibroblast growth factor in plasma from multiple endocrine neoplasia type 1: relation to pituitary tumor. J Clin Endocrinol Metab 1993;76:1182–7.

4
PITUITARY CARCINOMA

Definition. Classic definitions hold that benign tumors do not invade adjacent tissues or metastasize to different sites, whereas malignant tumors, or cancers, have the ability to do either or both. In the pituitary, however, the definition of malignancy is still the subject of some debate. Most investigators classify pituitary tumors that exhibit lymphatic or hematogenous spread as malignant.

The criterion of invasive growth, although relatively common in pituitary tumors (11–13), is not generally accepted as indicative of malignancy since invasive adenomas do not have the potential to metastasize. The biologic behavior of these lesions is more akin to that of a basal cell carcinoma or pleomorphic adenoma of salivary gland; they can invade aggressively and defy surgical cure, and ultimately precipitate a lethal outcome.

Clinical Features. Primary pituitary carcinoma is exceedingly rare. Since it can be diagnosed with certainty only when patients have metastatic tumor deposits, the initial clinical presentation is usually that of a pituitary adenoma. Pituitary carcinomas have been associated with a number of clinical syndromes including hyperprolactinemia (9,10,17), Cushing's disease (2,4,10), more rarely, acromegaly (14) and even hyperthyroidism due to thyroid-stimulating hormone (TSH) excess (7). In some cases, the tumors have been unassociated with clinical or biochemical evidence of hormone excess (5,6); one well-differentiated gonadotropic tumor behaved in a malignant fashion (16).

Due to the spectrum of clinical presentations associated with pituitary carcinomas, the biochemical features vary considerably. They may follow any of the patterns of functioning pituitary tumors with hormone excess of any type, or they may be unassociated with hormone excess and manifest with variable hypopituitarism.

Radiologic Findings. Radiologic investigation can confirm the presence of metastatic tumor deposits in a patient with a pituitary tumor. These may involve various sites, including widespread dissemination throughout the subarachnoid space (2,4,5), cervical lymph nodes (6), distant bony sites (7,17), liver and lungs (7,17), and other extracranial sites. Skull X rays and computerized tomography (CT) and magnetic resonance imaging (MRI) scans usually reveal a locally invasive lesion that may extend beyond the sella turcica and into parasellar structures. Cranial nerves and adjacent brain structures may be involved.

Morphologic Findings. Pituitary carcinomas have no well-defined morphologic criteria apart from the presence of metastases. They generally exhibit hypercellularity, nuclear pleomorphism, mitoses, necrosis, hemorrhage, and invasion but these are not reliable indicators of malignancy since they are found in pituitary adenomas; in particular, invasive adenomas are well recognized and yet appear to have no potential for malignant spread (12). A necessary criterion for the diagnosis is, therefore, metastasis to remote areas of the cerebrospinal subarachnoid space, brain parenchyma, or extracranial sites including lymph nodes, lungs, liver, or bone.

Immunocytochemistry and electron microscopy cannot diagnose malignancy, but play a role in characterizing pituitary carcinomas. They generally allow classification of the tumor according to the criteria described for adenomas. In some cases, the tumor cells may be poorly differentiated; immunohistochemical and fine structural features may only reveal endocrine differentiation of the tumor.

Pathogenesis. The rarity of these cases does not allow valid conclusions concerning the pathogenesis of pituitary carcinoma. Point mutations in the H-*ras* gene have been reported in metastatic deposits from three pituitary carcinomas, but not in their respective primary lesions (8), or in several other carcinomas examined (1,8). Transforming DNA sequences of the *hst* gene have been identified in prolactinomas (3), but the significance of *hst* expression is unknown. p53 immunoreactivity has been reported in pituitary carcinomas, but there is as yet no indication of whether this reflects mutation of this tumor suppressor gene (15).

Prognosis and Therapy. In general, patients who develop malignant tumors of the adenohypophysis have a poor prognosis. The number of published cases is insufficient to draw conclusions concerning appropriate therapy.

REFERENCES

1. Cai WY, Alexander JM, Hedley-Whyte ET, et al. Ras mutations in human prolactinomas and pituitary carcinomas. J Clin Endocrinol Metab 1994;78:89–93.

2. Frost AR, Tenner S, Tenner M, Rollhauser C, Tabbara SO. ACTH-producing pituitary carcinoma presenting as the cauda equina syndrome. Arch Pathol Lab Med 1995;119:93–6.

3. Gonsky R, Herman V, Melmed S, Fagin J. Transforming DNA sequences present in human prolactin-secreting pituitary tumors. Mol Endocrinol 1991;5:1687–95.

4. Kouhara H, Tatekawa T, Koga M, et al. Intracranial and intraspinal dissemination of an ACTH-secreting pituitary tumor. Endocrinol Jpn 1992;39:177–84.

5. Kuroki M, Tanaka R, Yokoyama M, Shimbo Y, Ikuta F. Subarachnoid dissemination of a pituitary adenoma. Surg Neurol 1987;28:71–6.

6. Luzi P, Miracco C, Lio R, et al. Endocrine inactive pituitary carcinoma metastasizing to cervical lymph nodes: a case report. Hum Pathol 1987;18:90–2.

7. Mixson AJ, Friedman TC, Katz DA, et al. Thyrotropin-secreting pituitary carcinoma. J Clin Endocrinol Metab 1993;76:529–33.

8. Pei L, Melmed S, Scheithauer B, Kovacs K, Prager D. H-ras mutations in human pituitary carcinoma metastases. J Clin Endocrinol Metab 1994;78:842–6.

9. Petterson T, MacFarlane IA, MacKenzie JM, Shaw MD. Prolactin secreting pituitary carcinoma. J Neurol Neurosurg Psychiatry 1992;55:1205–6.

10. Saeger W, Lübke D. Pituitary carcinomas. Endocr Pathol 1996;7:21–35.

11. Sautner D, Saeger W. Invasiveness of pituitary adenomas. Pathol Res Pract 1991;187:632–6.

12. Scheithauer BW, Kovacs KT, Laws ER Jr, Randall RV. Pathology of invasive pituitary tumors with special reference to functional classification. J Neurosurg 1986;65:733–44.

13. Selman WR, Laws ER Jr, Scheithauer BW, Carpenter SM. The occurrence of dural invasion in pituitary adenomas. J Neurosurg 1986;64:402–7.

14. Stewart PM, Carey MP, Graham CT, Wright AD, London DR. Growth hormone secreting pituitary carcinoma: a case report and literature review. Clin Endocrinol (Oxf) 1992;37:189–95.

15. Thapar K, Scheithauer BW, Kovacs K, Pernicone PJ, Laws ER Jr. P53 expression in pituitary adenomas and carcinomas: correlation with invasiveness and tumor growth fractions. Neurosurgery 1996;38:765–71.

16. Trouillas J, Beauchesne P, Barral F, Pialat J, Brunon J. Gonadotropic pituitary carcinoma [Abstract]. Endocr Pathol 1995;6:384.

17. Walker JD, Grossman A, Anderson JV, et al. Malignant prolactinoma with extracranial metastases: a report of three cases. Clin Endocrinol (Oxf) 1993;38:411–9.

❖❖❖

5

TUMORS OF THE HYPOTHALAMUS AND NEUROHYPOPHYSIS

The location of the pituitary gland makes it subject to involvement by lesions that arise in the central nervous system tissues adjacent to it. It is, therefore, the site of primary neuronal tumors, gliomas, and lesions of the dura and leptomeninges. In addition, the posterior pituitary is the site of the rare granular cell tumor. The morphologic features of tumors of the central nervous system are reviewed in detail in another Fascicle in this series (5) and the reader is referred to that text for further information. The unusual clinical or morphologic features peculiar to this location are discussed here.

NEURONAL TUMORS

Definition. Hypothalamic neuronal tumors are rare neoplasms that have been reported in the literature as "gangliocytomas" or "ganglioneuromas" (16). These lesions are composed of mature neurons resembling hypothalamic ganglion cells and are capable of producing hypothalamic peptides; this is the main reason for implying that they are hypothalamic in derivation. Some authors prefer to consider them hamartomas because they occur in children and it is thought that they represent developmental anomalies. In other instances, they are named ganglioneuromas or gangliocytomas because there is evidence that they represent neoplasms which may have their onset in adulthood and are capable of continued growth. Such tumors have also been described in other parts of the brain as extra-hypothalamic gangliocytomas (7). A few authors have used the term "choristoma" to describe collections of hypothalamic neurons within the adenohypophysis proper (19,20).

Clinical Features. The presentation of these lesions may be attributable to mass effects; they may present as sellar, suprasellar, or hypothalamic masses. Hypothalamic tissue destruction results in hypothalamic disturbances that affect temperature and appetite regulation and neurologic symptoms such as mental retardation or tonic-clonic seizures. Suprasellar masses can result in hypopituitarism with hyperprolactin-

emia and visual field defects; sellar lesions may result in partial or total hypopituitarism.

In some instances, these tumors are hormonally active and cause endocrinopathies that are usually mediated by the pituitary gland. They have been associated with acromegaly, precocious puberty, Cushing's disease, and amenorrhea-galactorrhea.

Radiologic Findings. The most common location of these peculiar neoplasms is in the hypothalamus or tuber cinereum, with different grades of involvement of the third ventricle. They may be outside the hypothalamus at the base of the brain but attached to the hypothalamus by a thin connection. They may also be found within the parenchyma of the adenohypophysis. In particular, hypothalamic hamartoma associated with acromegaly often presents as a solitary intrasellar mass that mimics a simple pituitary growth hormone-producing pituitary adenoma; microscopic examination reveals a gangliocytoma associated with a pituitary adenoma in such cases (2,3,13,19).

Gross Findings. The gross appearance of hypothalamic gangliocytomas is very heterogeneous. They may be nodular, pedunculated, sessile, solid, or cystic. They may be within, attached to, or completely detached from the hypothalamus. The color has been described as pinkish gray, brown, or red. Necrotic areas are occasionally found. They vary from microscopic lesions composed of only a few cells and measuring a few millimeters to masses that measure more than 5 cm.

Histologic Findings. Hypothalamic neuronal tumors are composed of randomly oriented, large, mature ganglion cells (fig. 5-1). The neurons vary in size and shape. They have large nuclei and very prominent nucleoli; binucleated and even multinucleated cells are seen. Most of the ganglion cells contain abundant cytoplasm, and Nissl granules are conspicuous at the periphery of the cell body. The Bodian stain highlights numerous processes that represent axons or dendrites. Some tumors have a glial stroma as well as calcification alternating with collagenous stroma and blood vessel proliferation.

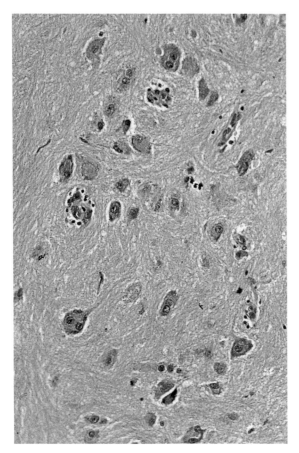

Figure 5-1
HISTOLOGY OF HYPOTHALAMIC
NEURONAL GANGLIOCYTOMA
This tumor is composed of randomly oriented large neurons that have abundant cytoplasm and Nissl substance at the periphery of the cell body. Cell processes are readily identified. Occasional binucleate forms confirm the tumorous nature of this tissue.

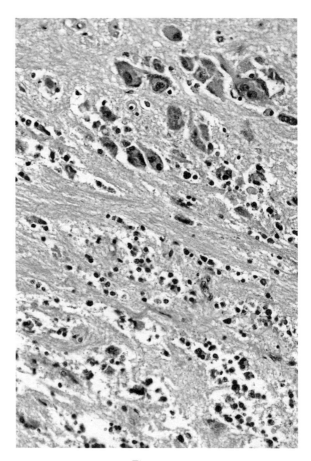

Figure 5-2
HISTOLOGY OF HYPOTHALAMIC
GANGLIOCYTOMA ASSOCIATED WITH
PITUITARY ADENOMA
This hypothalamic tumor was associated with a pituitary adenoma. At the junction between the two lesions there is some intermingling of the two tumor types.

Hypothalamic gangliocytomas can be found intermingled with nontumorous or hyperplastic adenohypophysis. Several have been adjacent to or intermingled with a frank adenoma of the pituitary (figs. 5-2, 5-3). In cases of intimate admixture within what appears to be a primary intrasellar lesion, the neuronal component of the tumor may be inconspicuous (fig. 5-4).

Immunohistochemical Findings. As neuronal cell tumors, these lesions are positive for synaptophysin and neurofilament (fig. 5-5). If glial elements are present they stain with glial fibrillary acidic protein (GFAP), and S-100 protein may be positive. Immunohistochemistry with specific antisera demonstrates the presence of peptides and hormones in the cytoplasm of the neoplastic neuronal cells. In patients with acromegaly, the ganglion cells may contain growth hormone-releasing hormone (GRH) (fig. 5-6), glucagon, somatostatin, vasoactive intestinal peptide (VIP), corticotropin-releasing hormone (CRH), gonadotropin-releasing hormone (GnRH), and gastrin (2,3,13,21); associated pituitary adenomas generally contain growth hormone (fig. 5-7). In patients with amenorrhea-galactorrhea, prolactin and VIP have been localized in the cytoplasm of ganglion cells of intrasellar gangliocytoma (13). Tumors associated with Cushing's disease contain CRH (1,17); some authors have detected adrenocorticotropic

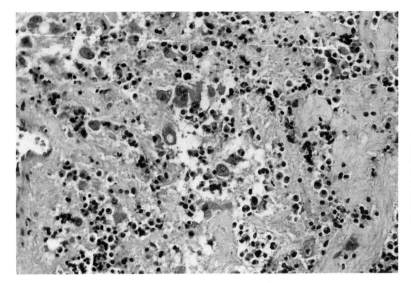

Figure 5-3
HYPOTHALAMIC
GANGLIOCYTOMA
ASSOCIATED WITH
PITUITARY ADENOMA

These lesions can present as a solitary sellar mass. Only microscopic examination confirms the presence of a hypothalamic tumor within the parenchyma of a pituitary adenoma. In this instance, the neuronal elements are conspicuous; multinucleate ganglion cells are readily identified and the neuropil provides stroma for the pituitary adenoma.

Figure 5-4
HYPOTHALAMIC
GANGLIOCYTOMA
ASSOCIATED WITH
PITUITARY ADENOMA

This pituitary adenoma contains only a few scattered neuronal cell bodies. A high index of suspicion is sometimes required to identify this neuronal component in a pituitary tumor.

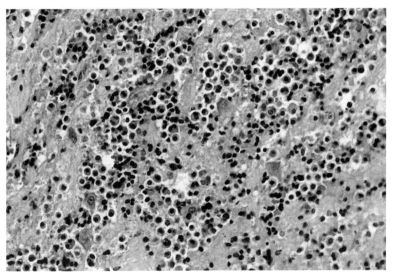

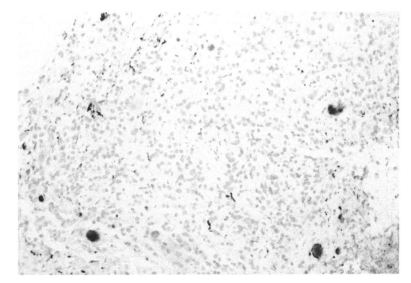

Figure 5-5
IMMUNOHISTOCHEMICAL
LOCALIZATION OF
NEUROFILAMENT IN
HYPOTHALAMIC GANGLIOCYTOMA

This patient had acromegaly and a sellar hypothalamic gangliocytoma associated with a pituitary adenoma. The ganglion cells are immunoreactive for the neurofilaments that decorate the neuronal cell bodies and axonal processes.

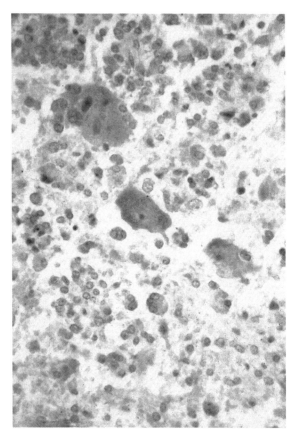

Figure 5-6
IMMUNOHISTOCHEMICAL LOCALIZATION OF
GROWTH HORMONE–RELEASING HORMONE
IN HYPOTHALAMIC GANGLIOCYTOMA

This patient had acromegaly and a sellar hypothalamic gangliocytoma associated with a pituitary adenoma. The ganglion cells are immunoreactive for growth hormone–releasing hormone (GRH); the pituitary adenoma cells are negative.

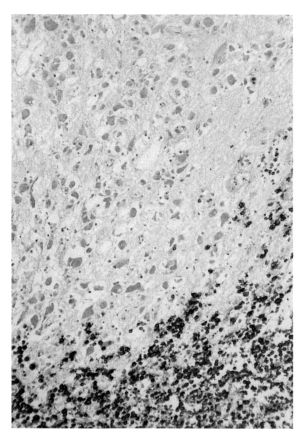

Figure 5-7
IMMUNOHISTOCHEMICAL LOCALIZATION OF
GROWTH HORMONE IN A PITUITARY
ADENOMA ASSOCIATED WITH A
HYPOTHALAMIC GANGLIOCYTOMA

In this patient, a hypothalamic gangliocytoma was associated with pituitary adenoma. The patient had acromegaly. The pituitary adenoma cells are immunoreactive for growth hormone while the neurons are not. The neurons in this tumor were positive for GRH.

hormone (ACTH), β-lipotropin, and somatostatin in the cytoplasm of the tumor cells. Children with precocious puberty have neuronal tumors that contain GnRH (6,9,11) but may also contain immunoreactivity for CRH, β-endorphin, and oxytocin (15). Some gangliocytomas unassociated with clinical evidence of hormone excess show multiple immunoreactivities, including positivity for VIP, galanin, α-subunit, somatostatin, and serotonin (22). Rarely, neuropeptides are not detected in these lesions.

Ultrastructural Findings. Ganglion cell tumors are characterized by the presence of large mature neurons with large nuclei containing prominent nucleoli (fig. 5-8). The cell bodies contain well-developed endoplasmic reticulum, abun-

dant mitochondria, and neurofilaments. The neuronal processes are filled with neurofilaments and neurotubules, and harbor numerous small membrane-bound secretory granules; there is not a well-recognized correlation between the size or shape of the secretory granules and the hormonal profile or clinical syndrome. Synaptic formations are noted in some tumors and a few contain membrane-bound autophagic vacuoles.

In a few cases there has been ultrastructural evidence of an intimate association between neurons and adenohypophysial cells, both adenomatous and nontumorous. Gangliocytomas associated with acromegaly display nerve terminals

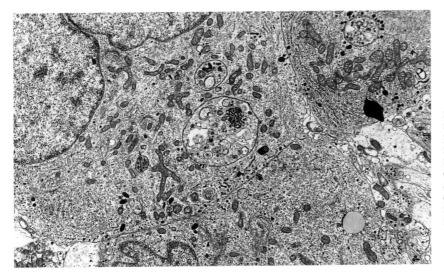

Figure 5-8
ULTRASTRUCTURE
OF HYPOTHALAMIC
GANGLIOCYTOMA

This tumor is composed of large neurons which have a binucleate morphology. The abundant cytoplasm contains well-developed rough endoplasmic reticulum and numerous mitochondria. While occasional small secretory granules are found within the cell body, the cytoplasm is punctuated by neuronal processes that contain accumulations of secretory granules.

Figure 5-9
ULTRASTRUCTURE OF
HYPOTHALAMIC
GANGLIOCYTOMA
ASSOCIATED WITH
PITUITARY ADENOMA

This tumor is composed of a mixture of neurons and somatotrophs. The neurons resemble those illustrated in figure 5-8 and the adenomatous somatotrophs have the characteristic morphology of cells of a sparsely granulated somatotroph adenoma. Note the juxtanuclear fibrous bodies. A striking feature is the interrelationship between the two cell types: neuronal processes interdigitate with the cytoplasm of adenomatous somatotrophs.

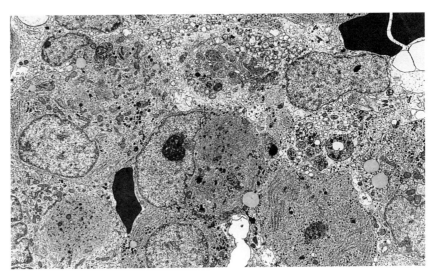

intimately attached to sparsely granulated adenomatous somatotrophs (figs. 5-9, 5-10) (2,3,19,20). An intrasellar gangliocytoma associated with Cushing's disease showed synaptic formation with hyperplastic corticotrophs (1).

Pituitary Morphology Associated with Hypothalamic Gangliocytoma. *Acromegaly.* The sparsely granulated somatotroph adenoma is the most common pituitary finding in patients with acromegaly and a hypothalamic hamartoma. Of 24 acromegalic patients in one review (16), only 6 did not have a pituitary growth hormone (GH)-containing adenoma. In two cases there were no abnormalities of the somatotrophs detected (2,8) and in two other cases, hyperplasia of somatotrophs was seen (10,19).

Galactorrhea-Amenorrhea. The pituitary morphology has not been thoroughly examined in patients with galactorrhea and amenorrhea associated with hypothalamic gangliocytoma (12, 14,18). One patient with these findings had a lactotroph adenoma (13); another had a mixed GH- and prolactin-producing pituitary adenoma (4).

Cushing's Disease. Cushing's disease associated with a CRH-containing intrasellar gangliocytoma has been associated with corticotroph hyperplasia (1). Two patients with Cushing's disease had gangliocytoma and corticotroph adenoma (13,17).

Precocious Puberty. The morphology of the pituitary in patients with hypothalamic gangliocytomas associated with precocious puberty has

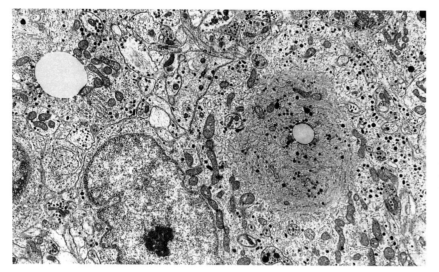

Figure 5-10
ULTRASTRUCTURE OF
HYPOTHALAMIC
GANGLIOCYTOMA
ASSOCIATED WITH
PITUITARY ADENOMA
Adenomatous sparsely granulated somatotrophs with fibrous bodies lie within the neuropil of neurons in a hypothalamic gangliocytoma, while neuronal processes are in direct contact with the cytoplasm.

not been described. Continuous stimulation of the adenohypophysis by GnRH should lead to downregulation of receptors; however, the increased level of plasma gonadotrophins does not support this theory.

Differential Diagnosis. Gangliocytomas are often of low cellularity and may be difficult to distinguish from normal tissue. Atypical pituitary adenomas, especially those composed of Crooke's cells which are large and contain abundant cytoplasm (see figs. 3-93, 3-94), can be mistaken for gangliocytoma.

Pathogenesis. The pathogenesis of these lesions is not known. Their association with pituitary adenomas in some patients suggests that there may be a common causative mechanism. It has been suggested that sellar gangliocytomas may arise by abnormal differentiation during neoplastic proliferation of adenohypophysial cells, however, it is more likely that these tumors have a true hypothalamic origin (16). The same tumorigenic stimulus may result in tumors of both hypothalamus and pituitary.

Prognosis and Therapy. These tumors are diagnosed at the time of surgery and cure has resulted from complete surgical resection (16). However, despite apparent cure of the endocrine disturbance, there may be radiographic evidence of residual tumor. The outcome of surgery in the small number of reported patients with these lesions is worse than that for pituitary adenomas, probably because of a higher incidence of extrasellar involvement.

When total resection of the lesion cannot be accomplished, the prognosis is varied. Most of these neuronal tumors have an extremely low proliferative potential and the overall prognosis is good; a few have caused severe hypothalamic destruction and have resulted in the death of the patient (16, 20). Radiotherapy appears to ameliorate hormone excess but it does not appear to prevent regrowth of the neuronal tumor (16); this is similar to the experience with radiotherapy in the treatment of ganglion cell tumors in the cerebral hemispheres. Medical therapy has been used infrequently and has been targeted specifically at correcting hormone excess syndromes.

GLIOMAS

Definition. Gliomas are neoplasms derived from and composed of neuroglial cells. They include astrocytomas and glioblastoma multiforme, oligodendrogliomas, and ependymomas. These tumors have a wide range of biologic behavior.

Clinical Features. Gliomas of the hypothalamus that selectively involve the pituitary or sella proper are rare (36,42). They can mimic pituitary adenomas, presenting as sellar mass lesions. Tissue destruction can result in hypothalamic hypopituitarism and decreased dopaminergic inhibition of prolactin may cause hyperprolactinemia. Aggressive and rapidly lethal gliomas occur following radiation therapy for pituitary adenoma, craniopharyngioma, or suprasellar germinoma (26–34,40,44). These tumors occur from

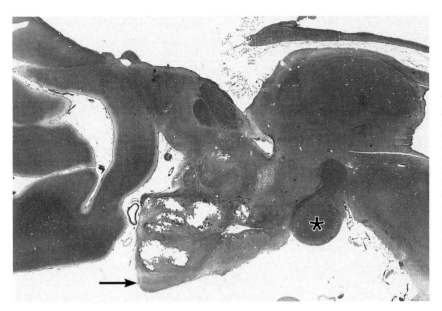

Figure 5-11
SUPRASELLAR
PILOCYTIC ASTROCYTOMA
Low-grade pilocytic astrocytoma arising in the suprasellar region can mimic a pituitary adenoma clinically. This parasagittal section stained with luxol fast blue/hematoxylin and eosin illustrates an adult type pilocytic astrocytoma in the hypothalamus anterior to the mamillary body (*). The walls of the third ventricle are involved and the optic chiasm (arrow) is compressed. The tumor was calcified and exhibits artefactual tearing. (Courtesy of Dr. J.M. Bilbao, Toronto, Canada.)

5 to 25 years after conventional radiation doses of 42.5 to 66 Gy.

Glioma of the optic nerve usually occurs in children or adolescents (23,38,43). These unusual lesions are usually found in patients with predisposing syndromes, such as neurofibromatosis or Beckwith-Wiedemann syndrome (35, 41). Patients usually present with visual loss, but a minority have associated endocrinopathy, usually hypopituitarism and diabetes but occasionally precocious puberty (38,43).

Radiologic Findings. The radiologic features vary with the type of tumor. With computerized tomography (CT), low-grade astrocytomas are lesions of low density and fail to enhance with contrast; contrast enhancement suggests malignant transformation, particularly if it is peripheral to a central hypodense area of necrosis, as seen in glioblastoma multiforme. With magnetic resonance imaging (MRI), astrocytomas characteristically have high signal intensity in the T2 mode.

The most common glioma in the sellar region is the pilocytic astrocytoma. Most common in children, hence the term "juvenile type," it is a relatively discrete, often cystic mass with prominent enhancement on CT scan (25). These tumors usually arise in the hypothalamus, in the wall of the third ventricle; they present as a suprasellar mass that displaces and compresses the optic chiasm. This glioma may also arise in the optic nerve, usually at the chiasm.

Morphologic Findings. Gliomas arising in the sellar region can be ependymomas or astrocytomas of any type. Most postradiation gliomas are malignant gliomas or glioblastoma multiforme; a single malignant oligodendroglioma has been reported (27). Glioma of the optic nerve is usually a low-grade pilocytic astrocytoma (fig. 5-11).

The low-grade juvenile pilocytic astrocytoma appears grossly well circumscribed but is usually infiltrative (24,25). It may have cysts and focal hemorrhages. Histologically, there is variation from field to field: compact fibrillary areas composed of polar or bipolar cells (fig. 5-12) are intermixed with looser cystic areas in which the cells are stellate. The polar cells account for the earlier name "polar spongioblastoma" used for these tumors that are now known to be astrocytic. Rosenthal fibers are usually conspicuous. The tumor cells may exhibit nuclear pleomorphism but mitoses are infrequent. Although the tumors are highly vascular, the vascular proliferation does not carry the malignant connotation that it bears in usual astrocytomas elsewhere.

The rare "adult" type of pilocytic astrocytoma (24,25) is more homogeneous, lacks microcysts, and tends to be more invasive than the juvenile variant. It is a slow-growing tumor and malignant transformation is rare.

Differential Diagnosis. The vascularity of the juvenile pilocytic astrocytoma resembles the vascular pattern of the neurohypophysis and the

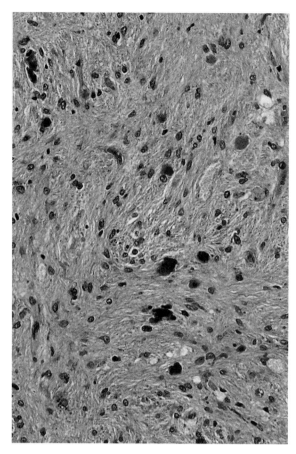

Figure 5-12
HISTOLOGY OF SUPRASELLAR
PILOCYTIC ASTROCYTOMA
This tumor is characterized by a fibrillary appearance
and elongated polar tumor cells. Rosenthal fibers are con-
spicuous. (Courtesy of Dr. J.M. Bilbao, Toronto, Canada.)

differential diagnosis includes nontumorous
neurohypophysis and reactive gliosis; the latter
is often difficult to distinguish from low-grade
glioma (25). Pituitary adenomas, particularly
prolactinomas and gonadotroph adenomas, can
mimic the architectural pattern of ependymoma
and the cytology is remarkably similar. Immunostains are critical to confirm the diagnosis;
ependymomas are strongly positive for glial
fibrillary acidic protein (GFAP).

Prognosis and Therapy. The low-grade lesions in children have a relatively good prognosis
because they grow slowly, but chiasmal lesions
can be more aggressive (23). In contrast, optic
gliomas that occur sporadically in adults are
usually rapidly fatal (37,39).

MENINGIOMAS

Definition. Meningiomas are tumors derived
from the meninges and their derivatives in the
meningeal spaces. They may arise from dural
fibroblasts or pial cells but the most common are
of arachnoid origin.

Clinical Features. Approximately 20 percent of these tumors of arachnoid and meningothelial cells occur in the sellar and parasellar
areas (53); they are most common in the sphenoid ridge and tuberculum sellae but also occur
rarely in the clivus. Suprasellar lesions often are
associated with visual field defects and other
neurologic deficits; they can cause endocrine
manifestations with hypopituitarism and
hyperprolactinemia due to stalk compression.
Biochemical testing reveals low levels of pituitary hormones but stimulation induces a response. Intrasellar involvement with tissue destruction and panhypopituitarism is rare and
usually occurs by downward extension; completely intrasellar tumors are rare (46).
Meningiomas occasionally arise in the sellar region following irradiation of the area for pituitary
adenoma or craniopharyngioma (48,51,55,56).

Meningiomas are more common in women
than men, possibly because of their expression
of progesterone and estrogen receptors (47).

Radiologic Findings. Radiologic investigation often distinguishes these lesions from pituitary adenomas, however, in some instances the
diagnosis is mistaken (50,54,57,58).

Morphologic Findings. Meningiomas are
histologically diverse tumors that have been
classified into 11 types according to the most
recent World Health Organization (WHO) International Histological Classification of Tumours
(49); the reader is referred to the Fascicle, Tumors of the Central Nervous System (45) for a
detailed review. The more familiar types and the
most common in the suprasellar area are the
meningothelial, fibrous or fibroblastic, and transitional variants (fig. 5-13). Papillary patterns
and anaplastic changes portend a more aggressive behavior and the possibility of metastasis.

Differential Diagnosis. Meningothelial
meningiomas are common in this region and are
likely to be confused with pituitary adenoma.
Features that aid in the diagnosis include
whorls, indistinct cell borders, and the presence

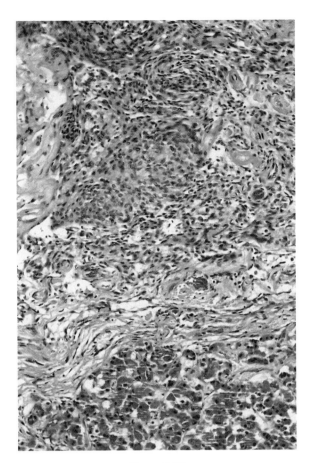

Figure 5-13
HISTOLOGY OF SELLAR MENINGIOMA
A sellar meningioma can mimic a pituitary adenoma clinically. The histology of this tumor is characteristic of meningioma. It is well demarcated from the adjacent adenohypophysis (bottom). This syncytial meningioma is characterized by architectural whorls and indistinct cell borders that help distinguish it from pituitary adenoma.

of psammoma bodies, a histologic hallmark of these tumors; the latter may also be present in pituitary adenomas, especially prolactin- and thyrotropin-producing tumors. In some cases, immunohistochemistry and even electron microscopy may be required to verify the diagnosis.

Prognosis and Therapy. The management of meningioma is generally surgical resection, but the surgical approach is critical (52). These highly vascular lesions can create problems with intraoperative bleeding. Because of their location, the surgical approach must attempt to resect the tumor as thoroughly as possible without compromising hypothalamic parenchyma, the optic nerves, or the pituitary stalk.

GRANULAR CELL TUMORS

Definition. Granular cells tumors of the infundibulum and posterior lobe of the pituitary resemble granular cell tumors of skin, tongue, breast, or gastrointestinal tract. These lesions have also been called *choristoma, granular cell myoblastoma, granular cell pituicytoma,* and *granular cell schwannoma.* Because they are not found in patients under the age of 20 years (62, 64), the term choristoma is not appropriate. They do not exhibit features of myocyte differentiation and some are negative for markers of schwannian and pituicyte differentiation (see below). It is therefore recommended that the term "granular cell tumor" be used for these tumors of uncertain histogenesis (59,67).

Clinical Features. Granular cell tumors are common but usually remain small lesions that do not give rise to symptoms; they are most frequently diagnosed as incidental findings at autopsy (62,64). Occasionally, they present as sellar masses causing visual field defects (60); curiously, given their location, only rarely is there associated diabetes insipidus (68). There are instances in which these lesions have been associated with pituitary adenomas (65) and they have occurred in patients with multiple endocrine neoplasia (MEN)-1 (66), but these are likely coincidental phenomena.

Radiologic Findings. Granular cell tumors are well-delineated, homogeneously dense, vascular masses that enhance with contrast on CT scan and produce a vascular blush on angiography (60). MRI detection has increased the sensitivity of diagnosis of small lesions. These isointense masses can resemble meningiomas (60), but a high intensity signal on T1-weighted images is a helpful diagnostic feature.

Morphologic Findings. These nodular lesions are firm, tan to grey, well-demarcated but unencapsulated nodules composed of closely apposed polygonal cells that have conspicuous, abundant, granular cytoplasm (figs. 5-14, 5-15). The cytoplasmic granules stain with the periodic acid–Schiff (PAS) technique and are diastase resistant. Immunohistochemical studies have shown that some of these tumors are negative for S-100 protein and glial fibrillary acidic protein (GFAP), casting doubt on both schwannian and pituicyte differentiation (67). They may show reactivity for

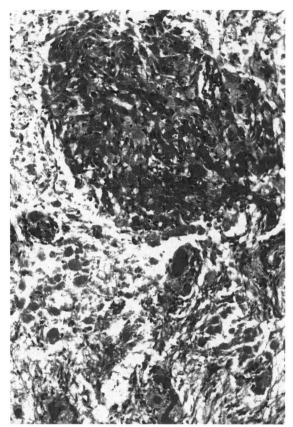

Figure 5-14
HISTOLOGY OF GRANULAR CELL TUMOR
A granular cell tumor is a well-circumscribed but unencapsulated nodular tumor in the neurohypophysis.

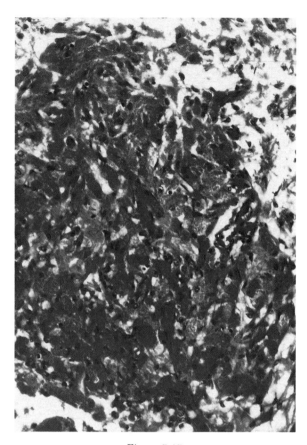

Figure 5-15
HISTOLOGY OF GRANULAR CELL TUMOR
This granular cell tumor is composed of large, closely apposed polygonal cells with abundant granular cytoplasm.

alpha-1-antitrypsin, alpha-1-antichymotrypsin, and cathepsin B, suggestive of histiocytic differentiation (63). Electron microscopy reveals cells containing phagolysosomes, with electron dense material and membranous debris (61).

Differential Diagnosis. Because of their location and radiologic appearance, these tumors may be confused with pituitary adenoma, meningioma, or even craniopharyngioma. On imaging studies or at autopsy gross examination, they can be distinguished from meningioma by lack of dural attachment, from craniopharyngioma by their solid nature, and from pituitary adenoma by their firm consistency. Although the histogenesis is unknown, their histologic appearance is remarkably characteristic.

Prognosis and Therapy. Since most of these lesions are not detected clinically, the approach to management has been determined by a few

cases only, and these have all been surgically resected (68). Although there have been rare reports of malignant granular cell tumors outside of the sella, in the pituitary they are considered benign neoplasms.

CHORDOMAS

Definition. Chordomas are rare lesions thought to be derived from remnants of the notochord (72,73). They occur in the midline, most often in the sacral region, but also in the region of the clivus, occasionally in vertebrae (75), and within the sella turcica (74).

Clinical Features. These slowly growing but locally aggressive neoplasms usually occur in patients over the age of 30 years; patients with unusual sphenoid lesions tend to be younger (76). Patients with chordomas of the clivus present

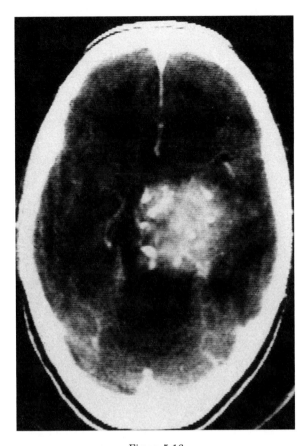

Figure 5-16
RADIOLOGIC FEATURES OF SELLAR CHORDOMA
This CT scan with contrast demonstrates the infiltrative, lobulated, and calcified appearance of a chordoma arising in the sellar region. (Courtesy of Dr. J.M. Bilbao, Toronto, Canada.)

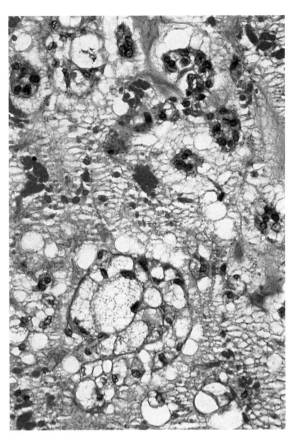

Figure 5-17
HISTOLOGY OF SELLAR CHORDOMA
The tumor is composed of large polyhedral "physaliphorous" cells that are characterized by a bubbly vacuolation of the cytoplasm and abundant mucinous matrix (Hematoxylin-phloxine-saffron stain). (Courtesy of Dr. J.M. Bilbao, Toronto, Canada.)

with pain, oculomotor disturbances, cerebellopontine angle syndrome, and intracranial hypertension. Parasellar involvement may manifest as anterior pituitary insufficiency.

Radiologic Findings. Chordomas are usually lobulated, calcified, and expansile osteolytic lesions (fig. 5-16). They may cause characteristic elevation of the periosteum, in which case they are suspected on the basis of the radiologic findings (71).

Morphologic Findings. These expansile or infiltrative tumors have a characteristic gross appearance: they are gelatinous and lobulated and may have areas of calcification.

Histologically, they are composed of large polyhedral cells with a characteristic bubbly appearance, hence the Greek term "physaliphorous" used to describe their vacuolation; vacuoles contain neutral mucins and glycogen (fig. 5-17). The cells are ar-

ranged in sheets or ribbons in an abundant stromal matrix that is rich in acidic mucopolysaccharides; scattered smaller cells and stellate cells are also present. The tumor cells have immunohistochemical markers of epithelial differentiation, low molecular weight keratins, and epithelial membrane antigen (EMA), as well as S-100 protein and vimentin. Some are positive for carcinoembryonic antigen (CEA). By electron microscopy, the tumor cells form desmosomes and microvilli, and have characteristic mitochondria surrounded by concentric lamellae of rough endoplasmic reticulum.

High-grade sarcomatous areas, resembling fibrosarcoma, osteosarcoma, or malignant fibrous histiocytoma, may herald dedifferentiation and are sometimes seen in metastatic deposits. These aggressive variants are rare in intracranial chordomas. In contrast, the spheno-occipital region is the preferred site of the "chondroid" variant, which exhibits areas of cartilaginous differentiation that may dominate the histologic picture. These chondroid chordomas lack keratin and EMA positivity and are considered by some to be chondrosarcomas (69,70). Patients with this variant have a better prognosis than those with the usual clival chordoma.

Differential Diagnosis. The differential diagnosis is usually not complicated, since these tumors have characteristic radiologic features, location, and gross and microscopic morphology. Some tumors may be difficult to distinguish from chondrosarcoma; in fact, as indicated above, the chondroid variant may in fact be a chondrosarcoma. The chordoma exhibits markers of epithelial differentiation, such as EMA and cytokeratins.

The distinction from adenocarcinoma may be difficult in some tumors since they form mucin and are positive for epithelial markers as well as CEA. The presence of S-100 protein in some chordomas is helpful. Nuclear pleomorphism can be prominent in both tumors; however, mitoses are less common in chordomas.

Prognosis and Therapy. Although surgery is the preferred initial therapeutic approach, the location and extent of tumor may make complete extirpation impossible. Radiotherapy is indicated for incompletely resected lesions. Mean survival is about 4 to 5 years, and metastases to lung, liver, bone, and lymph nodes occur rarely.

SCHWANNOMAS

Definition. These tumors are composed of spindle-shaped Schwann cells derived from cranial nerves. They are also known as *neurilemmoma* or *neurinoma*.

Clinical Features. Intrasellar and parasellar schwannomas occur rarely (77,79,80). The symptoms are those of a mass and mimic a clinically nonfunctioning pituitary adenoma. By impinging on the pituitary stalk or causing tissue destruction, they can result in hypopituitarism with or without hyperprolactinemia, respectively.

Radiologic Findings. On CT scan, these lesions are visualized as sellar or parasellar masses that enhance with contrast and can mimic pituitary adenoma. They are hypovascular on angiography.

Morphologic Findings. The morphology of these lesions in the pituitary region is identical to that of schwannomas elsewhere. The tumors are usually encapsulated and sometimes cystic lesions composed of spindle-shaped cells arranged in compact Antoni type A and loose Antoni type B areas; the former may exhibit palisading that leads to the formation of Verocay bodies. Immunohistochemical staining for S-100 protein is strong. Electron microscopic examination shows prominent basal lamina surrounding individual cells and the characteristic "long-spacing" collagen of the stroma. The reader is referred to the Fascicle, Tumors of the Soft Tissues (78) for further details.

Differential Diagnosis. The most relevant differential diagnosis of a schwannoma in this region is meningioma. Psammoma bodies and whorls indicate meningioma. Immunoreactivity for S-100 protein is characteristic of schwannoma but may be found in some meningiomas; EMA is identified in meningioma but only uncommonly in schwannoma.

Prognosis and Therapy. Similar to schwannomas elsewhere, these lesions are usually benign. They are amenable to surgical resection unless they involve critical structures in the parasellar region, in which case conservative surgical resection is indicated.

REFERENCES

Neuronal Tumors

1. Asa SL, Kovacs K, Tindall GT, Barrow DL, Horvath E, Vecsei P. Cushing's disease associated with an intrasellar gangliocytoma producing corticotrophin-releasing factor. Ann Intern Med 1984;101:789–93.

2. Asa SL, Scheithauer BW, Bilbao JM, et al. A case for hypothalamic acromegaly: a clinicopathological study of six patients with hypothalamic gangliocytomas producing growth hormone-releasing factor. J Clin Endocrinol Metab 1984;58:796–803.

3. Bevan JS, Asa SL, Rossi ML, Esiri MM, Adams CB, Burke CW. Intrasellar gangliocytoma containing gastrin and growth hormone-releasing hormone associated with a growth hormone-secreting pituitary adenoma. Clin Endocrinol (Oxf) 1989;30:213–24.

4. Burchiel KJ, Shaw CM, Kelly WA. A mixed functional microadenoma and ganglioneuroma of the pituitary fossa. J Neurosurg 1983;58:416–20.

5. Burger PC, Scheithauer BW. Tumors of the central nervous system. Atlas of Tumor Pathology, 3rd Series, Fascicle 10. Washington, D.C.: Armed Forces Institute of Pathology, 1994.

6. Culler FL, James HE, Simon ML, Jones KL. Identification of gonadotropin-releasing hormone in neurons of a hypothalamic hamartoma in a boy with precocious puberty. Neurosurgery 1985;17:408–17.

7. Felix I, Bilbao JM, Asa SL, Tyndel F, Kovacs K, Becker LE. Cerebral and cerebellar gangliocytomas: a morphological study of nine cases. Endocr Pathol 1994;88:246–51.

8. Greenfield JG. The pathological examination of forty intracranial neoplasms. Brain 1919;42:29–85.

9. Hochman HI, Judge DM, Reichlin S. Precocious puberty and hypothalamic hamartoma. Pediatrics 1981;67:236–44.

10. Jakumeit HD, Zimmermann V, Guiot G. Intrasellar gangliocytomas. Report of four cases. J Neurosurg 1974;40:626–30.

11. Judge DM, Kulin HE, Page R, Santen R, Trapukdi S. Hypothalamic hamartoma. A source of luteinizing-hormone-releasing factor in precocious puberty. N Engl J Med 1977;296:7–10.

12. Kamel OW, Horoupian DS, Silverberg GD. Mixed gangliocytoma-adenoma: a distinct neuroendocrine tumor of the pituitary fossa. Hum Pathol 1989;20:1198–203.

13. Li JY, Racadot O, Kujas M, Kouadri M, Peillon F, Racadot J. Immunocytochemistry of four mixed pituitary adenomas and intrasellar gangliocytomas associated with different clinical syndromes: acromegaly, amenorrhea-galactorrhea, Cushing's disease and isolated tumoral syndrome. Acta Neuropathol (Berl) 1989;77:320–8.

14. Müller W, Marcos F. Über das vorkommen von ganglienzellen in einem hypophysentumor. Virchows Arch Pathol Anat Physiol Klin Med 1954;325:733–6.

15. Nishio S, Fujiwara S, Aiko Y, Takeshita I, Fukui M. Hypothalamic hamartoma. Report of two cases. J Neurosurg 1989;70:640–5.

16. Puchner MJ, Lüdecke DK, Saeger W, Riedel M, Asa SL. Gangliocytomas of the sellar region—a review. Exper Clin Endocrinol 1995;103:129–49.

17. Puchner MJ, Lüdecke DK, Valdueza JM, et al. Cushing's disease in a child caused by a corticotropin-releasing hormone-secreting intrasellar gangliocytoma associated with an adrenocorticotropic hormone-secreting pituitary adenoma. Neurosurgery 1993;33:920–5.

18. Racadot OL, Vila-Porcile J, Racadot O. Adénomes hypophysaires et ganlioneuromes de la Selle turcique [Abstract]. J Microsc Biol Cell 1975;23:66.

19. Rhodes RH, Dusseau JJ, Boyd AS Jr, Knigge KM. Intrasellar neural-adenohypophyseal choristoma. A morphological and immunocytochemical study. J Neuropathol Exp Neurol 1982;41:267–80.

20. Scheithauer BW, Kovacs K, Randall RV, Horvath E, Okazaki H, Laws ER Jr. Hypothalamic neuronal hamartoma and adenohypophyseal neuronal choristoma: their association with growth hormone adenoma of the pituitary gland. J Neuropathol Exp Neurol 1983;42:648–63.

21. Slowik F, Fazekas I, Bálint K, et al. Intrasellar hamartoma associated with pituitary adenoma. Acta Neuropathol (Berl) 1990;80:328–33.

22. Yamada S, Stefaneanu L, Kovacs K, Aiba T, Shishiba Y, Hara M. Intrasellar gangliocytoma with multiple immunoreactivities. Endocr Pathol 1990;1:58–63.

Gliomas

23. Alvord EC Jr, Lofton S. Gliomas of the optic nerve or chiasm. Outcome by patients' age, tumor site, and treatment. J Neurosurg 1988;68:85–98.

24. Burger PC, Scheithauer BW. Tumors of the central nervous system. Atlas of Tumor Pathology, 3rd Series, Fascicle 10. Washington, D.C.: Armed Forces Institute of Pathology, 1994.

25. Burger PC, Scheithauer BW, Vogel FS. Surgical pathology of the nervous system and its coverings. 3rd ed. New York: Churchill Livingstone, 1991.

26. Dierssen G, Figols J, Trigueros F, Alvarez G. Gliomas astrocitarios asociados a radioterapia previa. Arch Neurobiol 1987;50:303–8.

27. Huang CI, Chiou WH, Ho DM. Oligodendroglioma occurring after radiation therapy for pituitary adenoma. J Neurol Neurosurg Psychiatry 1987;50:1619–24.

28. Hufnagel TJ, Kim JH, Lesser R, et al. Malignant glioma of the optic chiasm eight years after radiotherapy for prolactinoma. Arch Ophthalmol 1988;106:1701–5.

29. Kitanaka C, Shitara N, Nakagomi T, et al. Postradiation astrocytoma. Report of two cases. J Neurosurg 1989;70:469–74.

30. Liwnicz BH, Berger TS, Liwnicz RG, Aron BS. Radiation-associated gliomas: a report of four cases and analysis of postradiation tumors of the central nervous system. Neurosurgery 1985;17:436–45.

31. Maat-Schieman ML, Bots GT, Thomeer RT, Vielvoye GJ. Malignant astrocytoma following radiotherapy for craniopharyngioma. Br J Radiol 1985;58:480–2.

32. Marus G, Levin CV, Rutherfoord GS. Malignant glioma following radiotherapy for unrelated primary tumors. Cancer 1986;58:886-894.

33. Okamoto S, Handa H, Yamashita J, Tokuriki Y, Abe M. Post-irradiation brain tumors. Neurol Med Chir 1985;25:528–33.

34. Piatt JH Jr, Blue JM, Schold SC, Burger PC. Glioblastoma multiforme after radiotherapy for acromegaly. Neurosurgery 1983;13:85–9.

35. Riccardi VM. Neurofibromatosis. In: Gomez MR, ed. Neurocutaneous syndromes—a practical approach. 2nd ed. Boston: Butterworths, 1987:11–29.

36. Rossi ML, Bevan JS, Esiri MM, Hughes JT, Adams CB. Pituicytoma (pilocytic astrocytoma). J Neurosurg 1987;67:768–72.

37. Rudd A, Rees JE, Kennedy P, Weller RO, Blackwood W. Malignant optic nerve gliomas in adults. J Clin Neurol Ophthalmol 1985;5:238–43.

38. Rush JA, Younge BR, Campbell RJ, MacCarty CS. Optic glioma. Long-term follow-up of 85 histopathologically verified cases. Ophthalmology 1982;89:1213–9.

39. Taphoorn MJ, de Bries-Knoppert WA, Ponssen H, Wolbers JG. Malignant optic nerve glioma in adults. Case Report. J Neurosurg 1989;70:277–9.

40. Ushio Y, Arita N, Yoshimine T, Nagatani M, Mogami H. Glioblastoma after radiotherapy for craniopharyngioma: case report. Neurosurgery 1987;21:33–8.

41. Weinstein JM, Backonja M, Houston LW, et al. Optic glioma associated with Beckwith-Wiedemann syndrome. Pediatr Neurol 1986;2:308–10.

42. Winer JB, Lidov H, Scaravilli F. An ependymoma involving the pituitary fossa. J Neurol Neurosurg Psychiatry 1989;52:1443–4.

43. Wong JY, Uhl V, Wara WM, Sheline GE. Optic gliomas. A reanalysis of the University of California, San Francisco experience. Cancer 1987;60:1847–55.

44. Zampieri P, Zorat PL, Mingrino S, Soattin GB. Radiation-associated cerebral gliomas. A report of two cases and review of the literature. J Neurosurg Sci 1989;33:271–9.

Meningiomas

45. Burger PC, Scheithauer BW. Tumors of the central nervous system. Atlas of Tumor Pathology, 3rd Series, Fascicle 10. Washington, D.C.: Armed Forces Institute of Pathology, 1994.

46. Grisoli F, Vincentelli F, Raybaud C, Harter M, Guibout M, Baldini M. Intrasellar meningioma. Surg Neurol 1983;20:36–41.

47. Halper J, Colvard DS, Scheithauer BW, et al. Estrogen and progesterone receptors in meningiomas: comparison of nuclear binding, dextran-coated charcoal, and immunoperoxidase staining assays. Neurosurgery 1989;25:546–53.

48. Kasantikul V, Shuangshoti S, Phonprasert C. Intrasellar meningioma after radiotherapy for prolactinoma. J Med Assoc Thai 1988;71:524–7.

49. Kleihues P, Burger PC, Scheithauer BW. Histological typing of tumours of the central nervous system. World Health Organization international histological classification of tumours. 2nd ed. Berlin: Springer-Verlag, 1993.

50. Michael AS, Paige ML. MR imaging of intrasellar meningiomas simulating pituitary adenomas. J Comput Assist Tomogr 1988;12:944–6.

51. Okamoto S, Handa H, Yamashita J, Tokuriki Y, Abe M. Post-irradiation brain tumors. Neurol Med Chir 1985;25:528–33.

52. Probst C. Possibilities and limitations of microsurgery in patients with meningiomas of the sellar region. Acta Neurochir 1987;84:99–102.

53. Rohringer M, Sutherland GR, Louw DF, Sima AA. Incidence and clinicopathological features of meningioma. J Neurosurg 1989;71:665–72.

54. Slavin MJ, Weintraub J. Suprasellar meningioma with intrasellar extension simulating pituitary adenoma. Case report. Arch Ophthalmol 1987;105:1488–9.

55. Spallone A. Meningioma as a sequel of radiotherapy for pituitary adenoma. Neurochirurgia 1982;25:68–72.

56. Sridhar K, Ramamurthi B. Intracranial meningioma subsequent to radiation for a pituitary tumor: case report. Neurosurgery 1989;25:643–5.

57. Taylor SL, Barakos JA, Harsh GR IV, Wilson CB. Magnetic resonance imaging of tuberculum sellae meningiomas: preventing preoperative misdiagnosis as pituitary macroadenoma. Neurosurgery 1992;31:621–7.

58. Yeakley JW, Kulkarni MV, McArdle CB, Haar FL, Tang RA. High-resolution MR imaging of juxtasellar meningiomas with CT and angiographic correlation. Am J Neuroradiol 1988;9:279–85.

Granular Cell Tumors

59. Buley ID, Gatter KC, Kelly PM, Heryet A, Millard PR. Granular cell tumours revisited. An immunohistological and ultrastructural study. Histopathology 1988;12:263–74.

60. Cone L, Srinivasan M, Romanul FC. Granular cell tumor (choristoma) of the neurohypophysis: two cases and a review of the literature. Am J Neuroradiol 1990;11:403–6.

61. Landolt AM. Granular cell tumors of the neurohypophysis. Acta Neurochir 1975;(Suppl 22):120–8.

62. Luse SA, Kernohan JW. Granular cell tumors of the stalk and posterior lobe of the pituitary gland. Cancer 1955;8:616–22.

63. Nishioka H, Ii K, Llena JF, Hirano A. Immunohistochemical study of granular cell tumors of the neurohypophysis. Virchows Arch [B] 1991;60:413–7.

64. Shanklin WM. The origin, histology and senescence of tumorettes in the human neurohypophysis. Acta Anat (Basel) 1953;18:1–20.

65. Tomita T, Kuziez M, Watanabe I. Double tumors of the anterior and posterior pituitary gland. Acta Neuropathol (Berl) 1981;54:161–4.

66. Tuch BE, Carter JN, Armellin GM, Newland RC. The association of a tumour of the posterior pituitary gland with multiple endocrine neoplasia type I. Aust NZ J Med 1982;12:179–81.

67. Ulrich J, Heitz PU, Fischer T, Obrist E, Gullotta F. Granular cell tumors: evidence for heterogeneous tumor cell differentiation. An immunocytochemical study. Virchows Arch [B] 1987;53:52–7.

68. Vaquero J, Leunda G, Cabezudo JM, Salazar AR, de Miguel J. Granular pituicytomas of the pituitary stalk. Acta Neurochir 1981;59:209–15.

Chordomas

69. Burger PC, Scheithauer BW. Tumors of the central nervous system. Atlas of Tumor Pathology, 3rd Series, Fascicle 10. Washington, D.C.: Armed Forces Institute of Pathology, 1994.

70. Burger PC, Scheithauer BW, Vogel FS. Surgical pathology of the nervous system and its coverings. 3rd ed. New York: Churchill Livingstone, 1991.

71. Heffelfinger MJ, Dahlin DC, MacCarty CS, Beabout JW. Chordomas and cartilaginous tumors at the skull base. Cancer 1973;32:410–20.

72. Ho KL. Ecchordosis physaliphora and chordoma: a comparative ultrastructural study. Clin Neuropathol 1985;4:77–86.

73. Kleihues P, Burger PC, Scheithauer BW. Histological typing of tumours of the central nervous system. World Health Organization international histological classification of tumours. 2nd ed. Berlin: Springer-Verlag, 1993.

74. Mathews W, Wilson CB. Ectopic intrasellar chordoma. J Neurosurg 1974;39:260–3.

75. Sundaresan N. Chordomas. Clin Orthop Rel Res 1986;204:135–42.

76. Wold LE, Laws ER Jr. Cranial chordomas in children and young adults. J Neurosurg 1983;59:1043–7.

Schwannomas

77. Ishige N, Ito C, Saeki N, Oka N. Neurinoma with intrasellar extension: a case report. Neurol Surg 1985;13:79–84.

78. Lattes R. Tumors of the soft tissues. Atlas of Tumor Pathology, 2nd series, Fascicle 1. Washington, D.C.: Armed Forces Institute of Pathology, 1982.

79. Perone TP, Robinson B, Holmes SM. Intrasellar schwannoma: case report. Neurosurgery 1984;14:71–3.

80. Wilberger JE Jr. Primary intrasellar schwannoma: case report. Surg Neurol 1989;32:156–8.

6
CRANIOPHARYNGIOMA

Definition. The craniopharyngioma is thought to be derived from the remnants of Rathke's pouch. This interpretation and a description of the tumor was provided in 1904 by Erdheim (4) who made an extensive study of squamous epithelial cells in the region of the hypophysis. The name craniopharyngioma was introduced by Cushing in 1932 (4).

Clinical Features. Craniopharyngiomas represent 1 to 13 percent of intracranial neoplasms (4,12), although recent studies narrow that figure to 2 to 4 percent. As the most frequent sellar tumor of childhood, they represent 10 percent of central nervous system tumors in children (15). They occur at any age, from infancy (3) to old age (10), but the peak incidence is from 5 to 20 years. A second small peak occurs in the sixth decade. In some series males are more often affected (12).

The most common presenting symptoms are due to the effects of a mass in the region of the sella turcica. Approximately 75 percent of patients complain of headache and have visual disturbances (12). Less frequently, there are mental changes, nausea, vomiting, somnolence, or symptoms due to pituitary hormone deficiency. The hormone deficiency is due to destruction of hypophysial tissue or interruption of the pituitary stalk resulting in failure of hypothalamic regulation; the former is associated with a reduction in blood prolactin levels whereas the latter is characterized by mild hyperprolactinemia due to loss of hypothalamic dopaminergic inhibition of prolactin release. In children, dwarfism may be the presenting manifestation. In adults, sexual dysfunction is the most common endocrine complaint, with impotence in males and primary or secondary amenorrhea in females. Diabetes insipidus is found in approximately 25 percent of patients (5).

While these tumors can invade into the nasopharynx, there is a report of a primary nasopharyngeal craniopharyngioma arising in ectopic pharyngeal hypophysis (11).

Biochemical Findings. In addition to the mild hyperprolactinemia found in some patients, biochemical studies confirm variable degrees of hypopituitarism, with reduction of basal hormone levels or only subtle changes with normal hormone levels but reduced response to stimulation. In the case of pituitary stalk interruption, basal hormone levels may be low but administration of stimulating hormones may result in sluggish elevation of pituitary hormones in response. Patients with hypopituitarism also have reduced levels of thyroid hormones and glucocorticoids. Diabetes insipidus is characteristic.

Craniopharyngioma has been associated with a prolactinoma (6,7,16), in which cases there were two reasons for hyperprolactinemia. In addition, there have been cases of lymphocytic hypophysitis associated with craniopharyngioma; those patients had complete pituitary insufficiency (14).

Radiologic Findings. An enlarged or eroded sella turcica is found in approximately 50 percent of patients with this tumor; suprasellar calcification is also present in half. Craniopharyngiomas are usually cystic or may be cystic and solid; only 15 percent have no cystic component (15). Computerized tomography (CT) confirms the presence of a partially cystic lesion which may enhance with contrast. However, magnetic resonance imaging (MRI) appears to be the optimal technique for delimiting the extent of the lesion and the nature of the solid and cystic components; the lipid contents provide a high T1 signal intensity in the absence of contrast media (fig. 6-1) (13,16).

Gross Findings. The majority of tumors are suprasellar (12); only 15 percent have an intrasellar component. Although they may be as small as 1 cm, most are much larger at the time of diagnosis. They are well-circumscribed tumors (fig. 6-2) but there may be little or no capsule at the interface with brain parenchyma (fig. 6-3). The lesions usually contain a thick oil-like fluid which is described as "black sludge." Cholesterol crystals and calcification may be seen. Rarely, the tumors contain bone or teeth.

Microscopic Findings. Microscopically, the tumors are composed of cords or islands of epithelial cells in a loose fibrous stroma (figs. 6-4–6-6)

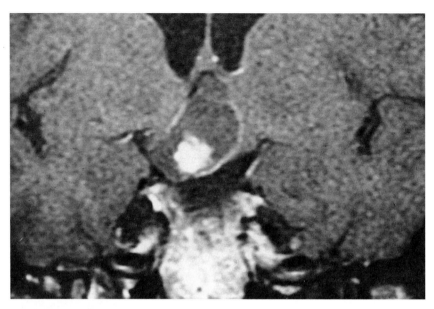

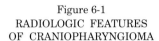

Figure 6-1
RADIOLOGIC FEATURES
OF CRANIOPHARYNGIOMA
MRI allows recognition of the solid and cystic components of sellar and suprasellar tumor; the lipid components provide high signal intensity in this T1-weighted image.

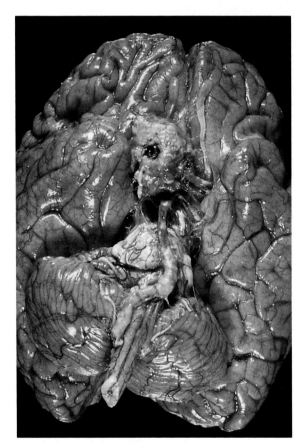

Figure 6-2
GROSS APPEARANCE OF CRANIOPHARYNGIOMA

At autopsy, this craniopharyngioma in a patient who had a longstanding history of blindness and panhypopituitarism, reveals a suprasellar tumor overlying the optic chiasm. Grossly it appears to be well delineated.

with intervening cysts. The epithelium usually has an outer palisaded layer, a mid-zone of stellate epithelial cells, and a superficial keratinizing layer. Cholesterol clefts are seen and extensive accumulation of cholesterol-containing fluid is the cause of the "machinery oil" seen grossly. Masses of keratin often form a nidus for calcification. Occasionally, there is an inflammatory component consisting of lymphocytes, plasma cells, and macrophages which may infiltrate the fibrous walls and septa of the tumor. Although the tumors are grossly well circumscribed, microscopically the borders are frequently irregular and may be associated with gliosis in the adjacent brain tissue.

Two subtypes of craniopharyngioma have been recognized (8), however, these tumors frequently refute subclassification because of overlap. The adamantinomatous type has a predominance of stellate components which results in a pattern resembling the dental ameloblastic organ and is similar to that seen in adamantinomas. The papillary variant is less common, is rare in children, and is said to have a better prognosis. It is characterized by solid or cystic growth of pseudo-papillary squamous epithelium and lacks the palisading, fibrosis, and cholesterol accumulation that characterize the typical craniopharyngioma.

Immunohistochemistry confirms the epithelial nature of the squamous component, which contains low and high molecular weight cytokeratins (fig. 6-7). However, the histology of these tumors is

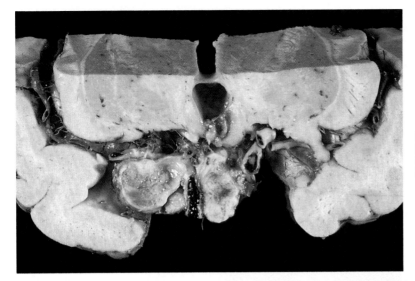

Figure 6-3
GROSS APPEARANCE OF
CRANIOPHARYNGIOMA
On cross section, the tumor illustrated
in figure 6-2 is seen to have a less well-de-
fined border. The tumor has a thick oily
appearance. (Plate IXB Fascicle 21, 2nd
Series.)

Figure 6-4
HISTOLOGY OF
CRANIOPHARYNGIOMA
In craniopharyngioma, the epithelium
usually has an outer palisaded layer and a
mid-zone of stellate epithelial cells. This
appearance mimics the features of dental
adamantinomas, hence the term "ad-
amantinomotous" craniopharyngioma.

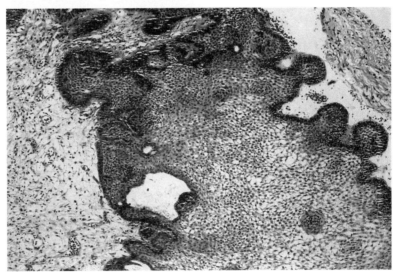

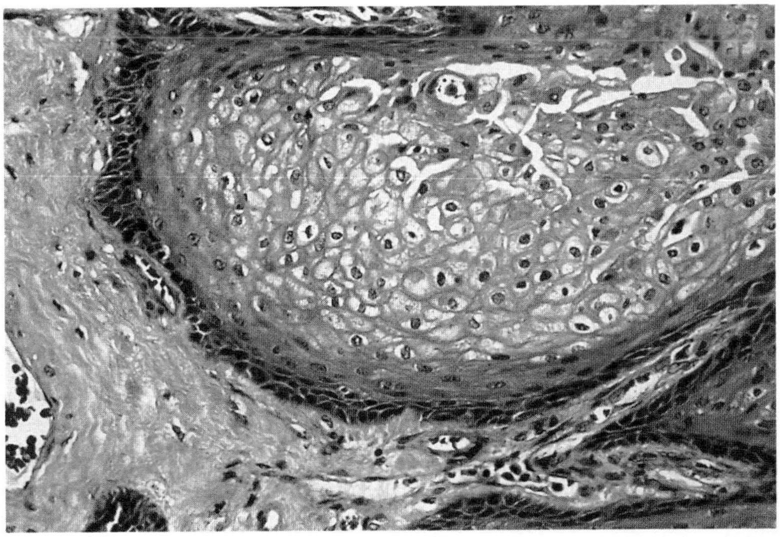

Figure 6-5
HISTOLOGY OF
CRANIOPHARYNGIOMA
In areas, the epithelium of a craniopharyngioma is squamoid with a palisaded basal layer (Hematoxylin-phloxine-saffron stain).

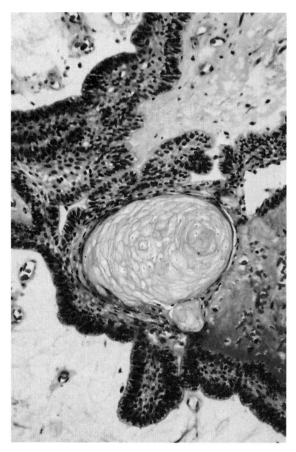

Figure 6-6
HISTOLOGY OF CRANIOPHARYNGIOMA

Palisading epithelium of craniopharyngioma forms keratin pearls containing ghost-like squamous cells; these areas may be a nidus for calcification. The surrounding stroma, stained with hematoxylin-phloxine-saffron, is very loose and edematous.

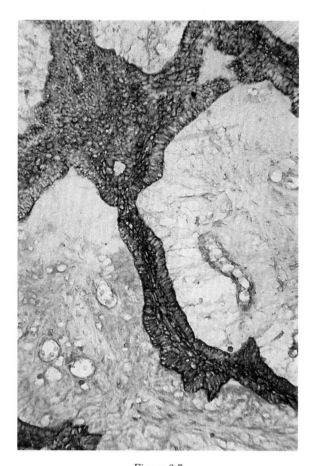

Figure 6-7
IMMUNOHISTOCHEMICAL LOCALIZATION
OF KERATINS IN CRANIOPHARYNGIOMA

These tumors generally contain abundant low and high molecular weight cytokeratins within the epithelial component.

generally sufficiently characteristic that special studies are not required to confirm the diagnosis.

Electron microscopy shows the characteristics of keratinizing epithelial cells with numerous tonofilaments, well-formed intercellular junctions, and no secretory granules (figs. 6-8–6-10).

Differential Diagnosis. These tumors may be confused with the epithelial cysts that occur in the sellar region (see chapter 11), particularly epidermoid cysts. The latter are unilocular cysts lined by orderly stratified squamous epithelium of uniform thickness overlying delicate fibrous connective tissue; this contrasts with the nodular, irregular appearance of the epithelial component of craniopharyngioma. Orientation artifact and inadequate sampling, however, may make the dis-

tinction difficult. Calcification is rare in epidermoid cysts and common in craniopharyngioma.

The infiltrating nature of craniopharyngioma provokes exuberant reactive gliosis that may be mistaken for pilocytic astrocytoma (see chapter 5). Reactive gliosis is usually of lower cellularity and lacks the cysts that are frequent in this glioma.

Pathogenesis. Craniopharyngiomas are thought to originate from nests of squamous epithelial cells commonly found in the suprasellar area surrounding the pars tuberalis of the adult pituitary (1). It has been accepted that these represent remnants of Rathke's pouch, however, there is evidence that they may represent metaplastic foci (1,2). It is intriguing that squamous nest are rarely seen in pituitaries of children, yet the incidence of craniopharyngiomas is higher in children than in adults.

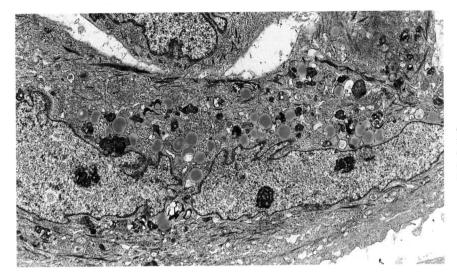

Figure 6-8
ULTRASTRUCTURE OF
CRANIOPHARYNGIOMA
The epithelial component of
craniopharyngioma is characterized by polygonal and elongated
cells that have well-formed intercellular junctions and contain
numerous tonofilaments.

Figure 6-9
ULTRASTRUCTURE OF
CRANIOPHARYNGIOMA
The stellate component of
craniopharyngioma has very
prominent intercellular junctions and large numbers of
cytoplasmic tonofilaments that
correspond to keratin.

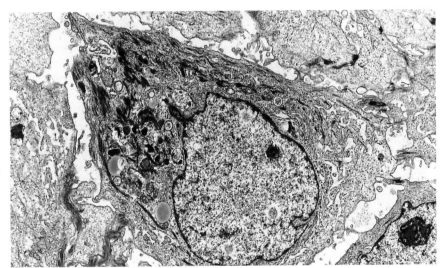

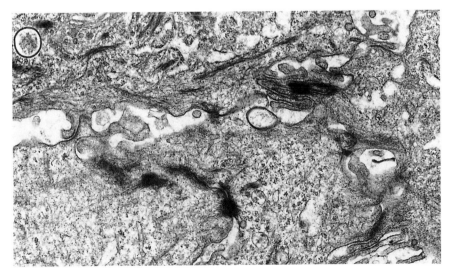

Figure 6-10
ULTRASTRUCTURE OF
CRANIOPHARYNGIOMA
Intercellular attachments
are extremely well formed in the
areas of complex interdigitation
of craniopharyngioma cells.

171

Prognosis and Therapy. If left alone, craniopharyngiomas are extremely infiltrative. They may cause extensive tissue damage, extending into the hypothalamus and as high as the third ventricle; obstruction of the ventricle may result in hydrocephalus. Uncommonly, craniopharyngiomas may spontaneously rupture or form abscesses.

Because of their highly infiltrative nature, they are often incompletely excised surgically. There is a 10 to 40 percent recurrence rate, particularly in younger patients. A subfrontal surgical approach is required in most patients; transsphenoidal surgery is suitable only for those rare patients with a mainly intrasellar tumor or for palliative subtotal removal or drainage for patients with failed previous surgery (9). Most surgeons advocate postoperative radiation to reduce recurrence (5,9). No medical therapy is currently known for these tumors, but often patients require hormone replacement for anterior pituitary insufficiency.

Malignant Craniopharyngioma. There is a single report of malignant transformation of a craniopharyngioma (15). This occurred on the fifth recurrence after a 35-year history of disease and 8 years following radiotherapy.

REFERENCES

1. Asa SL, Kovacs K, Bilbao JM. The pars tuberalis of the human pituitary. A histologic, immunohistochemical, ultrastructural and immunoelectron microscopic analysis. Virchows Arch [A] 1983;399:49–59.
2. Asa SL, Kovacs K, Bilbao JM, Penz G. Immunohistochemical localization of keratin in craniopharyngiomas and squamous cell nests of the human pituitary. Acta Neuropathol (Berl) 1981;54:257–60.
3. Azar-Kia B, Krishnan UR, Schechter MM. Neonatal craniopharyngioma. Case report. J Neurosurg 1975;42:91–93.
4. Banna M. Craniopharyngioma: based on 160 cases. Br J Radiol 1976;49:206–23.
5. Baskin DS, Wilson CB. Surgical management of craniopharyngiomas. A review of 74 cases. J Neurosurg 1986;65:22–7.
6. Cusimano MD, Kovacs K, Bilbao JM, Tucker WS, Singer W. Suprasellar craniopharyngioma associated with hyperprolactinemia, pituitary lactotroph hyperplasia, and microprolactinoma. Case report. J Neurosurg 1988;69:620–3.
7. Heffelfinger MJ, Dahlin DC, MacCarty CS, Beabout JW. Chordomas and cartilaginous tumors at the skull base. Cancer 1973;32:410–20.
8. Kleihues P, Burger PC, Scheithauer BW. Histological typing of tumours of the central nervous system. World Health Organization international histological classification of tumours. 2nd ed. Berlin: Springer-Verlag, 1993.
9. Laws ER Jr. Craniopharyngioma: diagnosis and treatment. Endocrinologist 1992;2:184–8.
10. Lederman GS, Recht A, Loeffler JS, Dubuisson D, Kleefield J, Schnitt SJ. Craniopharyngioma in an elderly patient. Cancer 1987;60:1077–80.
11. Lewin R, Ruffolo E, Saraceno C. Craniopharyngioma arising in the pharyngeal hypophysis. Southern Med J 1984;77:1519–23.
12. Petito CK, DeGirolami U, Earle KM. Craniopharyngiomas. A clinical and pathological review. Cancer 1976;37:1944–52.
13. Pigeau I, Sigal R, Halimi PH, Comoy J, Doyon D. MRI features of craniopharyngiomas at 1.5 Tesla. A series of 13 cases. J Neuroradiol 1988;15:276–87.
14. Puchner MJ, Lüdecke DK, Saeger W. The anterior pituitary lobe in patients with cystic craniopharyngiomas: three cases of associated lymphocytic hypophysitis. Acta Neurochir 1994;126:38–43.
15. Scheithauer BW. The hypothalamus and neurohypophysis. In: Kovacs K, Asa SL, eds. Functional endocrine pathology. Boston: Blackwell Scientific Publications, 1991:170–244.
16. Wheatley T, Clark JD, Stewart S. Craniopharyngioma with hyperprolactinaemia due to a prolactinoma. J Neurol Neurosurg Psychiatry 1986;49:1305–7.

❖❖❖

7
GERM CELL TUMORS OF THE SELLA TURCICA

Definition. These tumors are derived from germ cells that are residual along the midline; they are identical to germ cell tumors of the gonads and mediastinum.

Germ cell tumors represent less than 1 percent of intracranial neoplasms but in children, they constitute up to 6.5 percent of such lesions (12). The suprasellar region is the second most common site of involvement after the pineal. The tumors occur most often before the age of 20 years, more often in males than females.

Clinical Features. Intracranial germ cell tumors can be associated with hypopituitarism, diabetes insipidus, and visual disturbances; in severe cases, large lesions can cause intracranial hypertension, hydrocephalus, psychosis, and dementia (4–6,11–13). Hypothalamic destruction can result in bulimia or anorexia (5,12). Some tumors are associated with precocious puberty; although this has been attributed to hypothalamic destruction and release of gonadal inhibition, a more likely explanation is the production of β-chorionic gonadotropin (hCG) by the neoplastic germ cells. Elevated circulating levels of α-fetoprotein (AFP) indicate the presence of the yolk sac elements that characterize endodermal sinus tumors.

Radiologic Findings. The most common germ cell tumor, the germinoma, is usually a well-demarcated tumor that has high density on computerized tomography (CT) scan and enhances with contrast (11). Teratomas may exhibit fat densities and calcifications that are recognized radiologically. While the CT appearance of some of the other germ cell tumors may not be distinctive (3), magnetic resonance imaging (MRI) is more sensitive and can show features that are obscured on CT scan.

Morphologic Findings. The classification of parasellar and intrasellar germ cell tumors is similar to that of intracranial germ cell tumors of the pineal and other locations (7). Morphologically, the lesions are indistinguishable from their gonadal and extragonadal counterparts, however, there are immunohistochemical characteristics that appear to be unique to the intracranial tumors. Vimentin, keratin, and epithelial membrane antigen staining in these lesions has been interpreted as indicating mesenchymal and epithelial differentiation (9). The detailed morphologic descriptions of teratomas, germinomas (fig. 7-1), embryonal carcinomas (fig. 7-2), endodermal sinus tumors (figs. 7-3, 7-4), and choriocarcinomas can be found elsewhere (14).

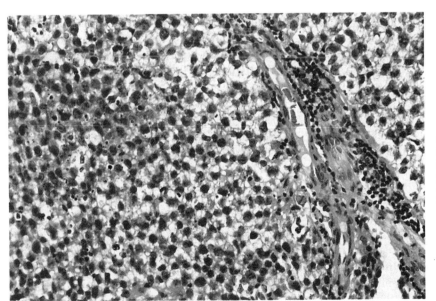

Figure 7-1
HISTOLOGY OF
SELLAR GERMINOMA
A germinoma of the sella turcica has characteristic histology, resembling germinomas and dysgerminomas in other sites. Two cell populations are identified, the larger tumor cells and smaller inflammatory cells.

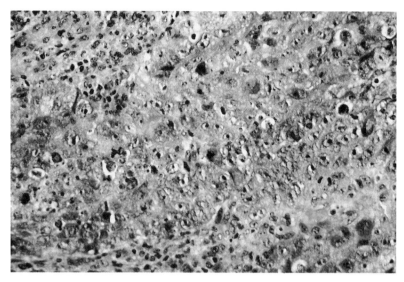

Figure 7-2
HISTOLOGY OF SELLAR
EMBRYONAL CARCINOMA
An embryonal carcinoma in the sella turcica resembles this germ cell tumor in other sites. It is composed of large cells with poorly defined borders and marked nuclear pleomorphism.

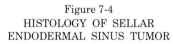

Figure 7-3
HISTOLOGY OF SELLAR
ENDODERMAL SINUS TUMOR
An endodermal sinus tumor of the sella turcica has a reticular architecture characterized by a meshwork of communicating spaces. Occasional papillary projections into the spaces are identified. (Courtesy of Dr. E. Silva, Houston, TX.)

Figure 7-4
HISTOLOGY OF SELLAR
ENDODERMAL SINUS TUMOR
Papillary projections into the spaces of this sellar endodermal sinus tumor resemble the Schiller-Duval bodies of gonadal endodermal sinus tumors. (Courtesy of Dr. J.M. Bilbao, Toronto, Canada.)

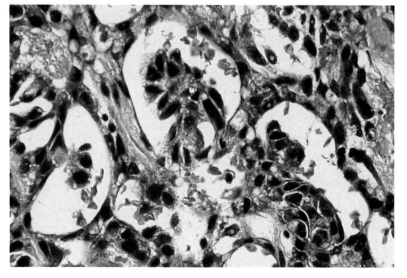

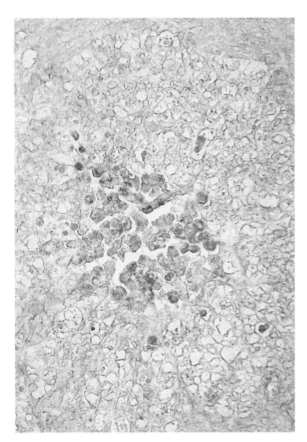

Figure 7-5
IMMUNOHISTOCHEMICAL LOCALIZATION OF
β-hCG IN SELLAR EMBRYONAL CARCINOMA
Production of β-hCG by this tumor can create a difficult clinical differential diagnosis since this marker is highly homologous to β-LH.

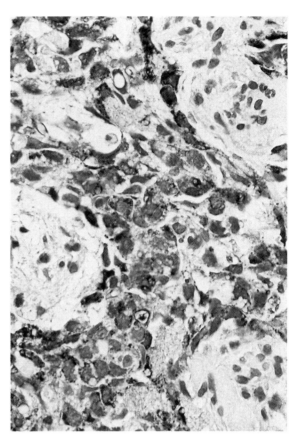

Figure 7-6
IMMUNOHISTOCHEMICAL LOCALIZATION
OF α-FETOPROTEIN IN
SELLAR ENDODERMAL SINUS TUMOR
Immunoreactivity for AFP characterizes the yolk sac elements that comprise endodermal sinus tumors. (Courtesy of Dr. J.M. Bilbao, Toronto, Canada.)

In the sellar region, germinomas and teratomas predominate and mixed germ cell tumors that show features of more than one tumor subtype are frequent, usually germinoma combined with one of the other tumor types or a combination of embryonal carcinoma and immature teratoma, known as teratocarcinoma. Recognition of even minor components that are characterized by more aggressive elements can predict a worse prognosis and may alter management; this underscores the need for complete tissue examination of truly representative biopsies.

Functionally, the hormonal activity of these lesions can be determined by immunohistochemistry. In general, syncytiotrophoblast elements are responsible for β-hCG, placental lactogen, and pregnancy glycoprotein (SP$_1$). Embryonal carcinomas contain AFP, SP$_1$, and β-hCG (fig. 7-5), whereas endodermal sinus tumors contain AFP only (fig. 7-6). Measurement of circulating markers such as β-hCG and AFP in blood is useful to detect recurrence. Germinomas are usually negative for these markers, but they are immunoreactive for placental alkaline phosphatase (PLAP); they may contain isolated β-hCG-reactive syncytiotrophoblast cells but these are not prognostically significant.

Differential Diagnosis. Germinomas are characterized by large clear cells and vesicular nuclei with prominent nucleoli, however, there is often a lymphocytic infiltrate and granulomatous inflammation that is abundant enough to mask the underlying neoplasm. The glycogen responsible for the cytoplasmic vacuolation is a potential source of confusion with metastatic malignancies. Immunostaining for PLAP can assist in confirming the correct diagnosis in both situations.

At the periphery of germ cell tumors there may be a reactive atypical gliosis that can mimic astrocytoma. Proper sampling will overcome this problem.

Prognosis and Therapy. Often the diagnosis is confirmed only at the time of surgery; rarely is surgery curative, however (2). If the diagnosis is suspected preoperatively, biopsy can type the lesion and determine whether surgery or other modalities such as radiation or chemotherapy are indicated. Germinomas are uniquely radiosensitive and long-term remission is achieved in approximately 70 percent of patients (13). The recognition of more aggressive elements in mixed tumors can predict failure of radiotherapy. Other tumors are more aggressive and despite surgery, radiation, and chemotherapy, they may recur or metastasize, both within and beyond the central nervous system (1). Seeding via a ventriculoperitoneal shunt may also result in dissemination (8,10).

REFERENCES

1. Allen JC, Kim JH, Packer RJ. Neoadjuvant chemotherapy for newly diagnosed germ-cell tumors of the central nervous system. J Neurosurg 1987;67:65–70.

2. Baskin DS, Wilson CB. Transsphenoidal surgery of intrasellar germinomas. Report of two cases. J Neurosurg 1983;59:1063–6.

3. Chang T, Teng MM, Guo WY, Sheng WC. CT of pineal tumors and intracranial germ-cell tumors. Am J Neuroradiol 1989;10:1039–44.

4. Furukawa F, Haebara H, Hamashima Y. Primary intracranial choriocarcinoma arising from the pituitary fossa. Report of an autopsy case with literature review. Acta Pathol Jpn 1986;36:773–81.

5. Jennings MT, Gelman R, Hochberg F. Intracranial germ-cell tumors: natural history and pathogenesis. J Neurosurg 1985;63:155–67.

6. Kageyama N, Kobayashi T, Kida Y, Yoshida J, Kato K. Intracranial germinal tumors. Prog Exp Tumor Res 1987;30:255–67.

7. Kleihues P, Burger PC, Scheithauer BW. Histological typing of tumours of the central nervous system. World Health Organization international histological classification of tumours. 2nd ed. Berlin: Springer-Verlag, 1993.

8. Kuzel TM, Benson AB, Gurley AM, Cerullo L. Intracranial teratocarcinoma with ventriculoperitoneal shunt metastases. Am J Med 1989;86:736–8.

9. Nakagawa Y, Perentes E, Ross GW, Ross AN, Rubinstein LJ. Immunohistochemical differences between intracranial germinomas and their gonadal equivalents. An immunoperoxidase study of germ cell tumours with epithelial membrane antigen, cytokeratin and vimentin. J Pathol 1988;156:67–72.

10. Paine JT, Handa H, Yamasaki T, Yamashita J. Suprasellar germinoma with shunt metastasis: report of a case with an immunohistochemical characterization of the lymphocytic subpopulations. Surg Neurol 1986;25:55–61.

11. Poon W, Ng HK, Wong K, South JR. Primary intrasellar germinoma presenting with cavernous sinus syndrome. Surg Neurol 1988;30:402–5.

12. Rueda-Pedraza ME, Heifetz SA, Sesterhenn IA, Clark GB. Primary intracranial germ cell tumors in the first two decades of life. A clinical, light-microscopic, and immunohistochemical analysis of 54 cases. Perspect Pediatr Pathol 1987;10:160–207.

13. Sakai N, Yamada H, Andoh T, Hirata T, Shimizu K, Shinoda J. Primary intracranial germ-cell tumors. A retrospective analysis with special reference to long-term results of treatment and the behavior of rare types of tumors. Acta Oncol 1988;27:43–50.

14. Scully R. Tumors of the ovary and maldeveloped gonads. Atlas of Tumor Pathology, 2nd Series, Fascicle 16. Washington, D.C.: Armed Forces Institute of Pathology, 1979.

❖❖❖

8

HEMATOLOGIC TUMORS OF THE SELLA TURCICA

LYMPHOMA AND LEUKEMIA

Definition. Tumors of lymphocytic or plasmacytic differentiation are usually systemic disorders. Rarely, lesions in the region of the pituitary and hypothalamus appear to be solitary and primary in that site (11).

Clinical Features. As in the central nervous system in general (4,5,13), where lymphoma or leukemia most often are meningeal and extradural, pituitary involvement in patients with systemic hematologic malignancies results in subcapsular infiltration; intraparenchymal deposits are rare (8). The clinical manifestations of pituitary involvement usually are dominated by diabetes mellitus but occasionally there is excessive secretion of vasopressin, resulting in the syndrome of inappropriate antidiuretic hormone (SIADH) (8,13). Primary lymphoma involving the hypothalamus can result in hypopituitarism (3) and has been associated with the chiasmal syndrome (6).

Rarely, lymphomas, leukemias, or plasmacytomas present as sellar masses (1,2,9,12,15,16). The majority of these can cause symptoms of a mass lesion with or without hypopituitarism due to adenohypophysial tissue destruction. In most patients, there is evidence of systemic disease, and only rarely is the lesion considered a truly solitary sellar disorder (7,14). There is single report of pituitary adenoma associated with a primary brain lymphoma with hypothalamic involvement (10).

Radiologic Findings. Lymphomas in the region of the sella and hypothalamus are seen on magnetic resonance imaging (MRI) as masses with signals of similar intensity to their surroundings on T1-weighted images but are hyperintense on T2-weighted views. They enhance with contrast media, usually in a uniform pattern.

Morphologic Findings. Histologically, the lymphomas of the central nervous system and the sellar region resemble systemic lymphomas (fig. 8-1). They are almost always non-Hodgkin lymphomas with a diffuse rather than follicular pattern; the majority are B-cell tumors. Plasmacytomas are composed of well-differentiated plasma cells (fig. 8-2). The classification of these lesions is

worthy of an entire Fascicle and the reader is referred accordingly to the text on Tumors of the Lymphoid System for further details (17).

Differential Diagnosis. Thorough morphologic assessment can readily distinguish these tumors from pituitary adenomas. Histologic analysis alone may not reveal the hematologic nature of the disorder: a plasmacytoma composed of well-differentiated plasma cells can mimic a chromophobe adenoma (fig. 8-2) and lymphoma can be difficult to distinguish from a bromocriptine-treated prolactin-producing adenoma. However, immunostaining for leukocytic markers and lack of hormone immunoreactivity (figs. 8-3, 8-4) can identify

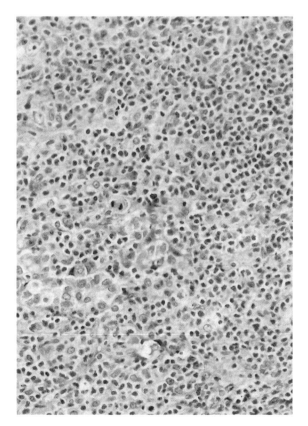

Figure 8-1
HISTOLOGY OF SELLAR LYMPHOMA

The pituitary is almost totally destroyed by an infiltrate of atypical lymphocytes with conspicuous mitoses. Scattered residual epithelial cells are still identifiable. (Courtesy of Dr. R.L. Apel, Brisbane, Australia.)

Figure 8-2
CYTOLOGY OF
SELLAR PLASMACYTOMA

A pituitary tumor can be diagnosed as plasmacytoma at the time of intraoperative consultation. These tumor cells have eccentric nuclei and binucleate forms are seen. The "clockface" chromatin pattern is characteristic. These lesions can mimic pituitary adenoma (see figure 2-1), however, the cytoplasmic basophilia and pale Golgi zone are inconsistent with pituitary cells; fibrous bodies that resemble the Golgi region of these plasma cells are not found in basophilic adenohypophysial cells. (Courtesy of Dr. J.M. Bilbao, Toronto, Canada.)

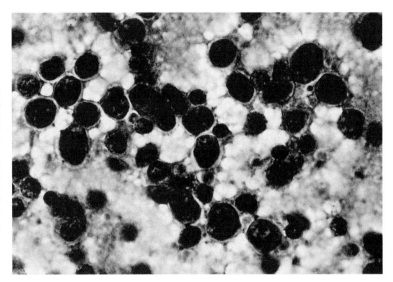

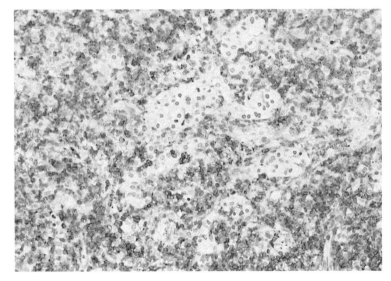

Figure 8-3
IMMUNOHISTOCHEMICAL
LOCALIZATION OF LEUKOCYTE
COMMON ANTIGEN
IN SELLAR LYMPHOMA

Staining for leukocyte common antigen decorates most of the cells in this field, identifying the infiltrating lymphocytes. Clusters of epithelial cells do not stain for this antigen. Stains for lymphocyte subsets reveal the monoclonal nature of this infiltrate in contrast to the polyclonal infiltrate of lymphocytic hypophysitis.

Figure 8-4
IMMUNOHISTOCHEMICAL
LOCALIZATION OF PITUITARY
HORMONES IN SELLAR LYMPHOMA

The trapped residual pituitary cells within a sellar lymphoma contain immunoreactive growth hormone.

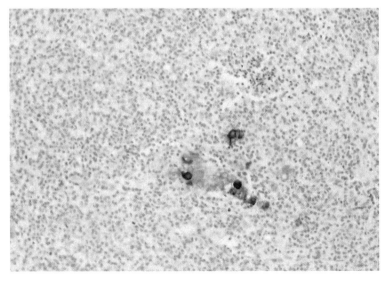

178

the tumor cells. In difficult cases, electron microscopy may be necessary to exclude epithelial differentiation.

The distinction from lymphocytic hypophysitis (see chapter 11) can be difficult. In hypophysitis, the infiltrate is cytologically benign and immunohistochemically polyclonal, whereas lymphomatous infiltrates are cytologically malignant and monomorphous, and show clonal restriction of immunologic markers.

Prognosis and Therapy. Since pituitary involvement with lymphoma or leukemia is usually reflective of systemic disease, the reader is referred to the Fascicle on Tumors of the Lymphoid System for a thorough review of prognostic and therapeutic considerations (17). Primary and isolated lymphomas of this region are too few to provide an intelligent approach to management.

LANGERHANS' CELL HISTIOCYTOSIS

Definition. The disorder formerly known as histiocytosis X, encompassing eosinophilic granuloma, Hand-Schüller-Christian disease, Letterer-Siwe disease, Langerhans' cell granuloma, and several other eponymic variants, is now classified as Langerhans' cell histiocytosis (25). This localized, multifocal or disseminated proliferation of epithelioid histiocyte-like Langerhans cells is currently thought to be a reactive rather than neoplastic process with an immunologic abberation underlying its etiology (25). The classic presentation of Hand-Schüller-Christian disease involves the hypothalamus (19,21,25) and the disorder may involve the pituitary gland itself (20,21).

Clinical Features. Lesions involving the hypothalamus and pituitary cause hypopituitarism and diabetes insipidus (19,20,27). Diabetes insipidus is the most common and usually the initial manifestation. Rarely, the hypopituitarism is due to adenohypophysial tissue destruction (20,27). More commonly, the disease is predominantly hypothalamic and the hypopituitarism is secondary to hypothalamic destruction; in this situation pituitary hypofunction is associated with hyperprolactinemia due to destruction of the dopaminergic neurons that maintain tonic inhibition of that hormone (19,21).

Radiologic Findings. Langerhans' cell histiocytosis is characterized on CT scan by ill-defined,

contrast-enhancing, hypodense masses with areas of edema. MRI can detect the small multifocal lesions of this disorder more readily than CT scan (18); the lesions may be hypointense (27) but can have slightly increased T1 contrast and intense T2-weighted images. Involvement of the pituitary stalk is characteristic (23,26) and may precede the clinical manifestations (24).

Morphologic Findings. Histologically the Langerhans cells are characterized by an epithelioid, histiocyte-like appearance (figs. 8-5, 8-6). The cells have kidney-shaped nuclei and abundant cytoplasm. They are admixed with chronic inflammatory cells, foamy macrophages, and eosinophils. Immunohistochemistry identifies human leukocyte antigen (HLA)-DR antigens, CD1, and S-100 protein as markers of Langerhans cells. The cells also react with peanut agglutinin. Pathognomonic Birbeck granules are seen by electron microscopy, allowing a definitive diagnosis (19,20,22,25).

Differential Diagnosis. Intrasellar lesions of this disorder mimic pituitary adenoma. The histologic appearance is usually sufficiently characteristic to allow distinction but in difficult cases immunohistochemistry distinguishes leukocyte common antigen (LCA)- and S-100-positive histiocytes from pituitary cells or from germinoma cells, which can also resemble Langerhans cells. Lymphocytic hypophysitis and granulomatous inflammation (see chapter 11) are important differential diagnoses, just as encephalitis must be excluded in the hypothalamus. Prominence of eosinophils is suggestive of Langerhans' cell histiocytosis. In all of these disorders, the lymphocytic infiltrate is polyclonal and immunohistochemistry may not be helpful; the detection of Birbeck granules by electron microscopy may be the only definitive diagnostic feature.

Prognosis and Therapy. The prognosis is variable. When involvement is systemic, the disorder is frequently lethal and apparently isolated lesions can progress rapidly to widely disseminated disease that is unresponsive to any form of therapeutic intervention. Surgery has been reported to be curative for localized lesions (20) and radiotherapy has been used postoperatively with success in cases with isolated involvement of the area (21).

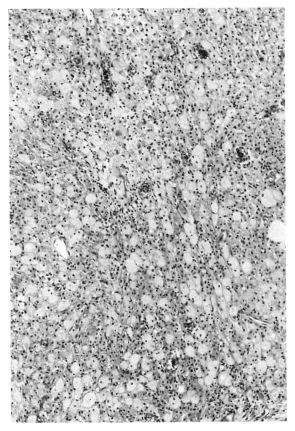

Figure 8-5
HISTOLOGY OF LANGERHANS'
CELL HISTIOCYTOSIS
Langerhans' cell histiocytosis is characterized by proliferation of epithelioid histiocyte-like cells admixed with chronic inflammatory cells.

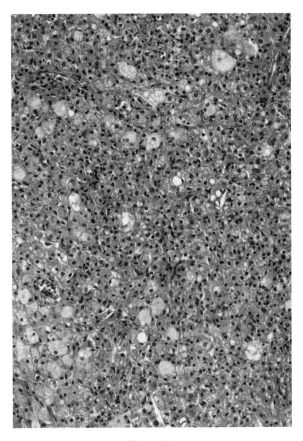

Figure 8-6
HISTOLOGY OF LANGERHANS'
CELL HISTIOCYTOSIS
The tumor cells have kidney-shaped nuclei and abundant foamy cytoplasm.

REFERENCES

Lymphoma and Leukemia

1. Bitterman P, Ariza A, Black RA, Allen WE III, Lee SH. Multiple myeloma mimicking pituitary adenoma. Comput Radiol 1986;10:201–5.
2. Buchmann E, Schwesinger G. The hypophysis and haemoblastoses. Zentralbl Neurochir 1979;40:35–42.
3. Duchen LW, Treip CS. Microgliomatosis presenting with dementia and hypopituitarism. J Pathol 1969;98:143–6.
4. Fine HA, Mayer RJ. Primary central nervous system lymphoma. Ann Intern Med 1993;119:1093–104.
5. Hochberg FH, Miller DC. Primary central nervous system lymphoma. J Neurosurg 1988;68:835–53.
6. Maiuri F. Primary cerebral lymphoma presenting as steroid-responsive chiasmal syndrome. Br J Neurosurg 1987;1:499–502.
7. Mancardi GL, Mandybur TI. Solitary intracranial plasmacytoma. Cancer 1983;51:2226–33.
8. Masse SR, Wolk RW, Conklin RH. Peripituitary gland involvement in acute leukemia in adults. Arch Pathol 1973;96:141–2.
9. Nemoto K, Ohnishi Y, Tsukada T. Chronic lymphocytic leukemia showing pituitary tumor with massive leukemic cell infiltration, and special reference to clinicopathological findings of CLL. Acta Pathol Jpn 1978;28:797–805.
10. Roggli VL, Suzuki M, Armstrong D, McGavran MH. Pituitary microadenoma and primary lymphoma of brain associated with hypothalamic invasion. Am J Clin Pathol 1979;71:724–7.
11. Samaratunga H, Perry-Keene D, Apel RL. Primary lymphoma of pituitary gland: a neoplasm of acquired MALT? Endocr Pathol 1997;8:335–341.
12. Sanchez JA, Rahman S, Strauss RA, Kaye GI. Multiple myeloma masquerading as a pituitary tumor. Arch Pathol Lab Med 1977;101:55–6.

13. Sheehan T, Cuthbert RJ, Parker AC. Central nervous system involvement in haematological malignancies. Clin Lab Haematol 1989;11:331–8.
14. Singh VP, Mahapatra AK, Dinde AK. Sellar-suprasellar primary malignant lymphoma: case report. Indian J Cancer 1993;30:88–91.
15. Urbanski SJ, Bilbao JM, Horvath E, Kovacs K, So W, Ward JV. Intrasellar solitary plasmacytoma terminating in multiple myeloma: a report of a case including electron microscopical study. Surg Neurol 1980;14:233–6.
16. Vaquero J, Areitio E, Martinez R. Intracranial parasellar plasmacytoma. Arch Neurol 1982;39:738.
17. Warnke R, Dorfman R, Weiss L, Cleary M, Chan J. Tumors of the lymph nodes and spleen. Atlas of Tumor Pathology, 3rd Series, Fascicle 14. Washington, D.C.: Armed Forces Institute of Pathology, 1995.

Langerhans' Cell Histiocytosis

18. Graif M, Pennock JM. MR imaging of histiocytosis X in the central nervous system. Am J Neuroradiol 1986;7:21–3.
19. Kepes JJ, Kepes M. Predominantly cerebral forms of histiocytosis-X. A reappraisal of "Gagel's hypothalamic granuloma," "granuloma infiltrans of the hypothalamus" and "Ayala's disease" with a report of four cases. Acta Neuropathol (Berl) 1969;14:77-98.
20. Nishio S, Mizuno J, Barrow DL, Takei Y, Tindall GT. Isolated histiocytosis X of the pituitary gland: case report. Neurosurgery 1987;21:718–21.
21. Ober KP, Alexander E Jr, Challa VR, Ferree C, Elster A. Histiocytosis X of the hypothalamus. Neurosurgery 1989;24:93–5.
22. Ornvold K, Ralfkiaer E, Carstensen H. Immunohistochemical study of the abnormal cells in Langerhans cell histiocytosis (histiocytosis X). Virchows Arch [A] 1990;416:403–10.
23. Peyster RG, Hoover ED. CT of the abnormal pituitary stalk. Am J Neuroradiol 1984;5:49–52.
24. Schmitt S, Wichmann W, Martin E, Zachmann M, Schoenle EJ. Primary stalk thickening with diabetes insipidus preceding typical manifestations of Langerhans cell histiocytosis in children. Eur J Pediatr 1993; 152:399–401.
25. The Writing Group of the Histiocyte Society. Histiocytosis syndromes in children. Lancet 1987;1:208–9.
26. Tien RD, Newton TH, McDermott MW, Dilon WP, Kucharczyk J. Thickened pituitary stalk on MR images in patients with diabetes insipidus and Langerhans cell histiocytosis. Am J Neuroradiol 1990;11:703–8.
27. Vadakekalem J, Stamos T, Shenker Y. Sometimes the hooves do belong to zebras! An unusual case of hypopituitarism. J Clin Endocrinol Metab 1995;80:17–20.

✧✧✧

9

VASCULAR AND MESENCHYMAL TUMORS
OF THE SELLA TURCICA

Definition. Vascular and mesenchymal tumors arise from vessel walls, fibrous connective tissue, fat, bone, and cartilage. They are, therefore, potentially found at almost any site, since these are components of every part of the body. There are benign and malignant variants of each type.

Clinical and Radiologic Findings. Although unusual, these tumors do occur in the sellar region. They usually present as mass lesions that may cause tissue destruction and variable degrees of functional impairment. The radiologic features, growth, and behavior vary with the tumor type.

Morphologic Findings. The morphologic features are not unlike those of tumors at other sites and the reader is referred to the Fascicles, Tumors of the Soft Tissues (12) and Tumors of the Bones and Joints (10) for detailed descriptions.

Vascular Tumors. Benign *cavernous hemangioma* is infrequent in the central nervous system and only a few examples involving the pituitary have been reported (6,7,15). These lesions may be incidental findings at autopsy.

Glomangioma of the sella is an interesting lesion from the point of view of histogenesis; it has been suggested that this curious tumor may arise from the gomitoli of the pituitary stalk (4) (figs. 9-1, 9-2).

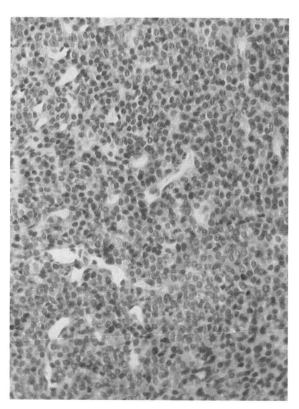

Figure 9-1
HISTOLOGY OF SELLAR GLOMANGIOMA

This tumor is composed of epithelial cells arranged in an organoid fashion around vascular channels. The tumor cells have indistinct cell borders and relatively monotonous round to oval nuclei.

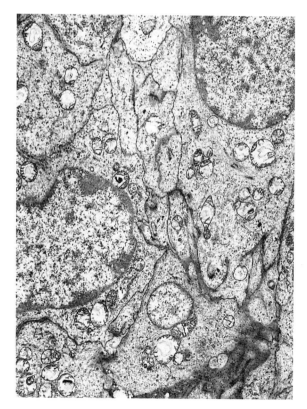

Figure 9-2
ULTRASTRUCTURE OF SELLAR GLOMANGIOMA

A glomangioma is composed of cells with smooth muscle differentiation. The tumor cells form a basement membrane which surrounds individual cells. Myofibrils within the cytoplasm show focal condensation into dense bodies. The features suggest origin in the gomitoli of the hypophysial portal vasculature.

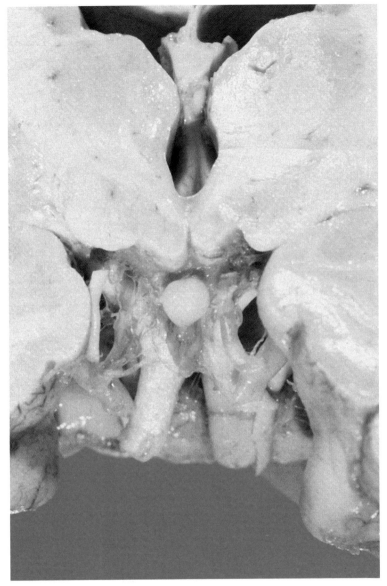

Figure 9-3
GROSS APPEARANCE
OF SELLAR LIPOMA

This benign tumor of adipocytes arises in the adipose tissue surrounding the pituitary stalk. Such a lesion can create symptoms of a sellar or suprasellar mass. (Courtesy of Dr. J.M. Bilbao, Toronto, Canada.)

A primary pituitary *hemangioblastoma* has been reported in a patient with von Hippel-Lindau disease (8).

Tumors of Fibrous Tissue, Fat, Bone, and Cartilage. These unusual tumors exhibit a wide range of differentiation. They include lipoma (fig. 9-3), giant cell tumors (19,20), *chondromyxoid fibroma* (18), *chondroma* (3,9), *enchondroma* (13), *chondrosarcoma* (16), and *alveolar soft part sarcoma* (5).

The development of sarcoma in the sella turcica may be sporadic, but more commonly is the result of previous ionizing irradiation. There are several reports in the literature of osteosarcoma and fibrosarcoma of the sella developing from 4 to 21 years after irradiation for pituitary adenoma or craniopharyngioma (1,2,11,14,17,21). These aggressive neoplasms result in rapid death of the patient.

REFERENCES

1. Ahmad K, Fayos JV. Pituitary fibrosarcoma secondary to radiation therapy. Cancer 1978;42:107–10.

2. Amine AR, Sugar O. Suprasellar osteogenic sarcoma following radiation for pituitary adenoma. Case report. J Neurosurg 1976;44:88–91.

3. Angiari P, Torcia E, Botticelli RA, Villani M, Merli GA, Crisi G. Ossifying parasellar chondroma. Case report. J Neursurg Sci 1987;31:59–63.

4. Asa SL, Kovacs K, Horvath E, Ezrin C, Weiss MH. Sellar glomangioma. Ultrastruct Pathol 1984;7:49–54.

5. Bots GT, Tijssen CC, Wijnalda D, Teepen JL. Alveolar soft part sarcoma of the pituitary gland with secondary involvement of the right cerebral ventricle. Br J Neurosurg 1988;2:101–7.

6. Castel JP, Delorge-Kerdiles C, Rivel J. Angiome caverneux du chiasma optique. Neurochirurgie 1989;35:252–6.

7. Chang WH, Khosla VK, Radotra BD, Kak VK. Large cavernous hemangioma of the pituitary fossa: a case report. Br J Neurosurg 1991;5:627–9.

8. Dan NG, Smith DE. Pituitary hemangioblastoma in a patient with von Hippel-Lindau disease. J Neurosurg 1975;42:232–5.

9. Dutton J. Intracranial solitary chondroma. Case report. J Neurosurg 1978;49:460–3.

10. Fechner RE, Mills SE. Tumors of the bones and joints. Atlas of Tumor Pathology, 3rd Series, Fascicle 8. Washington, D.C.: Armed Forces Institute of Pathology, 1993.

11. Gerlach H, Jänisch W. Intrakranielles sarkom nach bestrahlung eines hypophysenadenoms. Zentralbl Neurochir 1979;40:131–6.

12. Lattes R. Tumors of the soft tissues. Atlas of Tumor Pathology, 2nd series, Fascicle 1. Washington, D.C.: Armed Forces Institute of Pathology, 1982.

13. Miki K, Kawamoto K, Kawamura Y, Matsumura H, Asada Y, Hamada A. A rare case of Maffucci's syndrome combined with tuberculum sellae enchondroma, pituitary adenoma and thyroid adenoma. Acta Neurochir 1987;87:79–85.

14. Powell HC, Marshall LF, Ignelzi RJ. Post-irradiation pituitary sarcoma. Acta Neuropathol (Berl) 1977;39:165–7.

15. Sansone ME, Liwnicz BH, Mandybur TI. Giant pituitary cavernous hemangioma: case report. J Neurosurg 1980;53:124–6.

16. Sindou M, Daher A, Vighetto A, Goutelle A. Chondrosarcome parasellaire: rapport d'un cas opéré par voie ptériono-temporale et revue de la littérature. Neurochirurgie 1989;35:186–90.

17. Tanaka S, Nishio S, Morioka T, Fukui M, Kitamura K, Hikita K. Radiation-induced osteosarcoma of the sphenoid bone. Neurosurgery 1989;25:640–3.

18. Viswanathan R, Jegathraman AR, Ganapathy K, Bharati AS, Govindan R. Parasellar chondromyxofibroma with ipsilateral total internal carotid artery occlusion. Surg Neurol 1987;28:141–4.

19. Wolfe JT III, Scheithauer BW, Dahlin DC. Giant-cell tumor of the sphenoid bone. Review of 10 cases. J Neurosurg 1983;59:322–7.

20. Wu KK, Ross PM, Mitchell DC, Sprague HH. Evolution of a case of multicentric giant cell tumor over a 23-year period. Clin Orthop Rel Res 1986;213:279–88.

21. Yamamoto A, Hashimoto N, Yamashita J, Kikuchi H. A case of radiation-induced intracranial fibrosarcoma with repeated episodes of intratumoral hemorrhage. Neurol Surg 1989;17:193–6.

❖❖❖

10
METASTATIC NEOPLASMS OF THE SELLAR REGION

Definition. Blood-borne metastases from distant malignancies to the pituitary are the result of the high vascularity of this gland.

Epidemiology and Clinical Features. In patients with disseminated cancer, metastasis to the pituitary is common, in fact, it is more common than pituitary adenoma (7), ranging from 3 to 26.7 percent (7,13). Involvement of the posterior lobe is more frequent than the anterior lobe (7) and metastasis is the most common tumor of the neurohypophysis (4). The mechanism of spread is hematogenous, and the portal nature of the vascularization of the anterior lobe has been implicated as a protective barrier that accounts for the discrepancy in incidence.

The most common primary sites are lung, breast, and gastrointestinal tract (1–3,6,8). Among patients with breast carcinoma, pituitary metastases are statistically correlated with spread to other endocrine organs (3), suggesting a common mechanism that may implicate hormonal factors.

Most pituitary metastases are unassociated with symptoms and are therefore found incidentally at autopsy. Occasionally, however, patients may present with a sellar tumor and no prior history of malignancy (2). Posterior lobe involvement results in diabetes insipidus (4). Large tumors invade the cavernous sinus and its asso-

ciated structures, causing headache, visual field defects, ophthalmoplegia, and ptosis (6). Only rarely is there isolated anterior pituitary involvement, which can present as panhypopituitarism (2). Radiologically, these lesions are indistinguishable from pituitary adenoma.

A few cases of metastatic carcinoma involving a pituitary adenoma have been reported (5,9,11, 12,15,16). In this situation, the metastasis can be the cause of a sudden increase in size of the tumor and sudden worsening of symptoms of the mass.

Morphologic Findings. The diagnosis of a metastatic lesion is based on histologic, immunohistochemical, and ultrastructural findings. Most metastatic deposits exhibit a characteristic histology that suggests the type of differentiation (figs. 10-1, 10-2). In some instances, however, the pathologist may miss the diagnosis (figs. 10-3, 10-4) (8). In patients with no known primary lesion, thorough examination will provide evidence of the correct site of origin.

A melanoma in the sella should be considered most likely a metastasis; however, there are reports of sellar melanomas unassociated with evidence of a primary tumor elsewhere and these are considered to be primary sellar melanomas (10,14). The derivation of these lesions is not clear.

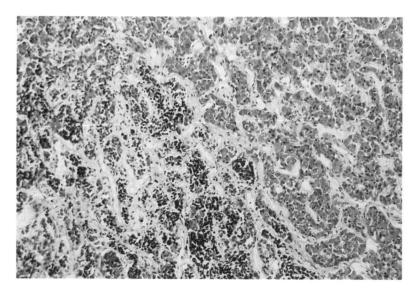

Figure 10-1
HISTOLOGY OF
METASTATIC CARCINOMA:
SMALL CELL CARCINOMA
Small cell carcinoma infiltrating and destroying the acini of the pituitary was found incidentally at autopsy in a patient with known small cell carcinoma of lung. (Courtesy of Dr. K. Kovacs, Toronto, Canada.)

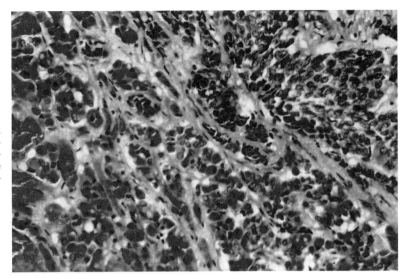

Figure 10-2
HISTOLOGY OF METASTATIC
CARCINOMA: BREAST
ADENOCARCINOMA

An incidental finding at autopsy of a
patient with disseminated breast carcinoma is the presence of pituitary metastasis; the monotonous tumor cells may be
very deceptive, unlike those of lung carcinoma (see figure 10-3).

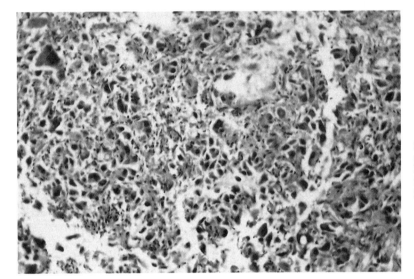

Figure 10-3
HISTOLOGY OF METASTATIC
CARCINOMA: PULMONARY
LARGE CELL CARCINOMA

This highly pleomorphic tumor was
found to involve the anterior and posterior pituitary of a patient with a previous
history of lung carcinoma. Analysis of this
tumor confirmed metastatic deposits
from the pulmonary primary.

Figure 10-4
HISTOLOGY OF METASTATIC
CARCINOMA: PULMONARY
LARGE CELL CARCINOMA

Pleomorphic tumor cells invade the
posterior lobe parenchyma in the pituitary of a patient with disseminated lung
carcinoma.

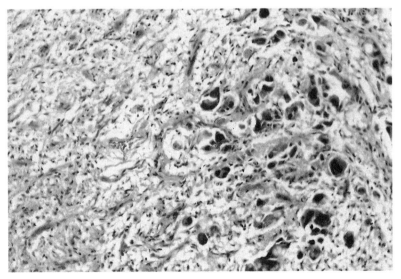

Differential Diagnosis. The major differential diagnosis involves the distinction of metastasis from pituitary adenoma. This problem arises rarely in patients with occult primary tumors who may present with manifestations of a pituitary mass. Mitotic activity, and cellular and nuclear pleomorphism are the hallmarks of malignancy, but these features may be present in pituitary adenomas. In particular, the sparsely granulated somatotroph adenoma (chapter 3) is notoriously worrisome histologically and may be mistaken for metastatic carcinoma, particularly if the history of acromegaly is not known by the pathologist or, in rare cases, if the tumor is clinically hormonally silent. In general, pituitary adenomas are readily characterized by their immunohistochemical profile, but tumors that are immunonegative for the usual hormones should be evaluated carefully, including ultrastructurally, in situations where the possibility of metastasis is raised by histologic criteria.

Prognosis and Therapy. Since these patients have disseminated malignancy, the therapy is aimed at palliation. Surgical decompression, with or without radiotherapy, can relieve symptoms (2).

REFERENCES

1. Allen EM, Kannan SR, Powell A. Infundibular metastasis and panhypopituitarism. J Natl Med Assoc 1989;81:325–30.

2. Branch CL Jr, Laws ER Jr. Metastatic tumors of the sella turcica masquerading as primary pituitary tumors. J Clin Endocrinol Metab 1987;65:469–74.

3. de la Monte SM, Hutchins GM, Moore GW. Endocrine organ metastases from breast carcinoma. Am J Pathol 1984;114:131–6.

4. Felix IA. Pathology of the neurohypophysis. Pathol Res Pract 1988;183:535–7.

5. James RL Jr, Arsenis G, Stoler M, Nelson C, Baran D. Hypophyseal metastatic renal cell carcinoma and pituitary adenoma. Case report and review of the literature. Am J Med 1984;76:337–40.

6. Kattah JC, Silgals RM, Manz H, Toro JG, Dritschilo A, Smith FP. Presentation and management of parasellar and suprasellar metastatic mass lesions. J Neurol Neurosurg Psych 1985;48:44–9.

7. Max MB, Deck MD, Rottenberg DA. Pituitary metastasis: incidence in cancer patients and clinical differentiation from pituitary adenoma. Neurology 1981;31:998–1002.

8. McCormick PC, Post KD, Kandji AD, Hays AP. Metastatic carcinoma to the pituitary gland. Br J Neurosurg 1989;3:71–9.

9. Molinatti PA, Scheithauer BW, Randall RV, Laws ER Jr. Metastasis to pituitary adenoma. Arch Pathol Lab Med 1985;109:287–9.

10. Neilson JM, Moffat AD. Hypopituitarism caused by a melanoma of the pituitary gland. J Clin Pathol 1963;16:144–9.

11. Post KD, McCormick PC, Hays AP, Kankji AD. Metastatic carcinoma to pituitary adenoma. Report of two cases. Surg Neurol 1988;30:286–92.

12. Ramsay JA, Kovacs K, Scheithauer BW, Ezrin C, Weiss MH. Metastatic carcinoma to pituitary adenomas: a report of two cases. Exper Clin Endocrinol 1988;92:69–76.

13. Roessmann U, Kaufman B, Friede RL. Metastatic lesions in the sella turcica and pituitary gland. Cancer 1970;25:478–80.

14. Scholtz CL, Siu K. Melanoma of the pituitary. Case report. J Neurosurg 1976;45:101–3.

15. van Seters AP, Bots GT, Van Dulken H, Luyendijk W, Vielvoye GJ. Metastasis of an occult gastric carcinoma suggesting growth of a prolactinoma during bromocriptine therapy: a case report with a review of the literature. Neurosurgery 1985;16:813–7.

16. Zager EL, Hedley-Whyte ET. Metastasis within a pituitary adenoma presenting with bilateral abducens palsies: case report and review of the literature. Neurosurgery 1987;21:383–6.

11
TUMOR-LIKE LESIONS OF THE SELLA TURCICA

HYPERPLASIAS

Definition. Hyperplasia is cell proliferation in response to a stimulus, as compared to the dysregulated cell proliferation of neoplasia. Hyperplasia can be physiologic, as in the pituitary during pregnancy when lactotroph hyperplasia is a normal response to the hormonal environment; alternatively, this process can be pathologic, the response to an abnormal excessive stimulus, as detailed in the following pages.

Clinical and Biochemical Findings. Hyperplasia of adenohypophysial cells can give rise to clinical syndromes indistinguishable from manifestations of pituitary adenomas. The reader is referred to chapter 3 for a review of the clinical features of growth hormone excess resulting in acromegaly and gigantism, hyperprolactinemia causing amenorrhea and galactorrhea in women and impotence in men, adrenocorticotropic hormone (ACTH) excess resulting in Cushing's disease with glucocorticoid excess, and thyrotropin hypersecretion which may be associated with hyperthyroidism, a euthyroid state, or hypothyroidism.

Radiologic Findings. The radiologic features of pituitary hyperplasia are varied. Computerized tomography (CT) and magnetic resonance imaging (MRI) may detect no abnormality (6,31) or may reveal a diffusely enlarged sella without evidence of a discrete tumor (fig. 11-1) (9). In some patients, however, the imaging results are interpreted as consistent with a pituitary adenoma (5,8,15,27,34). Occasionally, suprasellar extension is found (5,8,15,34).

Morphologic Findings. Adenohypophysial hyperplasia can be distinguished histologically from adenoma with a reticulin stain (17,28). The normal adenohypophysis is composed of acini with a well-developed reticulin fiber network; adenomas exhibit total breakdown of the reticulin pattern (see fig. 2-3); and hyperplasia results in expanded acini that preserve their reticulin (fig. 11-2). There are cases in which there is transition from hyperplasia to adenoma (fig. 11-3). In hyperplasia, other nontumorous cell types are recognized by their immunohistochemical profile of hormone content. Electron

microscopy is not useful in distinguishing hyperplasia from neoplasia (12,24).

The distinction between nodular and diffuse hyperplasia has been emphasized by some authors. The differences are usually based on the differential cell distribution of the various adenohypophysial cell types; the geographic localization of cells such as corticotrophs may lead to "nodules" of hyperplasia seen grossly by the surgeon or encountered histologically. Nevertheless, the criteria for the diagnosis of hyperplasia should be applied uniformly, whether the changes are seen focally or throughout the gland.

Somatotroph or *mammosomatotroph hyperplasia* has been reported mainly in patients with ectopic secretion of growth hormone–releasing hormone (GRH); chronic stimulation results in proliferation of these cells but adenoma rarely develops (9). Occasional cases of acromegaly are due to somatotroph hyperplasia (figs. 11-4–11-6) associated with hypothalamic gangliocytoma or

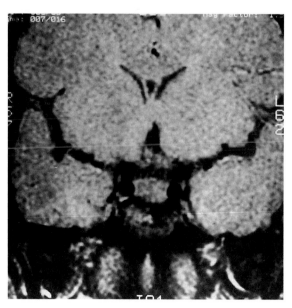

Figure 11-1
RADIOLOGY OF PITUITARY HYPERPLASIA
On T1-weighted MRI there is diffuse enlargement of the sella turcica but no discrete tumor is identified. (Courtesy of Dr. S. Ezzat, Toronto, Canada.)

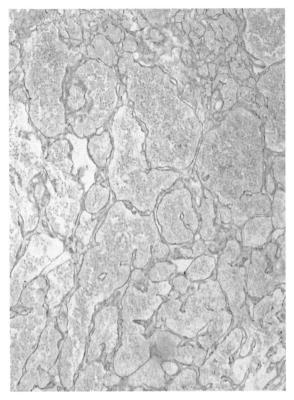

Figure 11-2
ADENOHYPOPHYSIAL
HYPERPLASIA: RETICULIN STAIN
The diagnosis of pituitary hyperplasia relies upon the documentation of an expanded acinar architecture as delineated by intact reticulin, compared to adenomas where there is total breakdown of the reticulin fiber network.

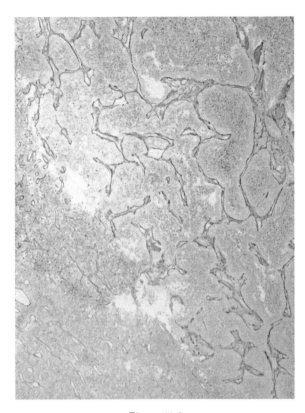

Figure 11-3
ADENOHYPOPHYSIAL HYPERPLASIA
WITH ADENOMA: RETICULIN STAIN
In this patient with adenohypophysial hyperplasia there is an associated adenoma with total reticulin disruption (bottom left). In some patients, continued stimulation of the pituitary results in transformation from hyperplasia to adenoma.

extrahypothalamic neoplasms that produce GRH (figs. 11-7, 11-8) (3,29). Mammosomatotroph hyperplasia unassociated with a known GRH-producing tumor has been reported in a young child with gigantism (24) and in association with McCune-Albright syndrome (19); the cause of the hyperplasia is unknown, but it may reflect excessive stimulation by GRH or, in some patients with McCune-Albright syndrome, mutations resulting in constitutive activation of the G proteins that mediate GRH stimulation (35).

Lactotroph hyperplasia is physiologic in pregnancy (2). The progressive increase in lactotrophs is associated with a gradual reduction in growth hormone mRNA. There is evidence that somatotrophs are recruited to produce prolactin as bihormonal mammosomatotrophs and possibly even convert to lactotrophs (33). The pathologic counterpart, *idiopathic lactotroph hyper-*

plasia, is characterized by enlarged but intact acini of adenohypophysial cells with a preserved but distorted reticulin fiber network (14,26). Most of the cells are chromophobic and contain prolactin immunoreactivity in a juxtanuclear globular distribution; occasional large, densely granulated cells contain diffuse cytoplasmic prolactin positivity. Other cell types are scattered throughout the tissue. By electron microscopy, stimulated lactotrophs with variable granularity predominate and other cell types are seen dispersed throughout the gland (14).

Corticotroph hyperplasia is associated with some cases of Cushing's disease, either alone or with a corticotroph adenoma (17,22,23). It also occurs in patients with untreated or inadequately treated Addison's disease (20). The distinction from adenoma relies on the pattern of reticulin staining as described above for other hyperplasias.

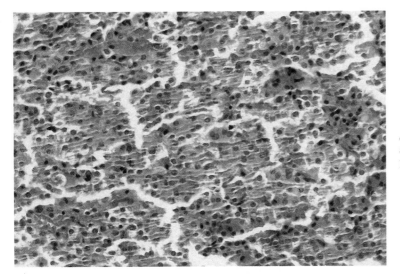

Figure 11-4
HISTOLOGY OF
SOMATOTROPH HYPERPLASIA
This pituitary exhibits hyperplasia of ad-enohypophysial cells. There are expanded acini of cells that are almost entirely acido-philic. The patient had growth hormone excess.

Figure 11-5
HISTOLOGY OF SOMATOTROPH
HYPERPLASIA: RETICULIN STAIN
Although the histology resembles somatotroph adenoma, the reticulin fiber network is intact; the acini are dilated by the cell proliferation.

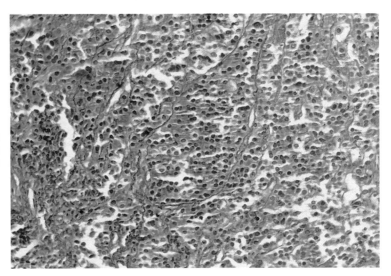

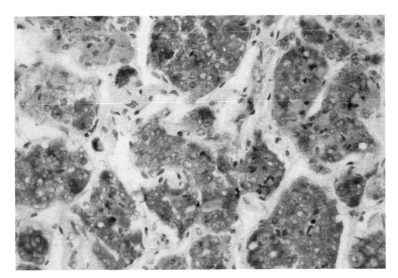

Figure 11-6
IMMUNOHISTOCHEMICAL
LOCALIZATION
OF GROWTH HORMONE IN
SOMATOTROPH HYPERPLASIA
Immunostaining reveals diffuse positivity for growth hormone in the majority of cells within this pituitary of a patient with acro-megaly but no evidence of adenoma. Inter-spersed cells were also positive for other ade-nohypophysial hormones.

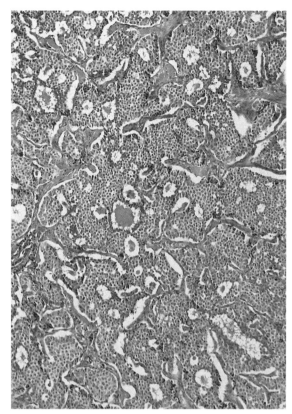

Figure 11-7
PULMONARY ENDOCRINE TUMOR PRODUCING
GROWTH HORMONE–RELEASING HORMONE
A patient with acromegaly and somatotroph hyperplasia was
subsequently diagnosed to have a pulmonary endocrine tumor.

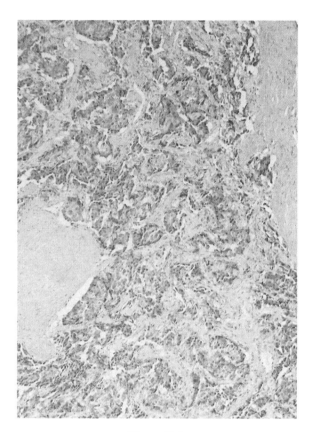

Figure 11-8
PULMONARY ENDOCRINE TUMOR PRODUCING
GROWTH HORMONE–RELEASING HORMONE
The pulmonary endocrine tumor contains immunoreactivity for growth hormone-releasing hormone. After resection of this tumor, the acromegaly subsided.

Thyrotroph hyperplasia occurs in cases of untreated primary hypothyroidism (4,8,10,15). The number and size of the thyrotrophs are increased (fig. 11-9). Periodic acid–Schiff (PAS) stains reveal positive droplets throughout the thyrotroph cytoplasm (fig. 11-10). Although these lesions clinically mimic pituitary adenoma, the reticulin stain confirms an intact reticulin fiber network (fig. 11-11). Thyroid-stimulating hormone (TSH) immunoreactivity is faint but diffuse (fig. 11-12). Thyrotroph hyperplasia often presents with hyperprolactinemia (12) since it is associated with lactotroph hyperplasia (fig. 11-13). Other cell types are distributed throughout the gland (fig. 11-14). By electron microscopy, the stimulated thyrotrophs, known as "thyroidectomy cells," have abundant, dilated rough endoplasmic reticulum and large Golgi complexes with reduced numbers of secretory granules (11) (see fig.

1-32). In the rat, there is evidence that at least some of the thyroidectomy cells may derive from a subset of altered somatotrophs which are bihormonal (13); the morphologic changes are reversible in the experimental animal.

Gonadotroph hyperplasia occurs in patients with longstanding primary hypogonadism. In these patients, "gonadectomy" or "gonad-deficiency" cells can be recognized by light microscopy as large, chromophobic, vacuolated cells with focal PAS-positive granules. The cytoplasm of these hyperplastic gonadotrophs is almost totally filled with dilated endoplasmic reticulum that contains flocculent material.

Pathogenesis. The proliferative effect of hypophysiotropic hormones on adenohypophysial cells has been well established. GRH is known to stimulate somatotroph proliferation (7) and transgenic mice overexpressing GRH develop

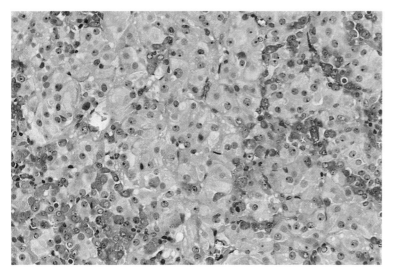

Figure 11-9
HISTOLOGY OF
THYROTROPH HYPERPLASIA
Hematoxylin and eosin staining reveals enlarged acini composed of cells with poorly defined cell borders and abundant pale eosinophilic cytoplasm. These represent hyperplastic thyrotrophs in a patient with primary hypothyroidism. Smaller basophilic and chromophobic cells intermingle with the hyperplastic cells.

Figure 11-10
HISTOLOGY OF
THYROTROPH HYPERPLASIA
The PAS stain documents the presence of numerous PAS-positive droplets throughout the cytoplasm of hyperplastic thyrotrophs. The thyrotroph hyperplasia was secondary to primary hypothyroidism.

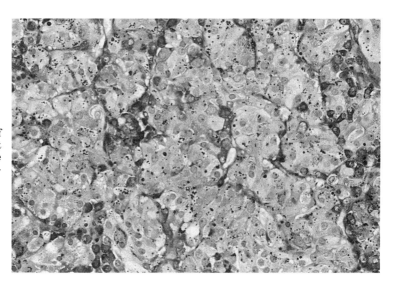

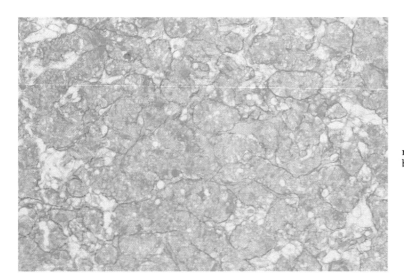

Figure 11-11
HISTOLOGY OF
THYROTROPH HYPERPLASIA
The reticulin stain documents an intact reticulin fiber network, in contrast to the total breakdown seen in a pituitary adenoma.

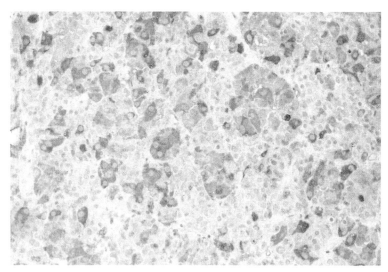

Figure 11-12
IMMUNOHISTOCHEMICAL
LOCALIZATION OF β-TSH IN
THYROTROPH HYPERPLASIA
There is diffuse pale cytoplasmic stain-
ing for β-TSH in the majority of cells in this
hyperplastic pituitary of a patient with pri-
mary hypothyroidism.

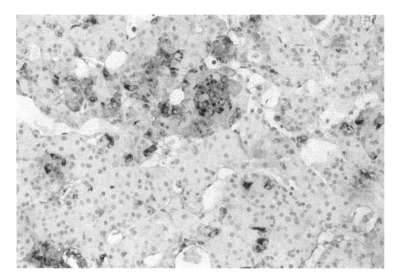

Figure 11-13
IMMUNOHISTOCHEMICAL
LOCALIZATION OF PROLACTIN IN
THYROTROPH HYPERPLASIA
Prolactin-immunoreactive cells are numerous and prominent in the pituitary of a
patient with primary hypothyroidism and
thyrotroph hyperplasia. Lactotroph hyperplasia usually causes associated hyperprolactinemia that can mimic prolactinoma.

Figure 11-14
IMMUNOHISTOCHEMICAL
LOCALIZATION OF ACTH IN
THYROTROPH HYPERPLASIA
ACTH-containing cells are present in
normal numbers and are scattered through-
out the adenohypophysial acini that contain
hyperplastic and hypertrophic thyrotrophs.
The same pattern is seen with stains for GH
or the gonadotropin β-subunits.

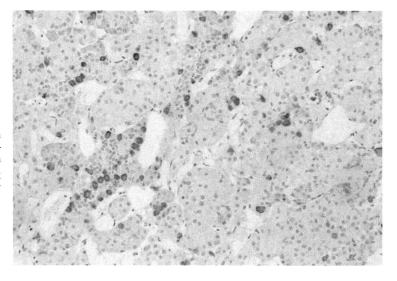

massive somatotroph and mammosomatotroph hyperplasia (21,32). Similarly, corticotropin-releasing hormone (CRH) stimulates corticotroph proliferation in vivo (1). The effects of hypothyroidism on thyrotrophs have been shown in animals (13) and man (30); the lack of feedback inhibition by thyroid hormones and chronic hypothalamic thyroid-releasing hormone (TRH) stimulation together are known to result in thyrotroph hypertrophy and hyperplasia with tumor formation. The essential role of TRH stimulation is suggested by the association of lactotroph hyperplasia with thyrotroph proliferation (4,8,10,15). Similarly, gonadotrophs are known to respond to loss of gonadal steroid regulation with proliferation (18,25).

The cause of idiopathic lactotroph hyperplasia remains unclear; although estrogen is known to cause lactotroph proliferation (16), the patients have no evidence of estrogen excess and the response of this lesion to bromocriptine suggests a possible loss of dopaminergic inhibition as an etiologic factor.

Prognosis and Therapy. These disorders are, with the exception of idiopathic lactotroph hyperplasia, attributed to hormonal imbalances that, when corrected, result in reversal of the pituitary lesion.

CYSTS

Non-neoplastic cysts occur in the region of the sella. These lesions can mimic the empty sella syndrome but unlike the arachnoid diverticulum of that entity, they do not communicate with the subarachnoid space. Cysts can be mistaken for pituitary adenoma due to similar clinical manifestations.

Rathke's Cleft Cysts

Definition. These cysts are thought to originate in the remnants of Rathke's pouch. As reviewed in chapter 1, Rathke's cleft arises from the oropharynx and migrates upwards, with anterior and posterior limbs that ultimately give rise to the anterior and intermediate lobes of the adenohypophysis, respectively. In the human the intermediate lobe is vestigial, and its remnants line small cystic cavities that are vestiges of the cleft. These cystic structures are very common but usually measure less than 5 mm in diameter (42). When they en-

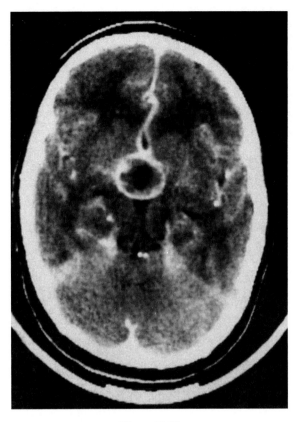

Figure 11-15
RADIOLOGIC FEATURES OF RATHKE'S CLEFT CYST
On CT scan with contrast, the pituitary contains a cystic lesion with rim enhancement at the periphery of the sella. (Courtesy of Dr. J.M. Bilbao, Toronto, Canada.)

large and become detectable, however, they can give rise to symptoms of a mass lesion.

Clinical Features. The cysts are usually detected clinically only when they expand to cause sellar compression (51,52), resulting in hypopituitarism and diabetes insipidus. They usually present in adults but do occur in infants and young children (39). Suprasellar extension results in visual field defects, oculomotor disturbances, and headaches; in severe cases, patients have developed hydrocephalus and even aseptic meningitis. There is a report of abscess formation within such a lesion (49). Rare cases of purely suprasellar Rathke's cleft cyst exist (37).

Radiologic Findings. Imaging usually discloses the cystic nature of these lesions (fig. 11-15). CT scans reveal low density cystic areas with capsular enhancement in most cases; the MRI appearance is variable (43,46,52).

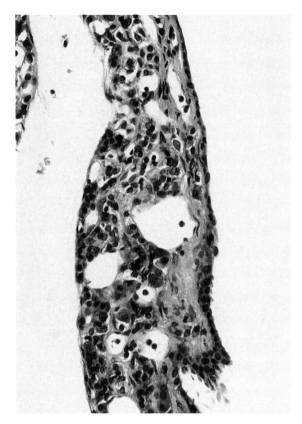

Figure 11-16
HISTOLOGY OF RATHKE'S CLEFT CYST
The cyst lining is composed of cuboidal epithelium. Immediately adjacent is nontumorous adenohypophysial parenchyma.

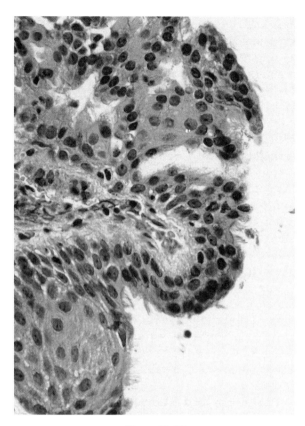

Figure 11-17
HISTOLOGY OF RATHKE'S CLEFT CYST
The lining of this Rathke's cleft cyst is composed of columnar epithelium with areas of squamous metaplasia.

Morphologic Findings. Morphologic examination reveals a cyst lining characterized by ciliated cuboidal (fig. 11-16) or columnar epithelium (fig. 11-17) resembling respiratory epithelium, with occasional goblet cells and occasional squamous elements (fig. 11-17). The degree of ciliation and the propensity for squamous metaplasia distinguish these cysts from the neuroepithelial-derived colloid cysts of the third ventricle.

Some pituitary adenomas have cystic elements that resemble Rathke's cleft cysts (41,47,48). It is impossible to determine if this represents a coincidental association of the two lesions or transition of differentiation in a single neoplasm.

Prognosis and Therapy. The management involves surgical drainage with or without partial excision; the recurrence rate is low (52). Most symptoms and signs are relieved postoperatively, but permanent hypopituitarism and diabetes insipidus require hormone replacement therapy.

Arachnoid Cysts

Definition. These lesions may be congenital anomalies or acquired cysts in the arachnoid of the sellar and parasellar regions (50).

Clinical Features. Arachnoid cysts arise within or above the sella turcica (40,45); they cause pituitary compression and hormonal insufficiency in the former and are associated with visual or neurologic defects in the latter.

Radiologic Findings. The cystic nature of these lesions are evident on CT and MRI scans. However, they may be difficult to distinguish from other cysts that occur in this area.

Morphologic Findings. The cysts are filled with clear, colorless fluid and are lined by arachnoid laminar connective tissue with a single layer of flattened epithelium.

Prognosis and Therapy. These cysts are adequately managed by drainage with partial cyst wall excision (40).

Dermoid and Epidermoid Cysts

Definition. Dermoid and epidermoid cysts arise from epithelial cells that are misplaced during embryologic development or rarely, traumatically. Epidermoid cysts are also known as *cholesteatomas.*

Clinical Features. Epithelial cysts can occur intracranially, most commonly at the cerebellopontine angle, but often in the suprasellar area where they cause hypopituitarism, often with hyperprolactinemia due to stalk compression, visual field defects, and nonspecific neurologic symptoms (53). There is a report of a dermoid cyst associated with an arachnoid cyst (38).

Radiologic Findings. Because of the cystic nature of these lesions, evident on CT and MRI scans, they may be difficult to distinguish from other cystic lesions of this area.

Morphologic Findings. Epidermoid cysts are lined by keratinizing squamous epithelium. Dermoid cysts are distinguished by the additional presence of skin appendages, including hair follicles and sweat glands.

Prognosis and Therapy. Management usually involves surgical resection. Complications of delayed treatment include rupture with chemical meningitis due to keratin debris (36) or the development of squamous carcinoma (44).

INFLAMMATORY LESIONS

Inflammatory lesions, of infectious or autoimmune etiology, also may mimic pituitary adenoma. These include sarcoidosis, the unusual giant cell granuloma, and lymphocytic hypophysitis; the latter is frequently associated with pregnancy and hyperprolactinemia and may be confused with lactotroph adenoma (56,76,113, 114). Careful clinical and biochemical assessment may avert the need for surgery in patients with inflammatory disorders.

Lymphocytic Hypophysitis

Definition. Lymphocytic hypophysitis is a rare chronic inflammatory lesion of the pituitary gland. Many reports strongly support the original suggestion of an autoimmune pathogenesis of this lesion; it is associated with other autoimmune disorders, primarily thyroiditis and ad-

renalitis and, less commonly, atrophic gastritis and lymphocytic parathyroiditis (120).

Clinical Features. More than 100 cases have been reported since the first description of the entity in 1962 (72). The disease shows a striking female predilection of approximately 8.5 to 1 and commonly affects young women during late pregnancy or in the postpartum period. The mean age of presentation in females is 34.5 years while in males it is one decade later (44.7 years) (120).

This disorder is frequently associated with pregnancy and hyperprolactinemia and may mimic prolactinoma (56). The inflamed gland is enlarged and may even extend beyond the sella, giving rise to mass effects such as headaches and visual field impairment.

Biochemical Findings. Most patients have partial or total adenohypophysial hypofunction. Neurohypophysial involvement manifesting as diabetes insipidus is rare but does occur.

Hyperprolactinemia is a normal finding during pregnancy and the postpartum period, and this explanation has been offered for the hyperprolactinemia that is frequently associated with lymphocytic hypophysitis. However, there are cases in which hyperprolactinemia occurred in males and in females who were not pregnant or breast feeding (120). This may be attributed to stalk compression by a suprasellar mass in some instances; alternatively, the inflammatory process may directly alter dopamine receptors and the tonic inhibitory effect of dopamine on prolactin release. An autoimmune mechanism involving the production of stimulating antibodies by plasma cells may lead to increased hormone secretion, analogous to the pathophysiologic mechanisms implicated in Graves' disease of the thyroid (93,105); this was the subject of speculation in one patient with elevated growth hormone (GH) levels and lymphocytic hypophysitis (77). Finally, diffuse destruction by the inflammatory process may in some cases result in escape of hormone into the circulation. One case of combined prolactin, GH, and thyroxine (T_4) hypersecretion in a young nulliparous woman has previously been described in the literature (89).

Isolated corticotropin deficiency is rare, but it represents the most common isolated type of anterior pituitary hormone deficiency encountered in patients with proven or putative lymphocytic hypophysitis (64,68,81,109,111,112,121). Isolated

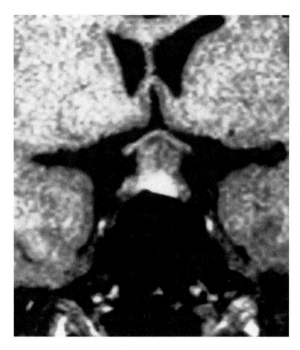

Figure 11-18
RADIOLOGIC FEATURES OF
LYMPHOCYTIC HYPOPHYSITIS
T1-weighted imaging of the sella in a patient with lymphocytic hypophysitis demonstrates a nonhomogeneous pituitary
mass with suprasellar extension that compresses the optic
chiasm upwards. This picture mimics pituitary adenoma.

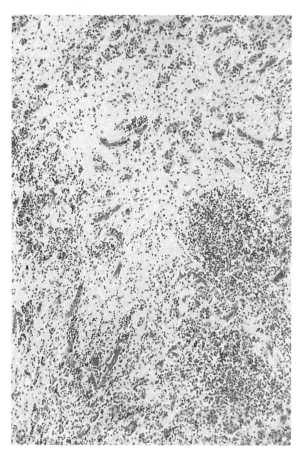

Figure 11-19
HISTOLOGY OF LYMPHOCYTIC HYPOPHYSITIS
The pituitary tissue is infiltrated by lymphocytes and
plasma cells which aggregate and result in tissue destruction. There is stromal fibrosis; small clusters of residual
epithelial cells are identified.

thyrotropin-stimulating hormone (TSH) deficiency has also been reported (64), and selective
absence of gonadotropins has been described (57).

Radiologic Findings. In patients with lymphocytic hypophysitis, CT or MRI has revealed
features of an enlarging pituitary mass in up to
95 percent of patients (83 percent in a current
series) with frequent evidence of suprasellar extension (120). The radiographic appearance cannot be easily distinguished from a pituitary adenoma (fig. 11-18). Recent reports, however, point
to some possible clues to the correct diagnosis on
MRI: loss of the hyperintense "bright spot" signal
of the normal neurohypophysis, thickening of
the pituitary stalk, and enlargement of the neurohypophysis in cases in which the latter is also
involved (54,79). These radiographic criteria
need to be prospectively evaluated.

Bromocriptine administration may improve
visual fields and reduce elevated prolactin levels, however, there is no evidence that it can alter
the size of the pituitary mass (120). Thus an attempt at therapeutic control of a presumed pro-

lactinoma may serve as a diagnostic clue in
patients with hypophysitis.

Morphologic Findings. *Gross Findings.*
Gross inspection of the pituitary gland at autopsy in patients with prolonged disease reveals
atrophy, associated with atrophy of pituitary target organs, the thyroid and adrenal glands.

Microscopic Findings. By light microscopy, this
disorder is characterized by a lymphoplasmacytic
infiltrate (fig. 11-19) which occasionally forms
lymphoid follicles and is accompanied by varying
numbers of neutrophils, eosinophils, and macrophages. The adenohypophysial parenchyma
shows variable destruction and oncocytic change.
The preserved cells are found in irregular islands
and small groups, isolated by a diffuse inflammatory infiltrate (figs. 11-20, 11-21) or fibrous

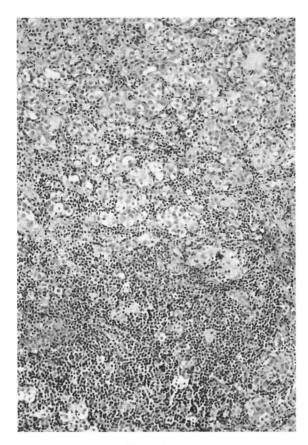

Figure 11-20
HISTOLOGY OF LYMPHOCYTIC HYPOPHYSITIS
A chronic lymphocytic infiltrate surrounds pituitary acini. Some of the epithelial cells show oncocytic change.

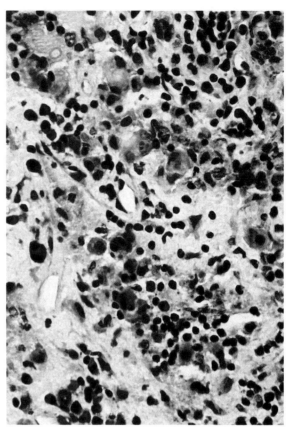

Figure 11-21
HISTOLOGY OF LYMPHOCYTIC HYPOPHYSITIS
Lymphocytes and plasma cells infiltrate the parenchyma of the adenohypophysis. There is destruction of adenohypophysial parenchyma with oxyphilic change of residual adenohypophysial epithelial cells.

tissue (fig. 11-18); the fibrosis is variable and likely correlates with the duration of disease.

Immunocytochemical analysis confirms the presence of lymphocytic markers such as leucocyte common antigen (LCA) in an infiltrate that is invariable polyclonal with L-26, UCHL, and kappa and lambda light chains. Cytokeratins and hormones identify the residual adenohypophysial cells (fig. 11-22); vasopressin, neurophysins, neurofilaments, S-100 protein, and glial fibrillary acidic protein (GFAP) indicate the presence of neurohypophysial elements in the inflamed tissue.

Electron microscopy reveals adenohypophysial tissue infiltrated by inflammatory cells (figs. 11-23, 11-24), mainly plasma cells and lymphocytes. In areas of severe inflammation, the inflammatory cells intermingle with damaged adenohypophysial cells that show degenerative changes, including oncocytosis and crinophagy (fig. 11-25).

Differential Diagnosis. The distinction from pituitary adenoma is clearly important but is usually not morphologically difficult. The differential diagnosis should include other inflammatory processes such as tuberculosis, sarcoidosis, syphilis, and giant cell granuloma, as well as germinoma, lymphoma, and plasmacytoma (see chapter 7). The presence of multiple granulomas composed of epithelioid cells and multinucleated giant cells generally distinguishes the other inflammatory conditions from lymphocytic hypophysitis. Sheehan's syndrome (postpartum pituitary necrosis), which may be associated with a similar clinical presentation of gradually progressive postpartum hypopituitarism, should also be considered in the differential diagnosis. This disorder can easily be excluded if there is no history

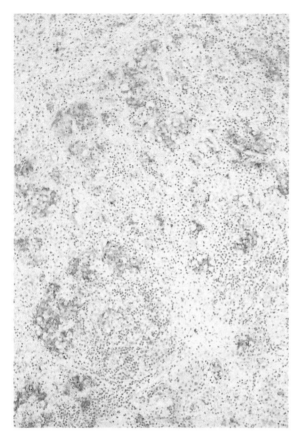

Figure 11-22
IMMUNOHISTOCHEMICAL LOCALIZATION
OF PITUITARY HORMONES
IN LYMPHOCYTIC HYPOPHYSITIS

Staining for growth hormone, as in this case, or any other pituitary hormone, localizes the residual adenohypophysial cells within the lymphocytic infiltrate.

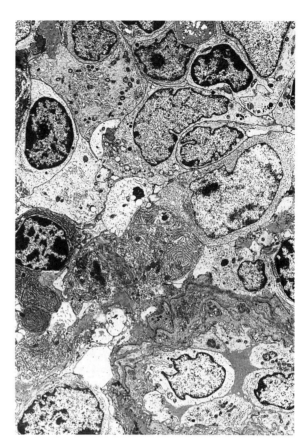

Figure 11-23
ULTRASTRUCTURE OF
LYMPHOCYTIC HYPOPHYSITIS

The pituitary is infiltrated by lymphocytes and plasma cells that interdigitate with adenohypophysial cells. The epithelial cells form nests and follicles but their ultrastructural appearance is significantly altered by the inflammatory process.

of a complicated delivery (116), and some patients with presumed Sheehan's syndrome but no clear history of postpartum hemorrhage or sepsis may have lymphocytic hypophysis (61,67).

Prognosis and Therapy. Preoperatively, a diagnosis of lymphocytic hypophysis is rarely suspected (69,99,102,108,120). This underscores the lack of any specific and reliable diagnostic clinical, biochemical, or radiographic markers that facilitate the correct preoperative diagnosis. For the time being, the majority of patients undergo surgery, at which time the diagnosis is established by histologic examination.

The natural history of lymphocytic hypophysitis is variable. Progressive severe and permanent hypopituitarism reflective of the degree of destruction of hypophysial cells can result in se-

vere complications and death. However, spontaneous partial or total pituitary function recovery and mass resolution has been described in some patients with morphologically documented or clinically suspected lymphocytic hypophysitis (59,78,80,94,96, 101,102,120). In these cases, the hypopituitarism may have been due to compression of hypophysial cells either by the inflammatory infiltrate or edema, rather than to irreversible cell destruction.

The majority of patients, however, require active treatment. Corticosteroid therapy has been advocated to reduce inflammation, and has been effective in some patients (60,90,100,117), however, its efficacy in this disorder remains uncertain (99,108,120). Surgery should be performed in cases associated with progressive compressive

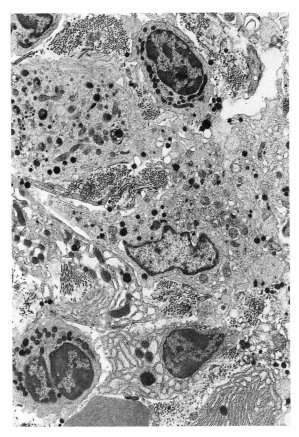

Figure 11-24
ULTRASTRUCTURE OF
LYMPHOCYTIC HYPOPHYSITIS
Plasma cells and lymphocytes infiltrate among dispersed adenohypophysial cells which show evidence of degeneration. There is stromal fibrosis with collagen accumulation.

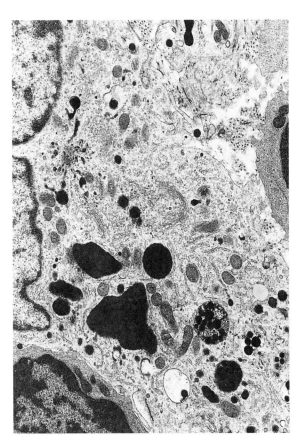

Figure 11-25
ULTRASTRUCTURE OF
LYMPHOCYTIC HYPOPHYSITIS
Degenerating adenohypophysial cells show crinophagy, uptake of secretory material within complex lysosomes.

features or those in which radiographic or neurologic deterioration is observed during conservative management with corticosteroids and hormone replacement (99,106). Transsphenoidal surgery is both diagnostic and therapeutic. It has resulted in amelioration of symptoms of a sellar mass in some patients (120). Hyperprolactinemia (87,91,92, 100,105,107) and reduced pituitary function (60,94,97) have also been reported to resolve following pituitary surgery in some cases. However, surgical intervention has been associated with further deterioration of visual field defects in one patient (103) and may result in diabetes insipidus and worsened hypopituitarism (120); it is therefore essential that a frozen section diagnosis of this entity should result in less aggressive resection of potentially viable pituitary tissue.

Pathogenesis. The pathogenesis of lymphocytic hypophysitis has been attributed to autoimmunity even from its first description (72). The disease is associated with other endocrine autoimmune phenomena. Circulating antipituitary antibodies have been detected in a minority of patients with the disease (88,90,102, 123). The association of lymphocytic hypophysitis with pregnancy has been explained by the documentation of antibodies that react with nonhormonal antigens in hyperplastic lactotrophs (63). Hyperplasia and hyperactivity of lactotrophs in female patients can be attributed to pregnancy; the association with pregnancy has been attributed to hyperplasia of lactotrophs that may trigger the immune response. Antipituitary antibodies have also been detected in patients with the "empty sella syndrome" (84), idiopathic GH deficiency (62,65), Cushing's syndrome (115), and different autoimmune isolated and polyendocrinopathies without hypophysitis (63). In an isolated case of ACTH deficiency, the presence of antibodies to corticotrophs were thought to be directed against an antigen that represents a cell-specific factor required for pro-opiomelanocortin (POMC) processing (112).

Specific subtypes of the major histocompatibility complex (MHCs) human leukocyte antigens (HLAs) that are correlated with a number of autoimmune endocrine disorders have been detected in patients with lymphocytic hypophysitis (56,69,73,90,95,98,103,104,118). It is likely that HLA-DR genes are not responsible for the genesis of the autoimmune response per se, but may be closely related, in some subjects, with the genes directly responsible (55).

Experimentally, subcutaneous injections of human anterior pituitary gland homogenates in Freund's adjuvant produce a disease histologically characterized by focal lymphoid aggregates and diffuse mononuclear cell infiltration of the pituitary. Interestingly, this adenohypophysitis was found to be more pronounced in pregnant and lactating rats (85,86). Similar results have been obtained by immunization of rabbits with homologous pituitary tissue in complete Freund's adjuvant (83).

Other Inflammatory Disorders

Infectious Lesions. Acute and chronic infections in the sella turcica are rare but they do occur, usually in association with sphenoid sinus infection. Infection also can result from cavernous sinus thrombosis, or may be attributable to spread of otitis media mastoiditis or peritonsillar abscess. Rarely, pituitary infection results from vascular seeding of distant or systemic infection (58).

Pituitary tumors have been associated with the development of pituitary abscess (71); the infection may not be detected clinically or may present as pituitary apoplexy. It has been suggested that bony erosion by the tumor predisposes such patients to the spread of sinonasal infection.

Granulomatous Hypophysitis: Giant Cell Granuloma and Sarcoidosis. Granulomatous inflammation of the pituitary can be caused by tuberculosis, syphilis, or fungal infections; presen-

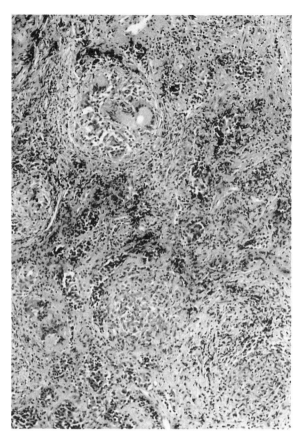

Figure 11-26
HISTOLOGY OF
GRANULOMATOUS HYPOPHYSITIS
The pituitary contains granulomas, aggregates of lymphocytes and epithelioid histiocytes with multinucleate giant cells. There is almost total destruction of adenohypophysial tissue.

tation in these cases as a primary pituitary mass is rare and the lesion is usually an incidental autopsy finding. In contrast, pituitary granulomatous inflammation as the primary manifestation of sarcoidosis or isolated localized granulomatous inflammation, known as giant cell granuloma, can present with sellar enlargement and hypopituitarism, mimicking a clinically nonfunctional pituitary adenoma (66,74,110,119,122).

Histologically, these lesions are characterized by the formation of granulomas, aggregates of lymphocytes and epithelioid histiocytes with multinucleate giant cells (figs. 11-26–11-28). In every case, the possibility of underlying infection must be excluded.

The etiology of isolated giant cell granuloma is unknown. It has been suggested that it represents

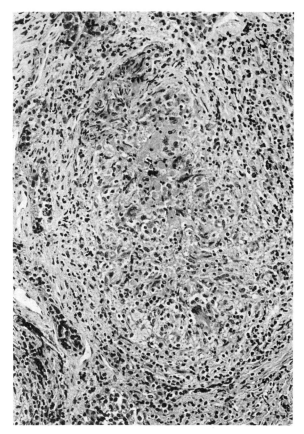

Figure 11-27
HISTOLOGY OF
GRANULOMATOUS HYPOPHYSITIS
A large granuloma exhibits early central necrosis in a patient with sarcoidosis.

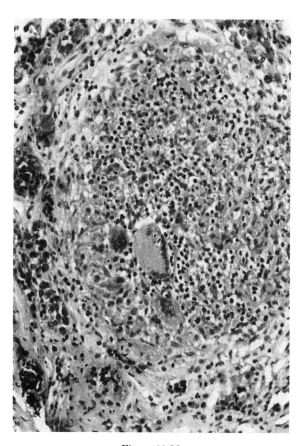

Figure 11-28
HISTOLOGY OF
GRANULOMATOUS HYPOPHYSITIS
A granuloma with giant cells is surrounded by trapped acini of residual adenohypophysial cells.

an autoimmune phenomenon, related to lymphocytic hypophysitis (74,82), but as yet there is no evidence to support this postulate.

Granulomatous hypophysitis has been associated with a prolactinoma in one case (75); it remains unclear if this was a coincidental association or if the inflammation represented a response to the tumor.

Inflammatory Pseudotumor. A lesion similar to orbital pseudotumor characterized by chronic inflammation and fibrosis has been reported to involve the sella turcica and parasellar tissues, causing hypopituitarism and mimicking a neoplastic process (70). The patient was subsequently found to have a similar mediastinal lesion, indicating that the sellar location is yet another site of the family of sclerosing lesions

that also include Riedel's thyroiditis, retroperitoneal fibrosis, and sclerosing cholangitis. The etiology and appropriate management of these disorders remains uncertain.

MISCELLANEOUS TUMOR-LIKE LESIONS

Aneurysms

Aneurysms of the carotid arteries can expand to give rise to masses in the suprasellar region (fig. 11-29), resulting in pituitary insufficiency and visual field defects that mimic pituitary adenoma (125). Angiography may be required to confirm the diagnosis (fig. 11-30). It is critical to distinguish these vascular malformations from pituitary tumors prior to surgery to avoid severe intraoperative bleeding.

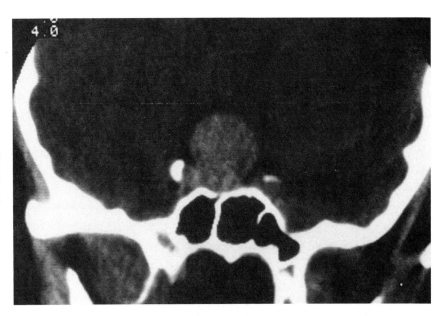

Figure 11-29
RADIOLOGIC FEATURES
OF INTERNAL CAROTID
ARTERY ANEURYSM
Conventional radiographic
techniques like this CT scan indi-
cate a parasellar mass that could
be mistaken for a pituitary tumor.
(Courtesy of Dr. J.M. Bilbao, To-
ronto, Canada.)

Meningoencephalocele

Encephaloceles in the sella turcica are rare
but have been reported to cause hypopituitarism
and a mass lesion (124). The diagnosis must be
made by radiography to prevent attempted biopsy which could result in major complications.

Hamartomas

Salivary gland rests occur in the posterior lobe
of the pituitary and are usually incidental autopsy
findings (129). They are attributed to the oropha-
ryngeal development of Rathke's pouch. Large lesions are symptomatic (127); they can cause hypopituitarism and mass effects with suprasellar
extension and cyst formation. A recent report suggests that these rests may rarely give rise to salivary gland-like tumors in the sella (126).

An unusual pituitary choristoma composed of
pituitary corticotrophs associated with heterotopic
adrenocortical cells has been reported as a sellar
mass associated with reduced adenohypophysial
function, mimicking a pituitary adenoma (128).

Parathyroid Bone Lesion ("Brown Tumor")

A patient with hyperparathyroidism and
chronic renal failure was found to have destruction
of the sella and parasellar structures associated
with hyperprolactinemia. This pattern suggested

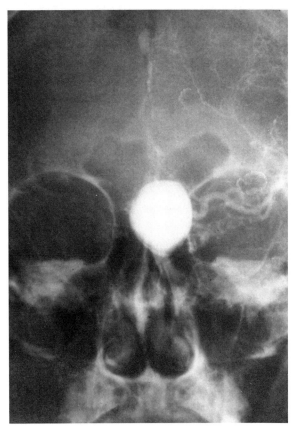

Figure 11-30
RADIOLOGIC FEATURES OF INTERNAL
CAROTID ARTERY ANEURYSM
Angiography of the lesion illustrated in figure 11-29
confirms that this is an aneurysm rather that a tumor.
(Courtesy of Dr. J.M. Bilbao, Toronto, Canada.)

an invasive pituitary prolactin-producing adenoma. However, at surgery no tumor was found and biopsy of the sphenoid bone revealed the characteristic changes of osteitis fibrosa cystica.

An ectopic pituitary adenoma was found in the clivus. This case indicates that a parathyroid bone lesion may be mistaken for pituitary adenoma in unusual circumstances (130).

REFERENCES

Hyperplasias

1. Asa SL, Kovacs K, Hammer GD, Liu B, Roos BA, Low MJ. Pituitary corticotroph hyperplasia in rats implanted with a medullary thyroid carcinoma cell line transfected with a corticotropin-releasing hormone complementary deoxyribonucleic acid expression vector. Endocrinology 1992;131:715–20.

2. Asa SL, Penz G, Kovacs K, Ezrin C. Prolactin cells in the human pituitary. A quantitative immunocytochemical analysis. Arch Pathol Lab Med 1982;106:360–3.

3. Asa SL, Scheithauer BW, Bilbao JM, et al. A case for hypothalamic acromegaly: a clinicopathological study of six patients with hypothalamic gangliocytomas producing growth hormone-releasing factor. J Clin Endocrinol Metab 1984;58:796–803.

4. Atchison JA, Lee PA, Albright AL. Reversible suprasellar pituitary mass secondary to hypothyroidism. JAMA 1989;262:3175–7.

5. Barkan AL, Shenker Y, Grekin RJ, Vale WW, Lloyd RV, Beals TF. Acromegaly due to ectopic growth hormone (GH)-releasing hormone (GHRH) production: dynamic studies of GH and ectopic GHRH secretion. J Clin Endocrinol Metab 1986;63:1057–64.

6. Berger G, Trouillas J, Bloch B, et al. Multihormonal carcinoid tumor of the pancreas secreting growth hormone-releasing factor as a cause of acromegaly. Cancer 1984;54:2097–108.

7. Billestrup N, Swanson LW, Vale W. Growth hormone-releasing factor stimulates proliferation of somatotrophs in vitro. Proc Natl Acad Sci USA 1986;83:6854–7.

8. Chan AW, MacFarlane IA, Foy PM, Miles JB. Pituitary enlargement and hyperprolactinaemia due to primary hypothyroidism: errors and delays in diagnosis. Br J Neurosurg 1990;4:107–12.

9. Ezzat S, Asa SL, Stefaneanu L, et al. Somatotroph hyperplasia without pituitary adenoma associated with a long standing growth hormone-releasing hormone-producing bronchial carcinoid. J Clin Endocrinol Metab 1994;78:555–60.

10. Grubb MR, Chakeres D, Malarkey WB. Patients with primary hypothyroidism presenting as prolactinomas. Am J Med 1987;83:765–9.

11. Horvath E, Kovacs K. Fine structural cytology of the adenohypophysis in rat and man. J Electron Microsc Tech 1988;8:401–32.

12. Horvath E, Kovacs K. The adenohypophysis. In: Kovacs K, Asa SL, eds. Functional endocrine pathology. Boston: Blackwell Scientific Publications, 1991:245–81.

13. Horvath E, Lloyd RV, Kovacs K. Propylthiouracil-induced hypothyroidism results in reversible transdifferentiation of somatotrophs into thyroidectomy cells.

A morphologic study of the rat pituitary including immunoelectron microscopy. Lab Invest 1990;63:511–20.

14. Jay V, Kovacs K, Horvath E, Lloyd RV, Smyth HS. Idiopathic prolactin cell hyperplasia of the pituitary mimicking prolactin cell adenoma: a morphological study including immunocytochemistry, electron microscopy, and in situ hybridization. Acta Neuropathol (Berl) 1991;82:147–51.

15. Khalil A, Kovacs K, Sima AA, Burrow GN, Horvath E. Pituitary thyrotroph hyperplasia mimicking prolactin-secreting adenoma. J Endocrinol Invest 1984;7:399–404.

16. Kontogeorgos G, Kovacs K, Horvath E, Scheithauer BW. Null cell adenomas, oncocytomas and gonadotroph adenomas of the human pituitary: an immunocytochemical and ultrastructural analysis of 300 cases. Endocr Pathol 1993;4:20–7.

17. Kovacs K, Horvath E. Tumors of the pituitary gland. Atlas of Tumor Pathology, 2nd Series, Fascicle 21. Washington, D.C.: Armed Forces Institute of Pathology, 1986.

18. Kovacs K, Horvath E, Rewcastle NB, Ezrin C. Gonadotroph cell adenoma of the pituitary in a woman with long-standing hypogonadism. Arch Gynecol 1980;229:57–65.

19. Kovacs K, Horvath E, Thorner MO, Rogol AD. Mammosomatotroph hyperplasia associated with acromegaly and hyperprolactinemia in a patient with the McCune-Albright syndrome. A histological, immunocytologic, and ultrastructural study of surgically-removed adenohypophysis. Virchows Arch [A] 1984;403:77–86.

20. Kubota T, Hayashi M, Kabuto M, et al. Corticotroph cell hyperplasia in a patient with Addison disease: case report. Surg Neurol 1992;37:441–7.

21. Mayo KE, Hammer RE, Swanson LW, Brinster RL, Rosenfeld MG, Evans RM. Dramatic pituitary hyperplasia in transgenic mice expressing a human growth hormone-releasing factor gene. Mol Endocrinol 1988;2:606–12.

22. McKeever PE, Koppelman MC, Metcalf D, et al. Refractory Cushing's disease caused by multinodular ACTH-cell hyperplasia. J Neuropathol Exp Neurol 1982;41:490–9.

23. McNicol AM. Patterns of corticotropic cells in the adult human pituitary in Cushing's disease. Diag Histopathol 1981;4:335–41.

24. Moran A, Asa SL, Kovacs K, et al. Gigantism due to pituitary mammosomatotroph hyperplasia. N Engl J Med 1990;323:322–7.

25. Nicolis G, Shimshi M, Allen C, Halmi NS, Kourides IA. Gonadotropin-producing pituitary adenoma in a man with long-standing primary hypogonadism. J Clin Endocrinol Metab 1988;66:237–41.

26. Peillon F, Dupuy M, Li JY, et al. Pituitary enlargement with suprasellar extension in functional hyperprolactinemia due to lactotroph hyperplasia: a pseudotumoral disease. J Clin Endocrinol Metab 1991;73:1008–15.

27. Ramsay JA, Kovacs K, Asa SL, Pike MJ, Thorner MO. Reversible sellar enlargement due to growth hormone-releasing hormone production by pancreatic endocrine tumors in an acromegalic patient with multiple endocrine neoplasia type I syndrome. Cancer 1988;62:445–50.

28. Saeger W, Lüdecke DK. Pituitary hyperplasia. Definition, light and electron microscopical structures and significance in surgical specimens. Virchows Arch [A] 1983;399:277–87.

29. Sano T, Asa SL, Kovacs K. Growth hormone-releasing hormone-producing tumors: clinical, biochemical, and morphological manifestations. Endocr Rev 1988;9:357–73.

30. Scheithauer BW, Kovacs K, Randall RV, Ryan N. Pituitary gland in hypothyroidism. Histologic and immunocytologic study. Arch Pathol Lab Med 1985;109:499–504.

31. Schulte HM, Benker G, Windeck R, Olbricht T, Reinwein D. Failure to respond to growth hormone releasing hormone (GHRH) in acromegaly due to a GHRH secreting pancreatic tumor: dynamics of multiple endocrine testing. J Clin Endocrinol Metab 1985;61:585–7.

32. Stefaneanu L, Kovacs K, Horvath E, et al. Adenohypophysial changes in mice transgenic for human growth hormone-releasing factor: a histological, immunocytochemical, and electron microscopic investigation. Endocrinology 1989;125:2710–8.

33. Stefaneanu L, Kovacs K, Lloyd RV, et al. Pituitary lactotrophs and somatotrophs in pregnancy: a correlative in situ hybridization and immunocytochemical study. Virchows Arch [B] 1992;62:291–6.

34. Thorner MO, Perryman RL, Cronin MJ, et al. Somatotroph hyperplasia: successful treatment of acromegaly by removal of a pancreatic islet tumor secreting a growth hormone-releasing factor. J Clin Invest 1982;70:965–77.

35. Weinstein LS, Shenker A, Gejman PV, Merino MJ, Friedman E, Spiegel AM. Activating mutations of the stimulatory G protein in the McCune-Albright syndrome. N Engl J Med 1991;325:1688–95.

Cysts

36. Abramson RC, Morawetz RB, Schlitt M. Multiple complications from an intracranial epidermoid cyst: case report and literature review. Neurosurgery 1989;24:574–8.

37. Barrow DL, Spector RH, Takei Y, Tindall GT. Symptomatic Rathke's cleft cysts located entirely in the suprasellar region: review of diagnosis, management and pathogenesis. Neurosurgery 1985;16:766–72.

38. Chhang WH, Sharma BS, Singh K, Suri S, Marwaha RK, Kak VK. A middle fossa arachnoid cyst in association with a suprasellar dermoid cyst. Indian J Pediatr 1989;26:833–5.

39. Christophe C, Flamant-Durand J, Hanquinet S, et al. MRI in seven cases of Rathke's cleft cyst in infants and children. Pediat Radiol 1993;23:79–82.

40. Jones RF, Warnock TH, Nayanar V, Gupta JM. Suprasellar arachnoid cysts: management by cyst wall resection. Neurosurgery 1989;25:554–61.

41. Kepes JJ. Transitional cell tumor of the pituitary gland developing from a Rathke's cleft cyst. Cancer 1978;41:337–43.

42. Keyaki A, Hirano A, Llena JF. Asymptomatic and symptomatic Rathke's cleft cysts. Histological study of 45 cases. Neurol Med Chir 1989;29:88–93.

43. Kucharczyk W, Peck WW, Kelly WM, Norman D, Newton TH. Rathke's cleft cysts: CT, MR imaging, and pathologic features. Radiology 1987;165:491–5.

44. Lewis AJ, Cooper PW, Kassel EE, Schwartz ML. Squamous cell carcinoma arising in a suprasellar epidermoid cyst. Case report. J Neurosurg 1983;59:538–41.

45. Meyer FB, Carpenter SM, Laws ER Jr. Intrasellar arachnoid cysts. Surg Neurol 1987;28:105–10.

46. Mize W, Ball WS Jr, Towbin RB, Han BK. Atypical CT and MR appearance of a Rathke cleft cyst. Am J Neuroradiol 1989;10:S83–4.

47. Nakasu S, Nakasu Y, Kyoshima K, Watanabe K, Handa J, Okabe H. Pituitary adenoma with multiple ciliated cysts: transitional cell tumor? Surg Neurol 1989;31:41–8.

48. Nishio S, Mizuno J, Barrow DL, Takei Y, Tindall GT. Pituitary tumors composed of adenohypophysial adenoma and Rathke's cleft cyst elements: a clinicopathological study. Neurosurgery 1987;21:371–7.

49. Obenchain TG, Becker DP. Abscess formation in a Rathke's cleft cyst. Case report. J Neurosurg 1972;36:359–62.

50. Spaziante R. Intrasellar arachnoid cysts [Letter]. Surg Neurol 1988;30:412–3.

51. Steinberg GK, Koenig GH, Golden JB. Symptomatic Rathke's cleft cysts. Report of two cases. J Neurosurg 1982;56:290–5.

52. Voelker JL, Campbell RL, Muller J. Clinical, radiographic, and pathological features of symptomatic Rathke's cleft cysts. J Neurosurg 1991;74:535–44.

53. Yamakawa K, Shitara N, Genka S, Manaka S, Takakura K. Clinical course and surgical prognosis of 33 cases of intracranial epidermoid tumors. Neurosurgery 1989;24:568–73.

Inflammatory Lesions

54. Abe T, Matsumoto K, Sanno N, Osamura Y. Lymphocytic hypophysitis: case report. Neurosurgery 1995;36:1016–9.

55. Asa SL. The pathology of autoimmune endocrine disorders. In: Kovacs K, Asa SL, eds. Functional endocrine pathology. Boston: Blackwell Scientific Publications, 1991:961–78.

56. Asa SL, Bilbao JM, Kovacs K, Josse RG, Kreines K. Lymphocytic hypophysitis of pregnancy resulting in hypopituitarism: a distinct clinicopathologic entity. Ann Intern Med 1981;95:166–71.

57. Barkan AL, Kelch RP, Marshall JC. Isolated gonadotrope failure in the polyglandular autoimmune syndrome. N Engl J Med 1985;312:1535–40.

58. Berger SA, Edberg SC, David G. Infectious disease in the sella turcica. Rev Infect Dis 1986;5:747–55.

59. Bevan JS, Othman S, Lazarus JH, Parkes AB, Hall R. Reversible adrenocorticotropin deficiency due to probable autoimmune hypophysitis in a woman with postpartum thyroiditis. J Clin Endocrinol Metab 1992;74:548–52.

60. Bitton RN, Slavin M, Decker RE, Zito J, Schneider BS. The course of lymphocytic hypophysitis. Surg Neurol 1991;36:40–3.

61. Bottazzo GF, Doniach D. Pituitary autoimmunity: a review. J Royal Soc Med 1978;71:433–6.

62. Bottazzo GF, McIntosh C, Stanford W, Preece M. Growth hormone cell antibodies and partial growth hormone deficiency in a girl with Turner's syndrome. Clin Endocrinol (Oxf) 1980;12:1–9.

63. Bottazzo GF, Pouplard A, Florin-Christensen A, Doniach D. Autoantibodies to prolactin-secreting cells of human pituitary. Lancet 1975;ii:97–101.

64. Burke CW, Moore RA, Rees LH, Bottazzo GF, Mashiter K, Bitensky L. Isolated ACTH deficiency and TSH deficiency in the adult. J Royal Soc Med 1979;72:328–35.

65. Crock P, Salvi M, Miller A, Wall J, Guyda H. Detection of anti-pituitary autoantibodies by immunoblotting. J Immunol Methods 1993;162:31–40.

66. Del Pozo JM, Roda JE, Montoya JG, Iglesias JR, Hurtado A. Intrasellar granuloma. Case report. J Neurosurg 1980;53:717–9.

67. Engelberth O, Jezková Z. Autoantibodies in Sheehan's syndrome. Lancet 1965;i:1075.

68. Escobar-Morreale H, Serrano-Gotarredona J, Varela C. Isolated adrenocorticotropic hormone deficiency due to probable lymphocytic hypophysitis in a man. J Endocrinol Invest 1994;17:127–31.

69. Feigenbaum SL, Martin MC, Wilson CB, Jaffe RB. Lymphocytic adenohypophysitis: a pituitary mass lesion occurring in pregnancy. Proposal for medical treatment. Am J Obstet Gynecol 1991;164:1549–55.

70. Gartman JJ Jr, Powers SK, Fortune M. Pseudotumor of the sellar and parasellar areas. Neurosurgery 1989;24:896–901.

71. Glauber HS, Brown BM. Pituitary macroadenoma associated with intrasellar abscess: a case report and review. Endocrinologist 1992;2:169–72.

72. Goudie RB, Pinkerton PH. Anterior hypophysitis and Hashimoto's disease in a young woman. J Pathol Bacteriol 1962;83:584–5.

73. Guay AT, Agnello V, Tronic BC, Gresham DG, Freidberg SR. Lymphocytic hypophysitis in a man. J Clin Endocrinol Metab 1987;64:631–4.

74. Hassoun P, Anayssi E, Salti I. A case of granulomatous hypophysitis with hypopituitarism and minimal pituitary enlargement. J Neurol Neurosurg Psychiatry 1985;48:949–51.

75. Holck S, Laursen H. Prolactinoma coexistent with granulomatous hypophysitis. Acta Neuropathol (Berl) 1983;61:253–7.

76. Horvath E, Kovacs K. The adenohypophysis. In: Kovacs K, Asa SL, eds. Functional endocrine pathology. Boston: Blackwell Scientific Publications, 1991:245–81.

77. Hughes JM, Ellsworth CA, Harris BS. Clinical case seminar: a 33-year-old woman with a pituitary mass and panhypopituitarism. J Clin Endocrinol Metab 1995;80:1521–5.

78. Ikeda H, Okudaira Y. Spontaneous regression of pituitary mass in temporal association with pregnancy. Neuroradiology 1987;29:488–92.

79. Imura H, Nakao K, Shimatsu A, et al. Lymphocytic infundibuloneurohypophysitis as a cause of central diabetes insipidus. N Engl J Med 1993;329:683–9.

80. Ishihara T, Nakatsu S, Hino M, et al. A case of pregnancy-induced lymphocytic adenohypophysitis complicated by postpartum painless thyroiditis. Nippon Naibunpi Gakkai Zasshi 1991;67:222–9.

81. Jensen MD, Handwerger BS, Scheithauer BW, Carpenter PC, Mirakian R, Banks PM. Lymphocytic hypophysitis with isolated corticotropin deficiency. Ann Intern Med 1986;105:200–3.

82. Klaer W, Nørgaard JO. Granulomatous hypophysitis and thyroiditis with lymphocytic adrenalitis. Acta Pathol Microbiol Scand 1969;76:229–38.

83. Klein I, Kraus KE, Martines AJ, Weber S. Evidence for cellular mediated immunity in an animal model of autoimmune pituitary disease. Endocr Res Commun 1982;9:145–53.

84. Komatsu M, Kondo T, Yamauchi K, et al. Antipituitary antibodies in patients with the primary empty sella syndrome. J Clin Endocrinol Metab 1988;67:633–8.

85. Levine S. Allergic adenohypophysitis: new experimental disease of the pituitary gland. Science 1967;158:1190–1.

86. Levine S. Allergic adrenalitis and adenohypophysitis: further observations on production and passive transfer. Endocrinology 1969;84:469–75.

87. Levine SN, Benzel EC, Fowler MR, Shroyer JV III, Mirfakhraee M. Lymphocytic hypophysitis: clinical, radiological and magnetic resonance imaging characterization. Neurosurgery 1988;22:937–41.

88. Ludwig H, Schernthaner G. Multiorganspezifische Autoimmunität bei idiopathischer Nebennierenrindeninsuffizienz. Wein Klin Wochenschr 1978;90:736–41.

89. Masana Y, Ikeda H, Fujimoto Y, et al. Lymphocytic adenohypophysitis. Case report. Neurol Med Chir 1990;30:853–7.

90. Mayfield RK, Levine JH, Gordon L, Powers J, Galbraith RM, Rawe SE. Lymphoid adenohypophysitis presenting as a pituitary tumor. Am J Med 1980;69:619–23.

91. Mazzone T, Kelly W, Ensinck J. Lymphocytic hypophysitis associated with antiparietal cell antibodies and vitamin B12 deficiency. Arch Intern Med 1983;143:1794–5.

92. McConnon JK, Smyth HS, Horvath E. A case of sparsely granulated growth hormone cell adenoma associated with lymphocytic hypophysitis. J Endocrinol Invest 1991;14:691–6.

93. McCutcheon IE, Oldfield EH. Lymphocytic adenohypophysitis presenting as infertility. Case report. J Neurosurg 1991;74:821–6.

94. McGrail KM, Beyerl BD, Black PM, Klibanski A, Zervas NT. Lymphocytic adenohypophysitis of pregnancy with complete recovery. Neurosurgery 1987;20:791–3.

95. Meichner RH, Riggio S, Manz HJ, Earll JM. Lymphocytic adenohypophysitis causing pituitary mass. Neurology 1987;37:158–61.

96. Mikami T, Uozumi T. Lymphocytic adenohypophysitis: MRI findings of a suspected case. No Shinkei Geka 1989;176:871–6.

97. Miura M, Ushio Y, Kuratsu J, Ikeda J, Kai Y, Yamashiro S. Lymphocytic adenohypophysitis: report of two cases. Surg Neurol 1989;32:463–70.

98. Miyamoto M, Sugawa H, Mori T, Hashimoto N, Imura H. A case of hypopituitarism due to granulomatous and lymphocytic adenohypophysitis with minimal pituitary enlargement: a possible variant of lymphocytic adenohypophysitis. Endocrinol Jpn 1988;35:607–16.

99. Nishioka H, Ito H, Miki T, Akada K. A case of lymphocytic hypophysitis with massive fibrosis and the role of surgical intervention. Surg Neurol 1994;42:74–8.

100. Nussbaum CE, Okawara SH, Jacobs LS. Lymphocytic hypophysitis with involvement of the cavernous sinus and hypothalamus. Neurosurgery 1991;28:440–4.

101. Ober KP, Elster A. Spontaneously resolving lymphocytic hypophysitis as a cause of postpartum diabetes insipidus. Endocrinologist 1994;4:107–11.

102. Ozawa Y, Shishiba Y. Recovery from lymphocytic hypophysitis associated with painless thyroiditis: clinical implications of circulating antipituitary antibodies. Acta Endocrinol (Copenh) 1993;128:493–8.

103. Pestell RG, Best JD, Alford FP. Lymphocytic hypophysitis. The clinical spectrum of the disorder and evidence for an autoimmune pathogenesis. Clin Endocrinol (Oxf) 1990;33:457–66.

104. Pholsena M, Young J, Couzinet B, Schaison G. Primary adrenal and thyroid insufficiencies associated with hypopituitarism: a diagnostic challenge. Clin Endocrinol (Oxf) 1994;40:693–5.

105. Portocarrero CJ, Robinson AG, Taylor AL, Klein I. Lymphoid hypophysitis. An unusual cause of hyperprolactinemia and enlarged sella turcica. JAMA 1981;246:1811–2.

106. Prasad A, Madan VS, Sethi PK, Prasad ML, Buxi TB, Kanwar CK. Lymphocytic hypophysitis: can open exploration of the sella be avoided? Br J Neurosurg 1991;5:639–42.

107. Quencer RM. Lymphocytic adenohypophysitis: autoimmune disorder of the pituitary gland. Am J Neuroradiol 1980;1:343–5.

108. Reusch JE, Kleinschmidt-De Masters BK, Lillehei KO, Rappe D, Gutierrez-Hartmann A. Preoperative diagnosis of lymphocytic hypophysitis (adenohypophysitis) unresponsive to short course dexamethasone: case report. Neurosurgery 1992;30:268–72.

109. Richtsmeier AJ, Henry RA, Bloodworth JM Jr, Ehrlich EN. Lymphoid hypophysitis with selective adrenocorticotropic hormone deficiency. Arch Intern Med 1980;140:1243–5.

110. Rickards AG, Harvey PW. Giant cell granuloma and the other pituitary granulomata. Quarterly J Med 1954;23:425–40.

111. Roosens B, Maes E, van Steirteghem A, Vanhaelst L. Primary hypothyroidism associated with secondary adrenocortical insufficiency. J Endocrinol Invest 1982;5:251–4.

112. Sauter NP, Toni R, McLaughlin CD, Dyess EM, Kritzmann J, Lechan RM. Isolated adrenocorticotropin deficiency associated with an autoantibody to corticotroph antigen that is not adrenocorticotropin or other pro-opiomelanocortin-derived peptides. J Clin Endocrinol Metab 1990;70:1391–7.

113. Scheithauer BW. Pathology of the pituitary and sellar region: exclusive of pituitary adenoma. Pathology Annual 1985;20(1):67–155.

114. Scheithauer BW. The hypothalamus and neurohypophysis. In: Kovacs K, Asa SL, eds. Functional endocrine pathology. Boston: Blackwell Scientific Publications, 1991:170–244.

115. Scherbaum WA, Schrell U, Glück M, Fahlbusch R, Pfeiffer EF. Autoantibodies to pituitary corticotropin-producing cells: possible marker for unfavourable outcome after pituitary microsurgery for Cushing's disease. Lancet 1987;i:1394–8.

116. Sheehan HL. Post-partum necrosis of the anterior pituitary. J Pathol Bacteriol 1937;45:189–214.

117. Stelmach M, O'Day J. Rapid change in visual fields associated with suprasellar lymphocytic hypophysitis. J Clin Neurol Ophthalmol 1991;11:19–24.

118. Supler ML, Mickle JP. Lymphocytic hypophysitis: report of a case in a man with cavernous sinus involvement. Surg Neurol 1992;37:472–6.

119. Taylon C, Duff TA. Giant cell granuloma involving the pituitary gland. Case report. J Neurosurg 1980;52:584–7.

120. Thodou E, Asa SL, Kontogeorgos G, Kovacs K, Horvath E, Ezzat S. Clinical case seminar: lymphocytic hypophysitis: clinicopathological findings. J Clin Endocrinol Metab 1995;80:2302–11.

121. Vandeput Y, Orth DN, Crabbe J. Combined primary and secondary adrenocortical failure. Ann Endocrinol (Paris) 1982;43:277–9.

122. Veseley DL, Maldonodo A, Levey GS. Partial hypopituitarism and possible hypothalamic involvement in sarcoidosis: report of a case and review of the literature. Am J Med 1977;62:425–31.

123. Wild RA, Kepley M. Lymphocytic hypophysitis in a patient with amenorrhea and hyperprolactinemia. J Repro Med 1986;31:211–6.

Miscellaneous Tumor-like Lesions

124. Durham LH, Mackenzie IJ, Miles JB. Transphenoidal meningohydroencephalocoele. Br J Neurosurg 1988;2:407–9.

125. Dussault J, Plamondon C, Volpe R. Aneurysms of the internal carotid artery simulating pituitary tumours. Can Med Assoc J 1969;101:51–6.

126. Hampton TA, Scheithauer BW, Rojiani AM, Kovacs K, Horvath E, Vogt P. Salivary gland-like tumors of the sellar region. Am J Surg Pathol 1997;21:424–34.

127. Kato T, Aida T, Abe H, et al. Ectopic salivary gland within the pituitary gland. Case report. Neurol Med Chir 1988;28:930–3.

128. Oka H, Kameya T, Sasano H, et al. Pituitary choristoma composed of corticotrophs and adrenocortical cells in the sella turcica. Virchows Arch 1996;427:613–7.

129. Schochet SS Jr, McCormick WF, Halmi NS. Salivary gland rests in the human pituitary. Light and electron microscopical study. Arch Pathol 1974;98:193–200.

130. Shenker Y, Lloyd RV, Weatherbee L, Port FK, Grekin RJ, Barkan AL. Ectopic prolactinoma in a patient with hyperparathyroidism and abnormal sellar radiography. J Clin Endocrinol Metab 1986;62:1065–9.

INDEX*

---

*Numbers in boldface indicate table and figure pages.

✧✧✧